Medicine: Preserving the Passion

Phil R. Manning, M.D.
Professor of Medicine
Paul Ingalls Hoagland Professor of Continuing Medical Education,
The Hastings Foundation
Associate Vice President for Health Affairs
Associate Dean for Postgraduate Affairs
Director, Development and Demonstration Center
in Continuing Education for Health Professionals
a Project of the W. K. Kellogg Foundation
University of Southern California
School of Medicine
Los Angeles, California

Lois DeBakey, Ph.D.
Professor of Scientific Communication
Baylor College of Medicine
Houston, Texas
Adjunct Professor, Tulane University School of Medicine
New Orleans, Louisiana

With 54 Figures

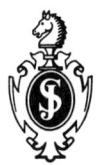

Springer-Verlag
New York Berlin Heidelberg
London Paris Tokyo

Also by Lois DeBakey, Ph.D.:
The Scientific Journal:
Editorial Policies and Practices

Allen County Public Library
Ft. Wayne, Indiana

This work was supported in part by a Special Scientific Project Grant (1 K10 LM 00068) from the National Library of Medicine.

Library of Congress Cataloging in Publication Data
Manning, Phil R., 1921–
  Medicine: preserving the passion.
  Includes bibliographies and index.
  1. Medicine—Study and teaching (Continuing education) I. DeBakey, Lois, co-author. II. Title.
[DNLM: 1. Education, Medical, Continuing—trends.
W 20 M284m]
R845.M36 1987   610'.7'15   86-11868

© 1987 by Springer-Verlag New York Inc.
All rights reserved. No part of this book may be translated or reproduced in any form without written permission from Springer-Verlag, 175 Fifth Avenue, New York, New York 10010, U.S.A.
The use of general descriptive names, trade names, trademarks, etc. in this publication, even if the former are not especially identified, is not to be taken as a sign that such names, as understood by the Trade Marks and Merchandise Marks Act, may accordingly be used freely by anyone.
While the advice and information in this book are believed to be true and accurate at the date of going to press, neither the authors nor the editors nor the publisher can accept any legal responsibility for any errors or omissions that may be made. The publisher makes no warranty, express or implied, with respect to the material contained herein.

Typeset by David E. Seham Associates, Inc., Metuchen, New Jersey.
Printed and bound by R.R. Donnelley & Sons, Harrisonburg, Virginia.
Printed in the United States of America.

9 8 7 6 5 4 3 2 1

ISBN 0-387-96357-8 Springer-Verlag New York Berlin Heidelberg
ISBN 3-540-96357-8 Springer-Verlag Berlin Heidelberg New York

Medicine:
Preserving the Passion

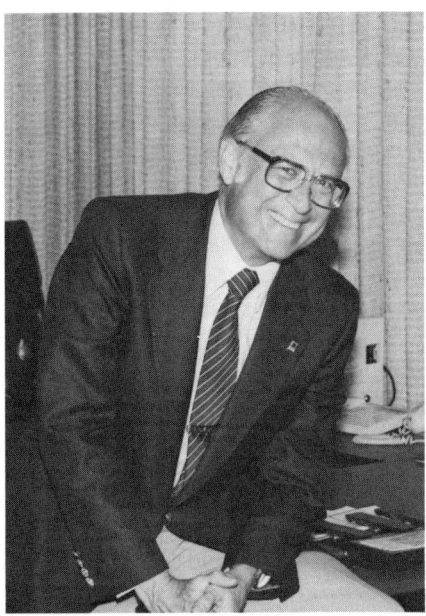 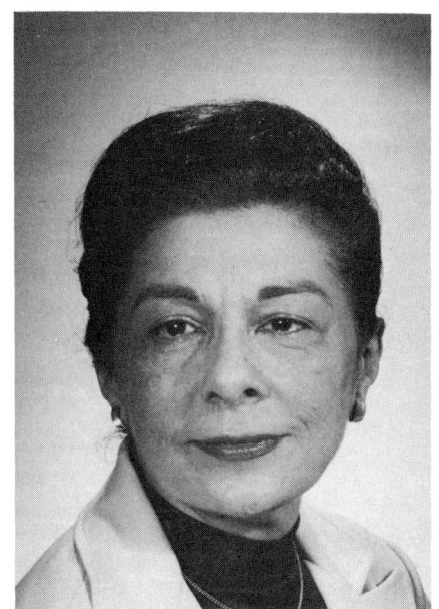

Continuing medical education is ripe for major changes that will encourage independent, practice-related study and will deepen the physician's involvement in his practice. The ultimate beneficiary will be the patient.

                Phil R. Manning, M.D.

An inquiring, analytical mind; an unquenchable thirst for new knowledge; and a heartfelt compassion for the ailing—these are prominent traits among the committed clinicians who have preserved the passion for medicine.

                Lois DeBakey, Ph.D.

Foreword

In *Medicine: Preserving the Passion,* Phil R. Manning, a pioneer and recognized authority in continuing medical education, and Lois DeBakey, a passionate advocate of critical reasoning and leading scholar in scientific communication, endeavor to shift the focus in lifelong learning from group exercises in a lecture hall to self-directed, practice-related activities. Although most experts have applauded this new concept, few publications have addressed methods for implementation. The Manning–DeBakey book describes such methods as devised by outstanding clinicians and academicians to obtain educational benefit from their clinical experience. Some techniques inspired by quality assurance, for example, these master clinicians have used successfully to improve their knowledge, skills, and patient care. This book not only identifies the primary concerns in continuing medical education, but also offers sound recommendations and effective solutions and suggests future directions and approaches.

The authors have analyzed the continuing educational practices of physicians in a wide range of environments, from small communities to the most acclaimed medical centers, and have extracted additional advice from the writings of past authorities like Osler. The resulting concepts will undoubtedly attract wide public attention. Office practice audit, self-directed learning, case indexing, patient education, computer-assisted education, and collegial networks, as well as regular reading, writing, and teaching, are among the successful methods described by physicians and surgeons who exemplify the highest standards of medical practice. Realizing that medical knowledge alone does not ensure excellent care, the authors have included a chapter on how outstanding clinicians avoid process problems such as omission and oversight. A wide variety of innovations in learning and teaching, including technologic advances, have been introduced to make continuing medical education more effective, and many have been adopted by some of today's most notable practitioners. Ways in which the computer can facilitate the implementation of these new concepts are also presented.

Continuing education for physicians has been a fundamental precept of the profession since the case descriptions of Hippocrates were used to understand prognosis. Physicians have thus always been expected to follow a personal plan for progressive learning throughout their practicing careers. The concepts expressed by the authors and their contributors illustrate the central focus of lifelong learning in the professional lives of successful physicians. For some, avocational interests involve recreational times spent with colleagues, not only to enjoy their camaraderie, but to exchange professional information and derive the benefits of mutual intellectual stimulation.

In the 1960s and 1970s legislatures became interested in methods that would maintain physicians' knowledge of medical advances. Legislative mandates sought to ensure the quality of health care provided to American citizens. Some states require a specified number of hours of continuing medical education for relicensure. But the accumulation of continuing education credits does not ensure incorporation of current medical knowledge into a physician's practice. Attendance at formal courses is of some value, but a direct beneficial effect on the quality of patient care is difficult to demonstrate. Future considerations for relicensure may therefore go beyond classroom instruction. Public concern in the 1980s about the cost and quality of health care has focused attention on continuing medical education, as reflected in the essays and commentaries of notable physicians.

Aware of the recent prominence of socioeconomic and ethical aspects of contemporary medicine, the co-authors and their influential interviewees reflect on the personal and moral traits of physicians that allow for humane considerations and compassion for the ailing, including attention to their patients' economic status. Their attention to these factors will undoubtedly focus greater emphasis on them in the medical curriculum.

Analysis of the current state of continuing medical education by Manning and DeBakey leads to new questions and expectations. Are physicians considering how their patients can assume more personal responsibility for maintaining their health? Has patient education become an integral part of medical practice? There is a growing public expectation that patients and their families should participate more fully in medical decisions and health care. In the future, physicians will be expected to have a personal plan of continuing education, which will determine in part how well they are prepared to provide optimal patient care. This book provides a blueprint for such a plan.

The principles of adult learning set forth here are sound and are applicable to disciplines other than medicine. This book about the personal and professional rewards of lifelong learning, although centering on physicians, has general applicability for adult education. Reading and consulting to obtain information to solve a question that arises in professional practice or work, for example, are productive in all fields. Discussions with peers and mentors, practice audits, teaching, writing, and reassessing information are all proven methods of remaining abreast of the latest

Dedicated to the practicing physician, who has invested many years in medical school and graduate training, often at great personal and financial sacrifice, and who places the highest priority on the health and welfare of his patients.

The education of the doctor which goes on after he has his degree is, after all, the most important part of his education.

>John Shaw Billings
>Boston, *Med Surg J* 131:140, 1894

The art of medicine cannot be inherited, nor can it be copied from books . . . .

>Paracelsus
>Foreword, *Das zweite Buch der Grossen Wundarznei,* 1536 (verso of leaf b, ed. 1562)

[T]he student begins with the patient, continues with the patient, and ends his studies with the patient, using books and lectures as tools, as means to an end.

>*William Osler*
>*Aequanimites, with Other Addresses,*
>"The Hospital as a College," 1903

available knowledge. Recent technologic advances will facilitate and expand the benefits of these approaches. The comprehensive scope and treatment of this subject, the expertise of the authors, essayists, and interviewees, and the interesting anecdotes related by renowned physicians not only present valuable information in an interesting way, but also provide a basis for future discussions and directions in this timely subject.

                          Robert D. Sparks, M.D.
                          President
                          Chief Programming Officer and Trustee
                          W. K. Kellogg Foundation
                          Battle Creek, Michigan

Preface

Medicine is a demanding profession that consumes inordinate time, attention, and effort. Physicians can, however, not only heighten their own satisfaction and enjoyment but also improve their patient care by observing certain principles that have guided master clinicians and academicians in their professional careers.

Evidence suggests that members of our society increasingly consider work only as a means of obtaining money for more enjoyable leisure time. Some, in fact, often expend more effort to avoid productivity than they would exert if they became deeply immersed in what they are doing. The result is a decline in the quality and quantity of their work and absence of fulfillment or enjoyment during working hours. Conscious involvement, on the other hand, might bring the joy they defer for leisure time.

Medical practitioners are fortunate that their profession permits enriched understanding of the medical and social sciences during their service to those in pain, discomfort, fear, or stress. For the physician seriously involved in medicine, the practice of medicine cannot ever become dull or boring, and even times that require "overwork" can bring satisfaction. The application of methods to enhance involvement and satisfaction in practice rewards the physician and his patients time and again.

To capture these rewarding principles, we interviewed or surveyed 621 physicians—academicians and private practitioners—as well as some spouses. The options for selection of interviewees and correspondents were numerous. We did not survey a randomly selected group to determine how physicians in general learn, but sought those who used professional techniques that other practitioners might find useful. We first interviewed distinguished medical school professors, leaders in medical societies, and practitioners who are recognized by their peers as outstanding. We asked this group to recommend other physicians who they thought might have useful methods to contribute. We then queried physicians attending postgraduate refresher courses sponsored by the University of Southern California School of Medicine. Our bibliographic research also yielded suggestions from renowned physicians of other periods. We fully realize that countless physicians whom we did not interview may use equally effective methods, but we hope that we have covered the techniques that are most practical and broadly applicable in medical practice.

This book, which synthesizes information derived from our interviews, other research, and experience, is intended to help physicians profit the most—intellectually, clinically, and emotionally—from their practice. Emphasis is on methods that link education to specific patients' problems. The preparation of the book was an uplifting experience, as we learned of the methods physicians have devised to continue their education— methods that mandatory formal continuing education does not encompass. No physician will want to adopt all the methods described, but each can choose those most amenable to his needs and circumstances. To preserve a sense of reality and identity, we have quoted some physicians directly. Because of repetition, however, not every physician interviewed was quoted verbatim. Those not mentioned specifically by name, however, made valuable contributions that we incorporated into the text, and we are indebted to all for their time and effort in providing us with information about their personal experiences. We have also included the personal essays of several leading physicians and one scientist because they contain interesting anecdotes and illustrate vividly many of the techniques we are advocating.

Although maintaining currency with the art and science of medicine requires general study, prompt access to specific information about an immediate problem is more effective in continuing medical education than memorization of facts that may not be used for some time. Toward this end, we describe techniques for access to utilitarian information, including the development of a personal information center and effective use of medical library services. We also relate how master physicians have used teaching and writing as practical mediums of self-education.

Formal courses and conferences, the traditional forms of continuing education, remain useful in special circumstances and are sometimes aided by technology. The valuable collegial network that often results provides not only an intellectual stimulus but a source of social enjoyment as well. We present ways of extracting the most from one form of such professional companionship, the medical consultation.

We also show how analysis of practice can help the physician profit maximally from his clinical experience and can help solve problems unrelated to medical knowledge—problems whose solutions require the physician to be the manager of the overall care of patients.

We illustrate the special problems of women physicians with multiple social roles and show how families can help physicians nurture their professional interests and hone their skills in medicine. We describe methods of strengthening the doctor–patient relationship, as well as of keeping abreast of social and ethical problems. Finally, we discuss the role of the computer in the implementation of the educational methods described.

Preface

Continuing medical education is ripe for major changes that will encourage independent, practice-related study and will deepen the physician's involvement in his practice. The ultimate beneficiary will be the patient. Computer technology will encourage and accelerate these changes, but since effective manual methods now exist, the physician need not and should not delay applying these techniques. It is more efficient, in fact, to gain experience with the concepts of active, practice-related learning before enlisting the help of the computer. The important point is not to delay, but to start *now*.

Phil R. Manning, M.D.
Lois DeBakey, Ph.D.

Acknowledgments

Phil R. Manning, M.D.

I wish to acknowledge the powerful influence of all my teachers and colleagues on my career in medicine and continuing education. Although there are too many to identify by name, several who had a special impact on me deserve special mention. I mention them not only to acknowledge their positive influences on me, but also to describe the human qualities that seem to me to be most important in medicine. Helen E. Martin, indomitable, hardworking, intelligent, and cultured, was a major force in my medical school training. Although overburdened (most other faculty members having been away in the Armed Services during World War II), Helen exerted a remarkable influence on medical students, interns, residents, and the practicing medical community, stressing an understanding of physiology and biochemistry in clinical medicine. She was totally unyielding in demanding that each patient receive the best care possible. Thomas H. Brem, a true gentleman, skilled in diagnosis and in stimulating students and residents to profit from their experience, has also had a major influence on me. In the thirty-five years I have known Tom, I cannot recall his speaking flippantly or angrily to any patient or physician-in-training. He always listens attentively and responds appropriately. His effect on the care of patients has been profound—through the hundreds of residents whom he has helped train and the colleagues whom he has influenced. He showed me, among innumerable other things, the benefits and satisfactions that derive from discussing clinical problems with colleagues.

Jesse Edwards, Howard Burchell, Raymond Pruitt, and Earl Wood showed me the virtue of the "brown-bag lunch conference." At these sessions, the subject was introduced by a case presentation, including bedside observations, electrocardiography, imaging, physiologic studies, and pathology. These four giants highlighted the discussions by challenging one another in a forceful, but friendly, way.

My colleague Telfer Reynolds has always vigorously pursued knowledge relating to patients under his care. To keep his experience from becoming memory-dependent, he records interesting cases on index cards. Demanding of himself and his co-workers, he is a physician's physician in every sense of the word. Another colleague who has influenced me positively is Peter V. Lee, whose interests in literature and art and whose participation in competitive swimming have enriched his life and broadened his influence. Most important to me has been his ability to understand problems and seek solutions.

I am indebted to George Miller for his writings and numerous stimulating conversations on medical education. The publications of John Williamson, Clement Brown, Patrick Storey, Richard Caplan, Berne Dyer, Tom Inui, and the McMasters group have been practical and valuable. Lawrence Weed has been a major stimulus, reinforcing and helping me clarify my thoughts on linking education to practice. Donald Lindberg, Marion Ball, and Edward Shortliffe have helped educate me on the use of computers in medical practice. Stephen Abrahamson, my colleague at the University of Southern California, has contributed regularly to my understanding of medical education. Suggestions have also been welcome from Donald Petit, David Covell, and Rochelle Bee. Thanks are also due to the staff of the National Library of Medicine for its assistance and support.

The writing of this book with Lois DeBakey was one of the most enjoyable experiences I have had. It was a magnificent illustration of the educational rewards of working with an estimable colleague, even though much of our collaboration was accomplished by telephone and correspondence. Lois sees through muddled and deceptive thought processes better than anyone I have met, and her ability to express concepts clearly and succinctly is incomparable. When we decided to collaborate on this book, we undertook a comprehensive review of previous publications. Then we elected to interview several hundred physicians. In discussions on the style of the book, we concluded that narrating some ideas in the words of the interviewees would be more interesting than an impersonal report.

I am indebted to several persons who assisted with the preparation of the manuscript. Barbara Silva organized my file system beautifully. Virginia Campen conscientiously helped verify references. David Arriola diligently typed several drafts and the final manuscript and, with Jane Burbank and Rochelle Bee, read the proofs, looking for errors that the gremlins always seem to insert. Diana Florence typed many of the original interviews. Each of these made my work easier.

It was my co-author Lois who insisted, throughout the project, on absolute accuracy at every point, constantly emphasizing the need for stringent verification of names, titles, quotations, and references cited and for painstaking proofreading. And it was her genius for detecting inconsistencies and errors inapparent to others that permitted their removal before publication. If any flaws remain, their responsibility lies with me, not her.

Finally, I appreciate the suggestions made by my family—my daughter, Carol J. Manning, M.D. (Mrs. Boettger); her husband, Mark Boettger, M.D.; my son, R. J. Manning, J.D.; and my wife Mary, a world class grandmother and potentially fine writer, who has devoted her life to her family rather than pursue a professional career.

Acknowledgments

Lois DeBakey, Ph.D.

The advantages of collegial associations are exemplified by the cooperative endeavor represented by this book. Phil Manning and I met a number of years ago when we served together on a national committee. A shared interest in academic activities and in excellence in medical education, coupled with mutual ethical and human values, drew us into a collegial relationship that has been productive through the years.

The idea for this book came from Phil, an internationally recognized leader in continuing medical education. When he broached the idea to me, his enthusiasm and eagerness to pass on to others the wisdom of the masters persuaded me to accept his invitation to collaborate. His plan of interviewing hundreds of physicians, including some of our most distinguished academicians and practitioners, offered a fresh perspective on continuing medical education. I have been the beneficiary of this collaborative effort, for I have learned a great deal from partnership with my clear-headed, highly informed co-author, and I am indebted to him for bringing me aboard this rewarding intellectual venture.

Since my family is responsible for my having chosen a scholarly career, my debt to them is deep and enduring. In my early childhood, my parents kindled the spark of learning and then helped me sustain the flame by stimulating my intellectual curiosity, encouraging the habit of reading, and making certain that our home was amply supplied with interesting books. Later, they provided the opportunity and support for my college and postgraduate education. I chose my parents well, for they were loving, intelligent, industrious, altruistic, and highly ethical. My brothers, Michael and Ernest, and sisters, Selena and Selma, also served as peerless models for me, and I am humbly and affectionately grateful for their encouragement and support of all my scholarly endeavors. I am especially indebted to my brother Michael, who directed me into such an exciting and fulfilling career. A man of vision, dedication, and ingenuity, he recognized the need for instruction in medical communication, and he encouraged my sister Selma and me to establish this new discipline. His lofty standards and noble character have been a lifelong inspiration. My eternal gratitude also goes to Selma—my preceptor, professional partner, and alter ego—not only for her sage counsel throughout the preparation of this and all my other publications, but for her unstinting support and sororal devotion throughout my life.

Our publisher, Springer-Verlag, has been most helpful and accommodating. We particularly thank Dr. Jerry L. Stone, Executive Editor, to whom Dr. Manning and I are sincerely grateful for the care with which our manuscript has been handled. To members of my staff, I express appreciation for their varied assistance, and to Linda Molten goes special recognition for her intelligent scrutiny of the proofs and astute detection of errors.

Most especially, we are indebted to all the physicians who were willing to grant us the benefit of their experience and wisdom. They provided much of the raw material for this book; we, the analysis, interpretations, and commentary. Finally, to our readers, we are grateful for your own intellectual curiosity; we hope you will feel rewarded for your investment in reading this book.

Contents

Foreword: Robert D. Sparks, M.D. — ix
Preface: Phil R. Manning, M.D. and Lois DeBakey, Ph.D. — xiii
Acknowledgments: Phil R. Manning, M.D. — xvii
Acknowledgments: Lois DeBakey, Ph.D. — xix
Photographs — xxiii
Introduction: Phil R. Manning, M.D. — xxv

Chapter 1. Enjoying the Struggle — 1
    Personal Essay: Michael E. DeBakey, M.D. — 15
    Personal Essay: J. Willis Hurst, M.D. — 25

Chapter 2. Reading: Keeping Current — 31
    Personal Essay: Eugene Braunwald, M.D. — 49
    Personal Essay: Philip A. Tumulty, M.D. — 53

Chapter 3. The Personal Information Center — 57
    Personal Essay: Joshua Lederberg, Ph.D. — 69

Chapter 4. The Institutional Medical Library — 73

Chapter 5. The Collegial Network — 81
    Personal Essay: Sherman M. Mellinkoff, M.D. — 97

Chapter 6. Learning from Formal Consultations — 101

Chapter 7. Formal Courses and Conferences — 111

Chapter 8. Technology in Traditional Continuing Education — 125

Chapter 9. Learning from Teaching	133
Personal Essay: Eugene A. Stead, Jr., M.D.	147
Personal Essay: Norton J. Greenberger, M.D.	151
Chapter 10. Analysis of Practice	153
Personal Essay: Ian R. Mackay, M.D.	173
Personal Essay: A. McGehee Harvey, M.D.	179
Chapter 11. Enlisting Help in the Analysis of Practice	181
Chapter 12. Social, Ethical, and Economic Problems in Medicine	193
Chapter 13. The Doctor–Patient Relationship, Physical Examination, and New Procedures	199
Chapter 14. Problems in Practice Unrelated to Medical Knowledge	213
Chapter 15. Women Physicians and Continuing Education	227
Chapter 16. Can Families Help?	239
Chapter 17. The Computer: Aid to Learning and Satisfaction from Practice	247
Chapter 18. The Computer: Guidance in Diagnosis and Therapy	261
Afterword: Phil R. Manning, M.D. and Lois DeBakey, Ph.D.	275
Interviewees and Correspondents	279
Index	287

Photographs

Stephen Abrahamson, 120
Ruth M. Bain, 83
Clarence J. Berne, 161
John E. Bethune, 75
Baruch S. Blumberg, 104
Eugene Braunwald, 48
Thomas H. Brem, 84
Kit Chambers, 242
Lois DeBakey, v
Michael E. DeBakey, 14
Saul J. Farber, 139
John P. Geyman, 205
Norton J. Greenberger, 150
A. McGehee Harvey, 178
J. Willis Hurst, 24
D. Geraint James, 243
Karin E. Jamison, 230
Harold Jeghers, 56
Joshua Lederberg, 68
Peter V. Lee, 208
Leo L. Leveridge, 257
Ceylon S. Lewis, Jr., 136
Donald A. B. Lindberg, 76
Ian R. Mackay, 172
Phil R. Manning, v
Helen E. Martin, 209

Margaret M. McCarron, 64
Sherman M. Mellinkoff, 96
George E. Miller, 143
Francis D. Moore, 89
Robert H. Moser, 36
Jack D. Myers, 267
Kunio Okuda, 202
Claude H. Organ, Jr., 119
Irvine H. Page, 196
Robert G. Petersdorf, 43
Robert E. Rakel, 197
Richard J. Reitemeier, 224
Telfer B. Reynolds, 160
Donald W. Seldin, 44
Dame Sheila Sherlock, 243
Edward H. Shortliffe, 264
Linda D. Shortliffe, 233
Lloyd H. Smith, 63
Eugene A. Stead, Jr., 146
George W. Thorn, 103
Philip A. Tumulty, 52
Lawrence L. Weed, 256
Warren L. Williams, 191
Marjorie Price Wilson, 90
James B. Wyngaarden, 142

Introduction

My first experience in continuing education was as a child, observing my father study nightly. Although he completed only the eighth grade of school and fully supported himself from the age of fourteen, he has read and studied each day to the present, as he approaches 100 years. He undertook educational projects that would help him in his real estate business, and he became a self-taught historian. Although deprived, himself, of schooling, he recognized its increasing importance and emphasized its indispensability to me, but he never stopped stressing by example the importance of independent study of problems arising in one's profession.

My maternal grandfather, after his father's early death, supported himself, his mother, younger brother, and sister from age eleven. Although not formally schooled, he, too, educated himself and rose to a high administrative post in a leading American firm. Reflecting on formal education, especially college, he contended that although college graduates had been taught facts, they often did not understand the significance of those facts, nor did they know how to continue their learning systematically beyond graduation. He was fond of saying that "the road to hell is crowded with people of good intention" and emphasized that performance, not intention, was important. Thus, from the beginning I learned by example that the struggle to remain informed must be continual, that systematic efforts in self-education are essential, that performance counts more than intention, and that continuing education in a profession is most profitable when linked to experience.

During college, this lesson was reinforced as I realized that it was possible to study hard, learn lessons well, perform well on a test, and still attain only a framework upon which to build. The need for experience to furnish challenges and opportunities for practical learning came home to me. These perceptions became clearer several years later, when I became acquainted with Alfred North Whitehead's *Aims of Education*,[1] in which he discussed the value of firsthand knowledge and the danger of "inert ideas." I also realized that Whitehead's "joy of discovery" was usually hard to come by in formal education, with its heavy reliance on facts and its paucity of opportunity for discovery.

Even in the active environment of my internship at the Los Angeles County General Hospital (now the Los Angeles County/USC Medical Center), the thrill of discovery was too often blunted by a resident spilling the beans about diagnosis with "Work up Mr. Jones, who has an epigastric mass that is most likely cancer of the stomach in view of the Virchow's node." The opportunity to gain firsthand information was thus often thwarted.

Since my residency days, I have been interested in individual methods of education for physicians to sustain the delight of learning and to improve their knowledge and skills by becoming more involved in daily clinical activities. My participation in continuing education at the University of Southern California has permitted me to become acquainted with effective techniques used by clinicians. Almost every outstanding physician I know has developed personal systematic methods of centering education on practice.

During my thirty years in formal continuing medical education, I have never heard anyone deny that physicians must be lifelong students. Self-directed and practice-linked learning are also well accepted in principle, but techniques that enhance their execution have not been emphasized in medical schools. By the time physicians enter residency training and practice, many have become too busy to develop their own methods. As a result, they lose the opportunity to profit maximally from their experience. Classroom instruction has therefore been called upon to perform functions that it is ill-equipped to do.

Since the turn of the century, the classroom has dominated continuing medical education in the United States. In 1906, the American Medical Association (AMA) sent Dr. J. N. McCormack to several states to stimulate interest in postgraduate education. Under this stimulus, several states began to organize courses. At the request of the AMA, Dr. John Blackburn, Director of the Bowling Green County Society in Kentucky, submitted a national plan and designed weekly programs on basic sciences and therapy for use by county medical societies.[2]

By 1909, about 350 county societies were sponsoring programs,[3] but because of a decline in attendance, these were ultimately discontinued. In 1916, Dr. W. S. Rankin, North Carolina state health officer, developed circuit courses that took education to rural physicians. The instructors traveled to various communities delivering lectures and discussing the diagnosis and treatment of patients brought in by class attendees.[4]

In 1927, the University of Michigan established the first department of postgraduate medicine within a medical school.[2] Eight years later, John B. Youmans, under the aegis of the Commonwealth Fund, made surprise visits to thirty physicians in small towns and rural communities of Tennessee who had completed formal postgraduate courses at Vanderbilt University School of Medicine and graded them against a standard developed to assess improved quality of practice.[5] Although there was no precourse visit for comparison, Dr. Youmans decided that practical programs dealing with patients and technical procedures were more beneficial than didactic lectures.

In 1932, the Commission on Medical Education of the Association of American Medical Colleges concluded that "Continued education of physicians is synonymous with good medical practice . . ." and called for cooperation of medical associations, medical schools, and hospitals in conducting comprehensive programs of postgraduate education.[6] In 1936, the University of Minnesota constructed the first permanent center to house continuing medical education. Four years later, in accordance with a resolution adopted by the Advisory Board for Medical Specialties, the Commission on Graduate Medical Education was organized. The Commission, led by Willard C. Rappleye, concluded that undergraduate medical education did not strongly motivate busy practitioners to pursue continuing education.[7]

After World War II, the W. K. Kellogg Foundation awarded grants to eighteen medical schools to broaden and innovate continuing medical education.[8] Since then, the growth of formal continuing medical education has been explosive, with hospitals, medical societies, and medical schools acting as the main sponsors. Mandatory continuing medical education and accreditation of organizations offering courses further stimulated the growth of postgraduate classroom instruction. Thus, the emphasis on formal classroom courses has overshadowed individual methods linking education more directly to the physician's own practice. The concept of lifelong learning, in fact, has seemed almost locked in the classroom.

Despite the continued emphasis on classroom education, various authorities, including Osler Peterson,[9] George Miller,[10] John Williamson,[11] and Clement Brown,[12] have demonstrated the limitations of formal continuing education. Miller and his followers have advocated that physicians analyze their practices to identify specific educational needs and thus direct their own education efficiently. In Miller's words, "the practitioner-learner must progress steadily from listener to questioner to participant to contributor."[10]

This book calls attention to the systematic methods that physicians have used to continue their learning, hone their skills, and benefit maximally from their experience. Although traditional classroom approaches will continue to be useful, we expect to see a major shift in emphasis, if not a revolution, away from the conventional classroom enterprise to individual techniques devised by the physician to address his own educational requirements.

Phil R. Manning, M.D.

References

1. Whitehead, Alfred North. *The Aims of Education and Other Essays.* New York: The MacMillian Company, 1959:1–3.
2. Bruce, James D. Postgraduate education in medicine. *J Mich State Med Soc* Jun 1937;36(6):369–377.
3. The American Medical Association, Council on Medical Education and Hospitals. *Graduate Medical Education in the United States: I—Continuation Study for Practicing Physicians 1937 to 1940.* Chicago: American Medical Association, 1940:216.
4. Adams, F. Denetee. The North Carolina extension plan: An experiment in postgraduate medical teaching. *JAMA* Jun 1923;80(23):1714–1717.
5. Youmans, John B. Experience with a postgraduate course for practitioners: Evaluation of results. *J Assoc Am Med Coll* May 1935;10(3):154–173.
6. Commission on Medical Education. Postgraduate medical education. In: *Final Report of the Commission on Medical Education.* New York: Office of the Director of Study, 1932:136.
7. Commission on Graduate Medical Education (W. C. Rappleye, Chm). *Graduate Medical Education.* Chicago: University of Chicago Press, 1940:168.
8. Shepherd, Glen R. History of continuation medical education in the United States since 1930. *J Med Educ* Aug 1960;35(8):740–758.
9. Peterson, Osler L.; Andrews, Leon P.; Spain, Robert S.; Greenberg, Bernard G. An analytical study of North Carolina general practice 1953–54. In 2 pts, pt 2. *J Med Educ* Dec 1956;31(12):1–8.
10. Miller, George E. Continuing education for what? *J Med Educ* Apr 1967;42(4):324.
11. Williamson, John W.; Alexander, Marshall; Miller, George E. Continuing education and patient care research: Physician response to screening test results. *JAMA* Sep 1967;201(12):118–122.
12. Brown, Clement R.; Uhl, Henry S.M. Mandatory continuing education: Sense or nonsense? *JAMA* Sep 1970;213(10):1660–1668.

1
Enjoying the Struggle

> Medicine has been called both a master and a mistress—a master when it is allowed to possess, oppress, and enslave; a mistress when it preserves the passion by remaining engrossing, intriguing, and exhilarating. It is as a mistress that medicine will delight and fulfill the physician.
>
> *Lois DeBakey*

At once one of the most demanding and most rewarding of all professions, medicine can be tyrannizing or exhilarating. If the pressing responsibilities, sensitive interpersonal relationships, and strenuous time pressures in caring for patients are allowed to create tedium or drudgery, the passion for medical practice will vanish. If patient care becomes overly demanding, onerous, or boring, enthusiasm and pleasure will fade, and both patient and physician will suffer. But that does not have to happen. The practice of medicine is admittedly a strict taskmaster, requiring daily decisions about puzzling, often life-threatening illnesses, and demanding constant awareness of the newest available information. But medicine also offers endless opportunities for enjoyment, satisfaction, and exhilaration through intellectual expansion and service to patients.

Can physicians organize their daily work to make the practice of medicine more gratifying? Our extensive interviews indicate that those who immerse themselves most deeply in clinical work enjoy the greatest fulfillment. Such engagement includes daily reading and interacting with colleagues about medical problems, continually examining the nature and results of practice, and modifying performance accordingly. Physicians who practice such immersion base their continuing education largely on the puzzling problems that arise in their practice (individual patients as well as aggregate practice) and the defects they uncover in their performance. And they take prompt remedial steps. The result is improved patient care, gratification, and gusto.

We are not advocating that physicians limit their potential for fulfillment and satisfaction to medical practice, since family, friends, the arts, sports, and hobbies all offer additional rewards. Physicians cannot, however, escape spending inordinate time in practice, so it behooves them to find ways to make the long hours more pleasurable and gratifying. Patients of physicians who enjoy their work, moreover, receive the best care. This book shows how some outstanding physicians have kept the flame of professional fervor alive despite excessive demands on their time and energy.

The Need for Lifelong Learning

Every good physician realizes he must perpetually supplement his knowledge base; he must discard and add continually. Underlying lifelong study are the need to remain aware of the state of medicine, the need to find solutions to specific problems in practice, and the desire for intellectual stimulation, with its attendant personal and social pleasure. The patient is the ultimate beneficiary of all.[1,2]

Rewards from Learning from Experience

Some of the benefits of lifelong learning are subtle, whereas others are more obvious.

Confidence, Self-respect, and Pride

A primary reward of an expanded intellect is greater self-confidence. As Osler wrote, "If you do not believe in yourself how can you expect other people to do so? If you have not an abiding faith in the profession you cannot be happy in it."[3] Paul Sanazaro agreed: "You need the motivation that stems from pride and security in your knowledge. You must know what you are doing and how it compares with the best you can do; any discrepancy should prompt you to do better." A driving force among the outstanding physicians whom we interviewed is their pride in performance—a desire never to be or seem professionally inadequate.

Enjoyment

Since people tend to invest more of themselves in what is enjoyable, the patient benefits when the physician likes his work. Emphasizing the salutary relationship of work and pleasure, George Bernard Shaw, in *John Bull's Other Island*, looked forward to a commonwealth where "work is play and play is life."[4] Osler was fond of quoting John Locke's definition

1. Enjoying the Struggle

of education as a relish for knowledge. "Get early this relish," Osler advised, "this clear, keen joyance in work, with which languor disappears and all shadows of annoyance flee away."[5]

Irvine Page described the engrossing quality of medicine thus: "Medicine makes life worthwhile. If you lose that attitude at any point in your life, you have essentially lost your life. You can combat that danger by remembering that medicine is a grand and rapidly possessive discipline that requires a lifelong interest in things human. If you give that up at any time in your practice, you are lost."

"The method a physician selects for lifelong learning must give pleasure or other rewards," said Eugene Stead, "because human beings will not continue a program that does not have tangible dividends." To make lifelong learning enjoyable, physicians need to organize their time and practice to allow for regular, but not necessarily rigidly scheduled, study in a pleasant, relaxed atmosphere—one that is comfortable, uninterrupted, and unhurried.

The merging of personal and professional pleasure is not uncommon among eminent physicians. To some physicians, the greatest pleasure in medicine comes from seeing a patient improve, and that pleasure is dependent on steady learning. As Michael DeBakey put it, "In medicine, helping others while solving complex intellectual puzzles is our special reward."

Attributes to be Nurtured

Curiosity

> Curiosity is, in great and generous minds, the first passion and the last. . . .
> *Samuel Johnson*[6]

"In research," said Baruch Blumberg, "and probably also in practice, maintaining and fostering curiosity—the ability to ask questions each time a new phenomenon occurs—is indispensable." Most physicians we interviewed considered an insatiable curiosity to be innate or to be established in early childhood, but they also recognized the need to nourish it. The drama and complexity of medicine, by providing opportunities for the thrill of discovery, can arouse curiosity despite the inhibitory effect of time pressures. Not being satisfied with an immediate answer, but wanting to go beyond is the mark of the intellectually curious.

Professor Jean Hamburger of Paris related an incident in medical history that illustrates how curiosity can guide genius, allowing a researcher to explain an experimental result that others may dismiss. "In 1879-1880,

Pasteur and his coworkers studied the fowl cholera germ. It was a most virulent agent, killing all exposed hens within 24 to 48 hours. After some time, however, some cultures of the germ were unable to kill the animals. 'I am possibly responsible for this failure,' said someone in the laboratory, 'since I left the cultures exposed to air for several days before using them. I shall not repeat this mistake, and the next experiment will be made with fresh cultures.' So the same hens were inoculated some weeks later with germs that were supposed to be very virulent. But Pasteur's coworkers were astonished to find that again the hens did not succumb. 'We are sorry,' they said to Pasteur. 'Something must be wrong with our technique or with the hens we use.' But Pasteur turned the negative results to advantage, and out of this 'failed' experiment came the discovery of vaccination with attenuated germs."

Alfredo Sadun recalled an incident involving David Glendenning Cogan, Chief at the Massachusetts Eye and Ear Infirmary of Harvard Medical School. "Dr. Cogan lived in a large townhouse on Beacon Hill, one of the most exclusive areas but not far from where the drunks reside. One evening the doorbell rang and when Mrs. Cogan opened the door, she found a drunk who was asking for money. He behaved obstreperously, and when she found it difficult to get rid of him, she enlisted Dr. Cogan's help. Mrs. Cogan then returned to the kitchen. An hour later, she realized that she had not heard from her husband. Unable to find him in the apartment, she feared he may have come to harm in turning away the drunk. Frantically, she left her apartment and raced down the stairs, only to find Dr. Cogan sitting on the street curb next to the drunk under a street light. Scattered around them were a variety of prisms, which Dr. Cogan was using to measure the extent of the drunk's alcohol-induced strabismus. Dr. Cogan was having the drunk fixate (on dollar bills) at varying distances and was then measuring the induced esotropia. He was carefully logging all the data. This incident illustrates the master clinician's child-like curiosity and the constant enthusiasm, which transcend the oddest situation. Even in the most unclinical setting, David Cogan saw an opportunity for gaining further understanding of a subject of interest."

STIMULATING CURIOSITY. Those we interviewed believe that you can promote curiosity by engaging in academic interests; relating knowledge to experience; associating with stimulating colleagues, mentors, and students; carefully delineating questions rather than seeking immediate answers to ill-defined problems; and developing pet interests in medicine. The burden of too much to do in too short a time, however, is sure to stifle curiosity.

Associating with intellectually curious people stimulates curiosity. Curiosity thrives in an open atmosphere that permits absolute intellectual honesty. Exposure to medical students, residents, fellows, and young colleagues who challenge traditional concepts can also excite curiosity.

Outstanding teachers foster curiosity, especially at the bedside, and teachers who continually ask "Why?" arouse curiosity in their students. Students and house officers who ask provocative questions can have a similar effect on their teachers.

The pursuit of knowledge in a field of special interest and the thrill of resolving previously unanswered or unasked questions are energizing. To formulate a theoretical answer and to later validate it scientifically provide rare moments of excitement. Concern about peer judgment and an intense desire to compete with peers for higher levels of knowledge also spur intellectual curiosity.

Discipline, Diligence, and Determination

Lifelong learning, like the study and training leading to an M.D. degree, requires discipline, diligence, and determination. The late Boy Frame stressed the importance of perseverance: "There is no better feeling than being filled with new knowledge and understanding before one relaxes; it intensifies the fun."

"No matter how much you read or know," said Norton Greenberger, "you have to keep refurbishing your information. In 1958, when I was a senior medical student at the Massachusetts General Hospital, I went on rounds with the Chief Resident, John Knowles. He seemed to know everything about everything. I asked him how he became so smart, and he replied that he had gotten into the habit of reading every day. If you read ten pages a day, that is about 3,000 pages a year, the equivalent of a textbook."

Although most physicians do not write books or review articles, the discipline required to write case reports,[7,8,9] reviews for hospital staff, and educational material for patients and office staff can pay tangible dividends. Claude Welch found that the discipline required to write advanced his education. "For many years, I wrote summary articles on advances in abdominal surgery for *The New England Journal of Medicine*. In preparation, I read all the articles in the major surgical journals as they appeared and noted the most important ones. The major collation and critiques, however, came during the summer, when all my spare time was devoted to reviewing the publications, writing the summaries in longhand, and then composing the article for the journal. The manuscript was subjected to peer review and, after publication, to criticism from readers. By that time, I had managed to retain a great deal of material that I had studied. I doubt that I could have remembered much of the material if I had used a simpler method."

The challenge of teaching stimulates the physician to study and to organize his thoughts. Having a target date encourages setting aside time to review and master a topic. In fact, the most effective way to ensure self-discipline, according to Saul Farber, is to make teaching a part of your daily life.

Compassion and a Sense of Service

In dedicated physicians, an encounter with sick or troubled patients triggers a sense of compassion and stimulates the desire to serve. Truly compassionate physicians are driven to hone their skills continually to serve their patients better. Willis Hurst considers competence to be an important sign of the physician's compassion, for the compassionate physician cares enough about the patient to seek answers to the clinical questions posed by the patient's illness. The methods described in this book permit the physician to channel his compassion into action benefiting his patients.

The importance of compassion becomes evident when one considers the vulnerability of the patient and the trust he places in his physician. As Sir Berkeley Moynihan wrote: "A patient can offer you no higher tribute than to entrust you with his life and health, and, by implication, with the happiness of all his family. To be worthy of this trust we must submit for a lifetime to the constant discipline of unwearied effort in the search of knowledge; and of most reverent devotion to every detail in every operation that we perform."[10]

When asked if he took his work home with him, Michael DeBakey responded: "Of course, I take my work home with me. Any doctor who doesn't should not be practicing medicine. I may have five or six open-heart operations scheduled tomorrow. They are all individual lives to me. I care about them. I worry about them. I think about all of them—their families and their hopes. I may be having dinner with you and talking about baseball, but my mind is with those patients. I wouldn't be a doctor if I didn't do that." We observed the same concern, compassion, and caring in all the outstanding physicians we interviewed, and we are convinced that because of these noble human qualities they are able to perform above the average in ministering to their patients.

Learning from Experience

> To study the phenomena of disease without books is to sail an uncharted sea, while to study books without patients is not to go to sea at all.
>
> *William Osler*[11]

All physicians have experiences from their own practices that reinforce Osler's views. Observations made under the pressure and excitement of patient care are usually remembered. Physicians can recall for decades lessons learned from specific patients and their problems. To be most reliable, the memory must, of course, be substantiated by a review of records and notes and must be integrated into current observations.

Robert Manning related an anecdote illustrating the value of such experience. "One of Dr. Richard Vilter's former residents mustered his courage, approached Dr. Vilter, and asked, 'Dr. Vilter, you are such a marvelous clinician. To what do you attribute your success?' Vilter replied, 'Good judgment.' The questioner thought for a moment and, not completely satisfied with the response, asked, 'But Dr. Vilter, to what do you attribute your good judgment?' Vilter replied 'Experience.' Still not satisfied, the questioner pursued it one step further. 'But Dr. Vilter, how does one gain experience?' Vilter's response: 'Bad judgment.' "

In subsequent chapters we describe conventional as well as idiosyncratic methods used by practicing physicians and academic clinicians to submerge themselves in their professional work and to gain maximal benefit from their experience. But, first, let us review the underlying philosophic principles. The methods used by our interviewees to gain the most from experience and from reading, conferences, and colleagues represent a blending of study and first-hand experience, as advocated by Osler.

First-hand Knowledge

> First-hand knowledge is the ultimate basis of intellectual life. To a large extent book-learning conveys second-hand information, and as such can never rise to the importance of immediate practice.
> *Alfred North Whitehead*[12]

Mortimer Adler underscored the importance of experience when he wrote: "[T]he difference between a man and a child is a difference wrought by experience, pain and suffering, by hard knocks. It cannot be produced by schooling."[13] William Osler echoed that idea when he admonished physicians: "Let not your conception of the manifestations of disease come from words heard in the lecture room or read from the book. See, and then reason and compare and control. But see first."[14] Oliver Wendell Holmes concurred that "The most essential part of a student's instruction is obtained . . . not in the lecture-room, but at the bedside. Nothing seen there is lost; the rhythms of disease are learned by frequent repetition; its unforeseen occurrences stamp themselves indelibly in the memory."[15]

W. Somerset Maugham, who studied medicine, emphasized his vivid memories of clinical experiences. "Even now that forty years have passed I can remember certain people so exactly that I could draw a picture of them. Phrases that I heard then still linger on my ears. I saw how men died. I saw how they bore pain. I saw what hope looked like, fear and relief; I saw the dark lines that despair drew on a face; I saw courage and steadfastness. I saw faith shine in the eyes of those who trusted in what I could only think was an illusion and I saw the gallantry that made a man greet the prognosis of death with an ironic joke because he was too proud to let those about him see the terror of his soul."[16]

MONITORING ONE'S OWN PRACTICE. The most fruitful education for a profession, Cyril Houle wrote, "occurs when its practitioners constantly monitor their own work, making judgments about success or failure and subsequently altering behavior as a consequence."[2] Such monitoring requires techniques that permit analysis of what the physician actually does in the aggregate and the lessons learned from puzzling individual patients. When the physician knows the types of problems seen, the drugs prescribed, and the procedures performed, he can direct his study for maximal benefit to his patients. Medical school faculties, despite lip service to the contrary, still emphasize the didactic transfer of information, and most physicians have therefore not been taught to organize their practices in a way to produce objective data that can direct their education. Fortunately, there are simple ways of organizing and analyzing everyday work, and we describe these throughout the book.

SELF-DIRECTED LEARNING. Malcolm Knowles cited accumulating evidence that "Whatever people learn through their own initiative, they understand better, internalize more effectively, apply more generally, and retain longer than anything they are taught didactically." Since the most valuable continuing education is linked to practical experience and since each physician has individual experiences, the physician can best direct his own learning guided by an analysis of his practice.

George E. Miller wrote: "There is ample evidence to support the view that adult learning is not most efficiently achieved through systematic subject instruction; it is accomplished by involving learners in identifying problems and seeking ways to solve them. It does not come in categorical bundles but in a growing need to know."[17]

Harold Jeghers summarized the basic premises of lifelong learning in medicine thus: "The secret is to learn to educate oneself. One remembers best what one learns by personal effort. Strong initiative and motivation are important. Reading should be directed primarily toward solving a problem with a specific goal in mind. Since patient care is basic to the practice of medicine, reading and learning are most effective when they involve discussion and solution of clinical problems. Beyond formal education, a well-developed personal medical library supports continued personal education."

Make the Most of Your Situation

Some physicians fail to become immersed in their practice because they allow it to become too routine. This is primarily an attitudinal problem, for almost any practice environment can be made stimulating. E. Mansell Pattison uses his regular resident clinical case conference to stimulate forays into "forgotten and new paths of clinical investigation." "My teacher, Dr. Maury Levine of Cincinnati," recalled Dr. Pattison, "used to admonish us that each clinical case is a research project. I similarly ask my residents to look for the unanswered research question in every routine case. The rewards have been ample. In just the past year, 'routine' cases uncovered interesting information. A depressed patient with porphyria led to a literature review and the discovery that porphyric psychosis is omitted from current textbooks of medicine; a case of pseudo-seizure led to the demonstration of a basic linkage in the thought-speech process; a case of self-mutilation led to the description of a new clinical syndrome; a case of dissociation led to the analysis of visceral brain components of consciousness. Four simple cases led to four major research projects. That is surely enough excitement in one year to keep a jaded administrator alive and enthusiastically on his toes to see what the next 'routine case' will turn up."

An incident involving Willis Hurst and Eugene Stead and related by William Waters, III, illustrates that any circumstance can take on investigative significance if you have a research bent. "When Dr. Stead was to serve as Visiting Professor, Dr. Hurst picked him up at the airport in his automobile. Dr. Hurst had a seatbelt installed only on the driver's side, since he used the car only for commuting. When both entered the car, Dr. Hurst buckled his seatbelt, and Dr. Stead looked around for his. Finding none, he asked facetiously, 'What am I? The control?'"

Companionship in Medicine

Self-directed learning does not, of course, require isolation. Adults almost always go to somebody for help in diagnosing, planning, evaluating, or obtaining content information.[18] In medicine, the collegial network provides strong support for physicians by allowing them to share experiences, knowledge, and inspiration in an atmosphere of fellowship while remaining responsible for their own learning. Discussions with colleagues about patients and medical problems afford excellent opportunities to gain information enjoyably.

"Encouragement of medical companionship is important," said Sherman Mellinkoff, "whether in group practice, participation in rounds, attendance at courses to update important subjects, or attendance at medical meetings. When a complicated problem needs clarification, I sometimes go to the library, but I usually turn to one of my colleagues for a consultation. It is so useful for doctors to have little groups or affinities that provide someone near at hand with whom to exchange ideas and discuss patients or published articles. Such interaction makes learning more vibrant and useful."

"One of the reasons we academicians like our work," noted Norton Greenberger, "is that we learn a lot by osmosis. We go to conferences, and we seek out people who have the answers to our questions. So my advice to young physicians is to surround yourself with people who can educate you."

Reducing Reliance on Memory

Acquiring knowledge when it is needed is more effective than memorizing facts that may not be used for weeks or months. "I have never tried to convert medical students into textbooks," said Eugene Stead. "If we did, we would clearly be forced to lower tuition, since the best composite of medical knowledge can be purchased for $150." Alfred North Whitehead, too, cautioned against the evil of "bare knowledge" and "inert ideas." He defined education as the art of the use of knowledge, whose importance lies in our active mastery of it—that is to say, it lies in wisdom. "Get your knowledge quickly, and then use it. If you can use it, you will retain it."[19] He wisely noted that "Knowledge does not keep any better than fish."[20]

Lawrence Weed has long objected to our expectation that physicians remember the details in the numerous textbooks they were required to memorize in medical school to pass their examinations. He laments that we further expect them to keep abreast of the newest medical information published and presented at meetings and to apply all this knowledge effectively in their practices. Failure, he believes, is built into those expectations.[21]

Using Information Sources Efficiently

Instead of describing methods that rely too heavily on memorization and learning facts unrelated to current problems, we shall emphasize manual and electronic methods that help physicians access and use information sources efficiently at times when problems arise.

Weed looks forward to the day when the computer will aid physicians in electronically implementing the current manual methods of managing information. He suggests that the computer will decrease reliance on memory. "What if information could be disseminated at the speed of light, and spread before the doctor readably, instantly, at office or hospital, so that he wouldn't have to do any more memorizing except the kind that happens automatically? What freedom to think, to judge, to analyze and synthesize facts, to give full and careful thought to the right pathway through a patient's difficulties, if the doctor can see a display of them all coupled with the medical information he needs to make decisions!"[21]

Framing the Right Questions

"One learns by asking oneself questions, then finding the answers," said Eugene Stead. The physician must decide what he knows and what he does not know. He must then formulate questions and consult the proper source to answer the questions. With emphasis on methods of organization, storing, and accessing pertinent information, the skill for for-

1. Enjoying the Struggle

mulating proper questions becomes essential. "I would be very happy if every student, every resident, and every cardiac fellow felt that it is more important to learn how to ask questions and pursue the answers, themselves, than it is for me to ask questions for them to answer," said Willis Hurst. "I believe that asking questions is what they should do all their lives."

Reading, conferences, and discussions with colleagues alert the physician to what he does not know. Associating with other physicians with similar interests helps in the delineation of the right questions, and an exchange of information leads to recognition of what needs to be answered. Unanswered questions should stimulate the physician, but he must guard against frustration from not being able to find all the answers alone.

Setting Priorities

Formulating clear, attainable goals not only enhances Harold Cross's satisfaction from his practice but improves his performance: "Defining goals for my practice never occurred to me until a few months before I entered private practice in 1958. Writing out specifically how I expected my practice to be run—to ensure a minimum standard of care for patients seeking a physical examination or being evaluated for a minor problem—greatly benefited me. A healthful life includes intellectual, emotional, and financial goals. To reach my intellectual goals, I initially set aside one half-day a week, and now I reserve one day a week—free of practice responsibility and calls—to pursue medical and other interests without taking any time from my family. Through this arrangement, I established and directed a blood gas laboratory, co-authored a book on problem-oriented practice, instructed hundreds of visitors to the PROMIS Clinic, trained nonsurgical orthopedic personnel, and am currently working on the use of the computer in solving medical problems."

Start Now

> The supreme value is not the future but the present. The future is a deceitful time that always says to us, 'Not yet,' and thus denies us.
> *Octavio Paz*[22]

Roy Behnke considers the complaint of some physicians that they are so far behind they can never catch up to be merely an excuse. "Many of my colleagues say that the task is so overwhelming, what is the use of trying to catch up? But you must start somewhere. Those who try to make continuing education too formal are the ones who never get it done; the system beats them. Medicine offers the advantage of informal education. You can pursue it at almost any hour of the day, and five minutes is time enough if you have arranged for the information to be easily accessible.'' So resist the temptation to procrastinate or defer the task. Remember:

> The Bird of Time has but a little way
> To fly—and Lo! the Bird is on the Wing.[23]

References

1. Richards, Robert K.; Cohen, Rita M. Why physicians attend traditional CME programs. *J Med Educ* Jun 1980;55(6):479-485.
2. Houle, Cyril O. *Continuing Learning in the Professions.* San Francisco: Jossey-Bass, 1980;208-209.
3. Osler, William. The reserves of life. Address delivered at St. Mary's Hospital, London, Oct 2, 1907. *St. Mary's Hospital Gazette* Nov 1907;13:97.
4. Shaw, Bernard. John Bull's Other Island. In: *Bernard Shaw Selected Plays with Prefaces*, Vol 2. New York: Dodd, Mead & Co., 1957:611.
5. Osler, William. After twenty-five years. An address at the opening of the session of the medical faculty, McGill University, September 21, 1899. *Montreal Med J* Nov 1899;28(11):832.
6. Johnson, Samuel. *The Rambler*, Vol 5, No. 150, Aug 24, 1751. London: J. Payne and J. Bouquet, 1752:120.
7. DeBakey, Lois. *The Scientific Journal: Editorial Policies and Practices.* St. Louis: The C. V. Mosby Company, 1976.
8. DeBakey, Lois; DeBakey, Selma: The Case Report. I. Guidelines for Preparation. *Int J Cardiol* Oct 1983;4(3):357-364.
9. DeBakey, Lois; DeBakey, Selma: The Case Report. II. Style and Form. *Int J Cardiol* Aug 1984;6(2):247-254.
10. Moynihan, Sir Berkeley. *Abdominal Operations*, Vol 1, revised, preface to the 4th ed. Philadelphia: W. B. Saunders Co., 1926:11-12.
11. Osler, William. Books and men. In: *Aequanimitas, with Other Addresses to Medical Students, Nurses and Practitioners of Medicine.* 3rd ed. Philadelphia: The Blakiston Company, 1945:210.
12. Whitehead, Alfred North. Technical education and its relation to science and literature. In: *The Aims of Education and Other Essays.* New York: The MacMillan Company, 1959:79.
13. Adler, Mortimer. Why only adults can be educated. In: Gross, Ronald, ed. *Invitation to Lifelong Learning.* Chicago: Follett Publishing Company, 1982:92.
14. Osler, William. In: Bean, William Bennett, ed. *Sir William Osler: Aphorisms from His Bedside Teachings and Writings.* Springfield, Illinois: Charles C. Thomas, 1968:36.
15. Holmes, Oliver Wendell. Scholastic and Bedside Teaching. In: *Medical Essays: 1842-1882*, Vol IX. Boston and New York: Houghton Mifflin Company, 1911:273.
16. Maugham, W. Somerset. *The Summing Up.* Garden City, New York: Doubleday & Company Inc., 1946.
17. Miller, George E. Continuing education for what? *J Med Educ* Apr 1967;42(4):322.
18. Tough, Allen. *The Adult's Learning Projects: A Fresh Approach to Theory and Practice in Adult Learning*, 2nd ed. Austin, Texas: Learning Concepts, 1979.

19. Whitehead, Alfred North. The rhythmic claims of freedom and discipline. In: *The Aims of Education and Other Essays*. New York: The MacMillan Company, 1959:57.
20. Whitehead, Alfred North. Universities and their function. In: *The Aims of Education and Other Essays*. New York: The MacMillan Company, 1959:147.
21. Weed, Lawrence L. *Your Health Care and How to Manage It*. Essex Junction, Vermont: Essex Publishing Company Inc., 1975:91.
22. Paz, Octavio. Development and other mirages. In: *The Other Mexico: Critique of the Pyramid*. Kemp, Lysander (trans). New York: Grove Press Inc., 1972:68.
23. Khayyam, Omar. *Rubaiyat of Omar Khayyam*. Fitzgerald, Edward (trans). London: John Lane the Bodley Head Ltd, 1922: quatrain 7.

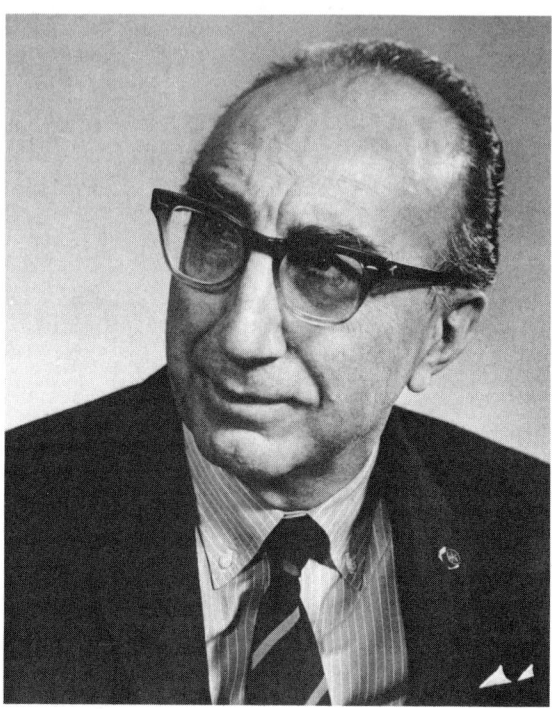

Medicine is an absorbing, even possessive, profession, but the intellectual rewards, humanitarian service, and fulfillment are unsurpassed.

Michael E. DeBakey, M.D.

The inscription on the bust of Michael E. DeBakey in The DeBakey Heart Center, which he directs, in the Texas Medical Center in Houston reads "Surgeon, Educator, Medical Statesman. In recognition of one who served so many." For his pioneering achievements in cardiovascular surgery, he has received countless honors from universities, medical and civic organizations, American Presidents, and heads-of-state throughout the world. As an undergraduate medical student, Dr. DeBakey devised a roller pump that later became an essential component of the heart-lung machine and thus made open-heart surgery possible. His vast contributions include the first successful excision and graft replacement of arterial aneurysms and obstructive lesions, the first successful carotid endarterectomy, the first successful use of an artificial heart-assist device in a patient, and the first successful coronary artery bypass. Inventor of numerous surgical instruments, author of more than 1200 articles and books, many now considered classics, he has served as editor and editorial board member of prestigious journals and as consultant to governmental agencies here and abroad.

Dr. DeBakey's total commitment to, and fascination with, medicine and its humanitarian aims have been an inspiration to patients, students, and associates alike.

Personal Essay

Michael E. DeBakey, M.D.
*Chancellor; Chairman, Department of Surgery; and
Olga Keith Wiess Professor of Surgery
Baylor College of Medicine
Houston, Texas*

Early Influences

Parents

I have been asked what inspired me to take the path I have pursued in life. The answer lies in my boyhood. My parents, with their keen intellects, natural curiosity, and high standards, were superb models because they sought excellence in everything they did. Anything worth their time, they felt, was worth doing well. By example, they inspired and encouraged me in that philosophy. They valued education highly and gave their children every opportunity to learn and to fulfill their potential, not only in school but in music, the arts, and athletics. All of us had music lessons as children. I learned to play several instruments and was a member of the school band. At home, we were surrounded by books, but we were also encouraged to read at least one book a week from the city library, in addition to our schoolwork. We learned early that books were wonderful companions.

At a very early age, we were also given an opportunity to experience gratification from some special achievement—whether it was mastering a subject in our schoolwork, learning to play a musical composition well, or excelling in gardening or a sport. Our parents helped us discover the *delight* of learning, and they often made our new knowledge more significant by relating it to some interesting story in their own lives or to some current or historical event. Although they did not prod or nag us about studying, they did encourage, direct, and support our learning. Almost every family event was a learning experience—whether it was a

---

Mike does a tremendous amount of surgery. Many people look upon this as a highly impersonalized, mechanical venture. But you ought to make rounds with Mike about ten o'clock in the evening and watch him go through and touch his people. No one else can do such technical work in a highly personal way as Mike can.

Eugene A. Stead, Jr., M.D.

Because of his warmth, compassion, and humanity that symbolize the finest ideals of his profession, he has been beloved by his students, colleagues, and many esteemed friends in every walk of life.

David C. Sabiston, Jr., M.D.

picnic, where we learned about nature; a hunting trip, where we learned sportsmanship; or a family meal, where conversations were always interesting. When we asked questions, our parents satisfied our immediate curiosity with an explanation, but then encouraged us to delve further into the subject by reading about it. If the children had disagreements about certain issues—and children can be extremely opinionated—our parents suggested we could settle the matter by consulting a dictionary, encyclopedia, or other authoritative source. They explained that our opinions would be respected more if we could support them with some evidence, and so we were discouraged from formulating firm opinions without a valid basis or, to express it differently, from developing raw prejudices. Reason and common sense were highly respected in our home.

One incident illustrates how our parents nurtured our education. When I was a young boy, my father took me with him on a hunting trip, and when he set me down in the field, he said, "Now stay right here; I won't be far away." He would go a short distance, glancing back at me often and returning every little while to bring back some ducks that he had shot. On one such occasion, he noticed that I had my hands behind my back, and he said, "What's wrong with your hands?" Eventually, I had to reveal my hands, which were bloody. He was immediately alarmed and asked, "What did you do? Did you cut yourself?" I confessed that I had taken a knife out of the pouch and had opened the ducks. "Why did you do that?" he asked. "I wanted to find out how they fly," I explained. Shortly after that, my father read me a book about birds flying. He noted my early curiosity, and he encouraged and stimulated it. Throughout my student years, he and my mother supported my fascination with medicine and surgery.

We hear much today about the disintegration of the American family, and my heart goes out to those who have missed the joys of belonging to a close-knit, loving family. Our parents' affection for us was evident in everything they did, but they also imposed discipline, often in subtle ways. We all had tasks assigned and were expected to show personal responsibility and self-reliance in performing them.

I feel fortunate in having received moral and spiritual guidance as a child, because I think it is valuable for everyone, and especially for physicians. Largely by parental example, we learned that honesty, integrity, compassion, and personal and social responsibility enrich life and enhance peace of mind. Intellectual development without these values is compromised, in my view. The family integrity that my parents cherished so deeply gave me a sense of purpose and gave my life direction. It is, perhaps, the greatest legacy anyone can receive, and for a physician it is indispensable.

Teachers

Having dedicated teachers who reinforced my parents' interest in education encouraged me to do my best in my assignments. I was fortunate to come under the guidance of a number of professors who took an interest in me, among them my zoology professor. I became so interested in zoology that when I went home on vacation, I set up a large aquarium in my parents' garage and filled it with various kinds of marine life so I could continue my study during the summer. That professor appointed me as a student assistant, and during subsequent summers I continued to work in his department. I gave courses, including graduate courses, and I had to read and study the material thoroughly in order to teach it. My professor of English Literature showed a similar interest in me and invited me to major in that subject. His guidance nurtured my literary bent.

Perhaps the professor who influenced me more than anyone else was Dr. Alton Ochsner, under whose influence I came as a medical student. At that time I was not sure I wanted to practice surgery, but he and his associate, Dr. Mims Gage, encouraged me to go into surgery and got me involved in research in the laboratory. I spent a lot of time in the laboratory, and so did Dr. Ochsner. I invented my first medical device when I was still in medical school—a roller pump, which later became an essential component of the heart-lung machine. I think my interest in inventions was whetted by watching my Father constantly improving devices he used and seeking, and usually finding, more efficient ways of accomplishing tasks.

Dr. Ochsner also got me involved in writing papers with him, and, as my early bibliography attests, we wrote a lot of papers together. So I was trained in academic work, and I liked it very much because it permitted continual learning. Dr. Ochsner suggested that I go abroad because he had been to Europe for some of his own training, and in those days, American physicians often studied in the great European universities. Although it was around the time of the Great Depression, my parents financed my stay abroad—another indication of how highly they valued education. I worked in the research laboratories of two eminent professors: René Leriche at the University of Strasbourg and Martin Kirschner at the University of Heidelberg. I learned to speak French and German, and I developed valuable associations. It was an extremely worthwhile period.

Self-discipline

Next to intellectual curiosity, perhaps self-discipline is most important for continuing education. I see a lot of young students who have not yet developed the self-discipline that is necessary for them to organize their studies and other activities effectively. They flit from one thing to another; they allow themselves to be distracted by matters that are not really helpful to them; they tend to associate diversion with passive entertainment. Television has probably been responsible, more than almost anything else, for promoting passivity. The enigma is that people can become glued to their television sets when the programming is generally so poor. Learning, however, is anything but passive; it is a highly active process that can also be extremely gratifying. Electronic devices represent a remarkable technologic advance, especially because of the speed with which they can provide masses of information, but they are no substitute for human reasoning. And reasoning is at the crux of the physician's daily work.

Reasoning

Few experiences are more enjoyable than reasoning and learning, whether your subject is nature, science, history, or the arts. The exhilaration of solving a difficult problem is hard to match. And when you put your whole heart and soul into whatever you do, your sense of self-worth soars. You gain self-confidence, and you are more at peace with yourself. Today entrepreneurs make millions selling books and giving courses on "self-actualization" and on finding out "who you are," but if you develop self-discipline and invest your full attention and effort in whatever you do, you will not need a course to tell you who you are. You will know.

Most physicians recognize the need for a good foundation in the sciences, but are less aware of the importance of the humanities. Since, however, literature deals with all aspects of the human experience—the happy and the tragic, the base and the ennobling—it teaches much about human nature and human life that is useful to the physician. Continuing to read good literature, including history, throughout life is an asset. For a while our educational system failed to give youngsters a knowledge or a sense of history, and that is unfortunate. I would urge every young physician to read the major works on medical history. Not only are the lives of the great achievers inspiring, but history puts the present in perspective, and so helps us better understand what is going on now and what the most judicious course might be for the future.

Philosophy, including ethics and logic, are also intriguing subjects, and those who study these subjects are likely to consider all aspects of an issue, including dissenting views, rather than to form dogmatic opinions. Because mathematics enhances reasoning ability, it is useful for physicians. Intellectual and cultural development should go hand in hand with physical development, and all are definite assets to the physician. Athletics improve a child's coordination and physical well-being, in addition to advancing his socialization by teaching cooperation and a sense of fair play. A diversity of activities not only affords balance, but provides a stable base for pursuits in adulthood.

Language

And then there is language—the crucial instrument of communication. The whole thinking process is entwined with language—terms and their meanings. Yet I see young people coming out of college today with little understanding of the need for clarity and precision in their speech and writing. Because of deficiencies in their education, they tend to be sloppy in their thinking. Medical students, in presenting a case, will say that a patient had a tumor of the breast without identifying which breast, or pain in the leg without indicating which leg. They know that the tumor was in the right breast, but they do not convey that information to their audience. In medicine especially, precision is paramount. To say that a patient has an infarction without precisely defining its site and extent is to withhold information crucial to effective treatment. Simplicity and clarity of expression are as important as precision for the physician, especially in communicating with patients. Taking the time to explain a patient's symptoms can relieve his anxiety about imagined grave health problems. The compassionate physician will sense a patient's anxiety and will try to assuage it. Moreover, the patient who understands his diagnosis and the prescribed treatment is likely to be more cooperative in that treatment and in following the physician's advice for remaining well after recovery.

Continuing Education

As every physician knows, the competent practice of medicine requires lifelong learning. I have been able to obtain the kind of information that meets my specific needs by keeping abreast of current publications, by studying topics of special interest more deeply, by arranging regular interdisciplinary discussions, including meetings on research, and by continually analyzing my own surgical results. In The DeBakey Heart Center, we hold weekly meetings at which the staffs in various basic and clinical research disciplines present their current work and bring up complex matters for general discussion. These regular meetings afford a remarkable educational opportunity.

Writing

Writing is also a superb method of continuing education, particularly in medicine, because it requires comprehensive, critical reasoning. Teachers and scientists have an obligation to disseminate new knowledge in this way. Since my early years, when my parents encouraged all of us to write letters and keep journals, I have had an interest in writing. When, as a grammar-school student, I went abroad with my family, I wrote letters about our trip to my teachers, and was pleased when the letters were published in the local newspaper. That, of course, further encouraged my literary efforts.

When I began collaborating on manuscripts with my chief, Dr. Alton Ochsner, I would retire to my office or laboratory at the medical school daily after completion of my routine teaching and clinical duties, and would remain there until midnight doing laboratory research, reading published articles, and preparing reports of our own results. One long counter in my office was always stacked high with library books, and I spent hours abstracting articles, verifying references, documenting statements, and reverifying statistics. I learned early to take personal responsibility for every step in the preparation of a manuscript for publication or presentation. That self-discipline has been most rewarding.

When I write articles for presentation or publication, I read material that I might not otherwise see in journals I routinely review. At meetings throughout the world in which I participate, I have been able to learn what research is being done and how medicine is practiced in different regions. As a member of various editorial boards over the years, I have also had the opportunity of reviewing manuscripts of research work at the forefront of medicine and have thus been kept informed of the latest scientific developments.

Analysis of Clinical Experience

Another excellent method of continuing education for the physician is periodic analysis of his clinical experience for presentation at meetings or for publication. In my own analyses, I try to determine the factors that affect survival, complications, and mortality. If I am analyzing my clinical results for aortic valve replacement, for example, I do a bibliographic search for articles on different kinds of valves and then compare my experience with the results of others. Such a study may lead me to use a certain valve. After a time, I will do another comparative analysis of my results with that valve and of results obtained by others. In this way, you can determine whether your techniques are better or worse than those of your peers.

Reviewing accumulated clinical cases can disclose extremely useful information. The analysis of angiograms of my patients with occlusive arterial disease, for example, led me to recognize certain patterns of disease and their segmental nature. That recognition permitted me to devise an effective surgical treatment for these patients, even though the cause of the disease remained obscure.

One technique that I use for follow-up is to write the physicians of patients, or the patients themselves, at regular intervals to inquire about their progress and state of health. Not only does this assure patients of my personal interest and concern, but it also provides valuable feedback about treatment or progress of the disease.

In the practice of medicine, you must continually expand your knowledge if you are to give your patients the best available care. When a new surgical technique is introduced, my colleagues and I first study it, and if we decide it shows promise as a safe and effective procedure, we try it, sometimes modifying and improving it. Continually seeking better ways of treating patients is every physician's obligation, and in my specialty that has sometimes led me to design a new surgical instrument or develop a new operative technique.

From time to time every physician will have an extraordinarily difficult case about which he would like a little more information. There are two ways to get it. One is to review previous publications to see if anyone has had such a case and, if so, how he dealt with it. The other is to review your own clinical experience to see if you have had that particular problem before and what the results were. I have complex problems referred to me from throughout the world, and a continual study of my clinical experience has been invaluable to me in handling those problems. Patterns emerge as your series increases, and recognition of such patterns led me to devise the surgical treatment for aneurysms before the cause of the underlying disease was fully understood.

We found, also, that the most common cause of death in patients with certain types of vascular disorders was coronary disease. In analyzing that experience, we focused upon coronary disease as an important factor contributing to death, and this led us to do specific studies on patients with vascular disease to determine whether they had coronary disease. That analysis showed that in some patients it is important to deal with the coronary disease before you deal with the other vascular disease. We did the same type of study with carotid arterial occlusive disease.

Keeping Current

The physician can facilitate his continuing medical education by developing a routine for keeping abreast of scientific publications. He can regularly review selected journals related to his particular practice, and he can have in his personal medical library, for his ready reference, books and articles dealing with his special medical discipline. Further, he can attend meetings related to the clinical problems he sees in his practice. And if he can set aside several hours a week to participate in hospital or medical-school activities, he will not only find them intellectually stimulating, but he will also learn of new developments almost as they occur. In most centers such as ours, activities of this kind are well organized. Every hospital, even in small communities, should have a continuing education program, with regular meetings for its medical and allied health staffs. Preparing presentations for such meetings is certainly educational for the speaker, and the information disseminated is useful to the listeners.

When such discussions center on patients under consideration at the time, they have a special impact. The interchanges with colleagues and students are invaluable.

In our Surgery Department, we have regular weekly conferences, at which the staff presents an analysis of various cases. If a faculty member goes to a medical meeting elsewhere to give a talk, he will summarize the proceedings for the staff, and a discussion will follow. We also have conferences dealing with complications and deaths, in which the clinical data are thoroughly discussed; another conference at which unusually interesting cases are presented; and a journal conference, which is largely for residents. For those of us interested in cardiovascular disease, the cardiology and cardiovascular surgery units hold combined conferences. Basic science personnel engaged in cardiovascular work often participate in such conferences. When I designed our Cardiovascular Research and Clinical Center, I insisted on having basic scientists and clinicians from all pertinent disciplines housed in the Center, and this interdisciplinary nature of our Center has been one of its most important and productive features.

My hope is that formal medical education will not become too rigid—that the emphasis will not focus on structure more than on the actual educational process. Continuing education means *active* learning, and whereas guidance, counseling, and direction are helpful, education should not be rigidified. If, for example, a student's purpose in studying is solely to pass an examination, he is not going to retain a great deal of knowledge—or gain very much wisdom. The examination should be a means of evaluating one's own state of knowledge, and the emphasis should be on the *knowledge*, not on the test. I would hope that medical education would not be restricted to the absorption of facts, but that it would encourage critical thinking, would include ethical issues, and would foster a humanitarian approach to the care of patients. All learning benefits the learner by expanding his mind and enlarging his world and benefits others when the acquired knowledge is applied for their advantage. In the case of physicians, the application of knowledge often yields dramatic humanitarian results, and we are therefore uniquely motivated, and obligated, to continue our education throughout life. In medicine, helping others while solving complex intellectual puzzles is our special reward.

Pleasure in Work

Finally, I consider it essential for each person to select a career that greatly appeals to him instead of taking the line of least resistance and cavalierly or fortuitously entering a path to which he must then commit himself for life. If your work is not to your liking, you will look for any diversion or distraction you can find; you will rarely do your best; and you will feel no pride or satisfaction in your performance. If, on the other hand, the career you have chosen is enjoyable, as mine is to me, you will look forward to going to work each day, and you will feel no desperate need to "escape" periodically. Medicine is an absorbing, even possessive, profession, but the intellectual rewards, humanitarian service, and fulfillment are unsurpassed.

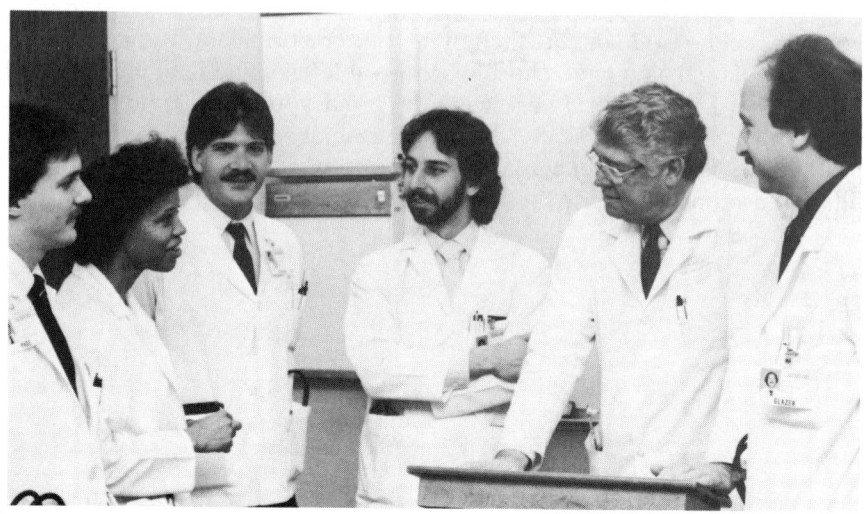

I would be very happy if every student, every resident, and every cardiac fellow felt that it is more important to learn how to ask questions and pursue the answers, themselves, than it is for me to ask questions for them to answer. I believe that asking questions is what they should do all their lives.

J. Willis Hurst, M.D. (second from right)

That Dr. Willis Hurst is a master teacher has been validated by his numerous awards for this skill, including the Master Teacher Award and the Gifted Teacher Award of the American College of Cardiology, as well as the Distinguished Teacher Award of the American College of Physicians. He has received both the Golden Heart Award and the Herrick Award from the American Heart Association. He has published countless articles, and is Editor of the classic textbook of cardiology, *The Heart*, as well as of *Medicine for the Practicing Physician*. He has served as Chairman of the Subspecialty Board of Cardiovascular Diseases, as a Member of the National Advisory Heart, Lung, and Blood Council, as President of the American Heart Association, and as President of the Association of Professors of Medicine.

Willis Hurst's interest in teaching and his genius for instruction are as fresh and powerful today as they were 26 years ago. I have many vivid pictures of Willis striding to the podium with several worn and aged books, ready to read the words of past masters to us. Willis brings to his medicine and his teaching a first-rate mind and a potent style. He has an unerring focus on the fundamentals of medicine. Every action, mannerism, and felicitous phrase are in the service of his teaching. He is a striking role model, exemplifying the best qualities to be found in physicians: compassion; clear thinking; and concern for patients, students, and house officers.

Kenneth Walker, M.D.

Personal Essay

J. Willis Hurst, M.D.
Candler Professor of Medicine (Cardiology)
Emory University School of Medicine
Chief of Cardiology, Emory University Hospital and Clinic
Atlanta, Georgia

Early Influences

Some of us are fortunate enough to have had excellent models in early life. My father, who was a school superintendent, greatly influenced my interest in, and keen desire for, knowledge and excellence. When I was a child, we lived in a large, dormitory-like house near the school where my father worked. My aunt, who taught the first three grades at the school, lived in the same building and taught me before I started school. I recall that when, as my first-grade teacher, she called on me in class to read and I did so, the entire class laughed. I suppose my class members thought it was a joke on the teacher. I was exposed to this superb teacher all day long and at night as well. She taught me through the third grade. My father recognized the ability of my next teacher and transferred her from the fourth to the fifth to the sixth grades as I progressed each year. So, I had only two teachers during the first six grades.

I was also blessed with good high-school teachers. Many of them were an inspiration to me, but my father's interest in education probably had the greatest influence on me. When I was about 15 years old, he gave up teaching to work for the Federal Savings and Loan Association because he could not support his family on the low salary teachers received during the Depression. But he always loved teaching; he read a great deal and encouraged me to read. I recall my great joy when we purchased our first encyclopedia. I spent many hours on cold winter days simply turning the pages of the encyclopedia. I am pleased to state I remember many of the pages until this day.

Compassion as an Important Component of Competence

Today, when so much is being said about compassion, we overlook competence as an important sign of the physician's compassion. If he cares enough about the patient to ask the necessary questions and is self-disciplined enough to seek the answers, competence becomes a component of compassion. The most competent physicians are usually compassionate.

Because they have great concern about being wrong, they make a concerted effort to be right. The most competent, most compassionate physicians have no psychological problem requesting consultation or admitting that they do not know something.

Teaching and Learning

Teaching and learning go hand in hand. Physicians should live up to their title, *doctor*, which means teacher. One can always find someone to teach. Practicing physicians should teach patients, just as they should interact instructively with colleagues.

Instead of giving details, the teacher should discuss concepts. The purpose of lectures should be to create interest, stimulate students' curiosity, and motivate them to seek further information. The teacher must also have a good sense of timing and know when to bring up each subject. Part of a teacher's success depends on personality, and the common denominator in the personality of good teachers is their ability to stimulate students to work on problems when the teacher is not there. The teacher then checks the ability of the student to *think* rather than regurgitate facts.

Asking the Right Question

Most physicians are stimulated to learn as a result of questions that arise about the care of their patients. When a specific question arises about one of my patients, I try to define the question early. Without a specific question, I would have to read one or more chapters in a textbook to solve the problem, whereas with a carefully circumscribed problem I need to look up only that specific information. In other words, the answer to the question starts with a clear and simple statement of the specific problem. The next step is to look up the answer in an authoritative general textbook of medicine and then bring the information up-to-date by reviewing the index issues of journals that have been published since publication of the latest edition of the textbook.

I encourage students, residents, and fellows to learn to ask the right questions rather than to expect me to pose the questions to them. In so doing, I hope to initiate in them a practice that will become habitual. Good teachers should guide students, not simply ask questions and elicit answers. If I could change one thing, I would like to correct that deficiency in our educational system. In the early years of schooling, students ask questions all day. Young children are curious and do not hesitate to ask questions, but as they grow older, the child-like questioning is blocked by external forces, and students are expected only to answer the teachers' questions. I have no objection to testing students by having them answer questions if they are also permitted and encouraged to *ask* questions of their teachers and, more important, of themselves. If the student phrases questions properly and has the self-discipline to pursue specific answers in textbooks, journals, or consultations with others, then the teacher has succeeded.

In medicine, as Kipling admonished reporters, we need to ask who, what, when, where, and how.* Remember, however, that many obstacles will interfere with asking those simple questions. Residents or fellows often have difficulty describing the discomfort of angina pectoris, and they may discuss the irrelevant. Finally, I will say: "*What* does it feel like to the patient? *When* does it occur? *Where* is the discomfort? *How* does it occur (pathophysiology)?" Not a bad set of guidelines for the description of ischemic coronary atherosclerosis.

When my publisher wanted me to prepare a book on self-assessment to help readers test their knowledge of my textbook, *The Heart*, I enlisted the cooperation of second-year cardiac fellows. They had been residents for three years, so they had been out of medical school for five years. I had them formulate questions about each chapter in *The Heart*. I was astounded because the fellows I thought would do a good job did not do well, and vice versa. We had the usual problems with grammar and with clear delineation of the questions—deficiencies that are well-known to all teachers. But more than that, some of them wrote questions that were of no teaching value, such as: What is the important item on the page? It took about four times longer than I had anticipated to complete this project. I learned that people who are skilled at answering a teacher's questions may not be skilled at asking questions, and vice versa. Those capable of asking themselves important questions, I believe, will be the leaders if they also have the self-discipline to pursue the answers.

Education outside Specialty

All specialists should participate at least once a week in discussions in the general field of medicine. Cardiologists need to talk with other cardiologists, but they also need to listen to gastroenterologists, surgeons, ophthalmologists, dermatologists, obstetricians, and other specialists. This is vital to physicians who wish to make good decisions about the problems exhibited by their patients. We must all concentrate on what *should* be done for a patient rather than what *can* be done. We can do many things today, but this does not mean that we *should* do them. The excellent subspecialist must make decisions about patients after reviewing *all* the problems the patient has.

---

*Kipling, Rudyard. The Elephant's Child. In: *Just So Stories*. New York: Magnum Easy Eye Books, Lancer Books, 1968:47.

Data and Problem Formulation

I have always appreciated the emphasis that Larry Weed gives to linking the patient problem to a clear set of questions. If you determine in advance the kind of data you are going to collect (data base), you should be able to state the problem clearly (problem formulation). The next question is "How do I attack this problem initially?" What diagnostic, therapeutic, and educational plans are needed? Larry Weed would say "Don't be pompous; nobody is smart enough to hit the nail on the head every time." The data should be recorded.

If you look more deeply at what Weed said, you will find that he is trying to bring to medicine some of the clear thinking and questioning that started with the Greek scholars. Weed and I both believe that we should observe and record our observations on patients as carefully as scientists record their observation in the research laboratory. From my perspective, I would consider the three great people in clinical internal medicine in this century to be William Osler, Paul White, and Eugene Stead.

Residency and Paul Dudley White

During my residency in internal medicine, I was fortunate enough to have contact with Dr. Paul Dudley White, who visited our school. Dr. Harry Harper, the cardiologist at the medical college and another superb teacher, was a friend of Dr. White's. He recommended me to Dr. White. When Dr. White offered me a position as a cardiac fellow at the Massachusetts General Hospital, I quickly accepted it. From that point on, Dr. White stimulated me in every conceivable fashion. My friendship with him and Mrs. White continued for many years, and I was honored to be asked to give the eulogy at Cambridge when he died.

Paul White used to say that the excitement of medicine had to do with the fact that you could link science to humanism in one profession. He was a kind, gentle man who did not urge, cajole, or plead with people to perform. But he was a recognized authority in his field who had worked with Sir Thomas Lewis and had known Sir James MacKenzie and all the leading cardiologists of the world. Because of his own standard of excellence, he inspired others to do their very best. He did more for cardiology then anyone else in this country.

Indexing Interesting Patients

From about 1912 to 1918, Dr. White collected data on patients on 4-by-6-inch cards. During part of that time, physicians did not know what types of heart diseases we had in this country. It was Dr. White who began to discuss etiology, anatomy, physiology, and function of the heart, and this information was later picked up by the New York Heart Association. By analyzing the material he had recorded on cards, he was able to determine the frequency of rheumatic heart disease and hypertension, among other conditions. He took this collection of cards, along with his bride, Ina, to the Isle of Capri, and wrote his first book. He exemplifies the way a scholar works: carefully collecting data on enough patients, interpreting those data, and reporting the results. I think it was that mammoth effort behind the first edition of his book that put cardiology ahead of many other disciplines. Dr. Paul White's first book on cardiology made the field a recognized specialty in this country, and it remains good reading today. The first edition contained innumerable old references that, regrettably, had to be eliminated in the later editions because of limited space.

Writing

I am sure that I acquired my interest in writing from Dr. White, for he expected his trainees to teach and write. Many of us have the misconception that teaching has to be oral. But think of how much we learn from reading the works of others. Writing textbooks and articles for journals is the finest method of teaching. Because physicians communicate to their colleagues primarily through the written word, the written document should be as clear as possible.

Writing the first edition of *The Heart* was somewhat of a trip into the unknown for me, but I knew that it would help me organize my thoughts and remember things. We are now completing the sixth edition of the book. I file items according to the chapters listed in the previous edition, although that does not mean that edition will have the exact organization of the previous one. Rather than tear out articles in my journals, I circle titles, and my secretary makes a photocopy of the articles, which I file in the appropriate chapter folder. As I create the table of contents for a new edition, I can readily transfer that information to this new table of contents.

For the chapters that I write, I first make an outline with no more than four headings. It took a long time to restrict myself to four, but I am convinced it provides better teaching. I review the publications of the past few years to determine what new information should be included. I make this decision on the basis of what is usable and what seems promising. Appropriate references must be carefully selected because no textbooks today can be documented like Paul White's first edition. In determining which references to include, I must read several and make a choice.

I write a chapter in longhand on legal pads, so that I can look at the entire manuscript and make corrections before it is typed. The manuscript is then typed on a word processor so that I can easily revise as much as is necessary. I rewrite some manuscripts more than 10 times.

Writing the book has been a self-imposed challenge. Each edition has been difficult, but has also been great fun. *The Heart* has always been written with the clinician in mind. I am happy that the book, which has been one of the most exciting projects I have done, has been translated into five other languages.

Now I am also engaged in developing the second edition of the textbook of medicine—*Medicine for the Practicing Physician*. The book is a message to all subspecialists that we must view our patients as a "whole" and not as "parts."

I learned early that one should work for others at the office and hospital. Accordingly, I begin my day, writing and thinking, at 4:00 a.m. The hours from 4:00 a.m. to 6:00 a.m. are mine—with few interruptions. My office and hospital work begins at 6:30 a.m.

2

Reading: Keeping Current

> All that goes on in medicine is to be the chief matter of interest to you. Hence you must be busy readers; and, as habits form, you will learn to look to medical journals with avidity, and new publications will be examined with keen relish. But to become distinguished, nay, to become even respectable in your profession, you must be something more than readers, you must become active thinkers and sifters of knowledge, learn, as Bacon counsels, to weigh and consider books.
> *Jacob M. Da Costa*[1]

Reading is the primary source of physicians' medical information. Print is not only the most highly developed and plentiful medium for medical information, but is also relatively economical, convenient, and easily accessible.

Beyond new developments in medical care, the need to review fundamental principles necessitates a lifelong plan of reading. In the words of Robert Moser, "Reading is as important a habit for a physician as brushing his teeth and watching his waistline. It becomes a part of his lifestyle, for it is needed to screen useful advances in theory, diagnosis, and therapy and to solve specific clinical problems confronting the practicing physician. If properly engrained, the habit never wanes for the duration of his practice." Just as nonphysicians get their pleasure from reading novels and magazines, many practitioners get pleasure from reading medical journals. Joseph Van Der Meulen enjoys making new associations with previous knowledge: "The insight that comes with such associations provides the pleasure. I spend leisure time reading practical material in science and medicine that reinforces my medical knowledge."

Physicians who take for granted the accessibility of reading material may find that the words of Shen Jiaqi of Shanghai will give them a better appreciation of their opportunities for enlarging their knowledge.

"Throughout his lifetime," Dr. Shen stated, "a doctor needs to be informed about new developments in medicine. And there is no shortcut to it beyond reading, but conditions sometimes suppress reading. That the tyrant of the Qin Dynasty burned books and buried intellectuals is a historical fact. During the last disastrous so-called cultural revolution, the 'Gang of Four' spread a fallacy that the more knowledge you have, the more reactionary you are. They duped virtuous people for years into reading little, and the education of a whole generation of youngsters was therefore delayed. Luckily, the horror is over, and the People's Republic of China is now setting off an upsurge of intellectualism. Everyone, old and young, has been moving into the tide of reading to make up for what has been lost in the past.

"With the rehabilitation of Confucius, China's great ancient philosopher and educationist, I would again recommend his famous quotations about reading. 'Reading without thinking is null and void, whereas thinking without reading is critical and riskful.' 'Reviewing old articles yields new ideas.' 'To read constantly is a great happiness.' I think these proverbs are still instructive as guidelines for reading."

Guiding Principles

"Read with two objects," advised Osler, "first, to acquaint yourself with the current knowledge on a subject and the steps by which it has been reached, and secondly, and more important, read to understand and analyse your cases."[2] General undirected reading helps the physician stay current with the state of the art, whereas reading about puzzling individual cases (or a series of cases seen in practice) has an immediate, specific, and practical purpose.

Relating Reading to Experience

Both types of reading, general and specific, will be more valuable if you have an objective in mind or can relate what you read to your clinical experience. Experienced physicians gain the most from general reading because they can associate much of what they read with their clinical observations. As Gerald Plitman noted, "After a certain time practicing medicine, you can hardly pick up a journal without being able to relate an article to some patient you have had. I think all physicians should try to apply the title of each article they read to a patient they have seen."

Screening

John Shaw Billings made an apt observation that illustrates the importance of screening: "There is a vast amount of this effete and worthless material in the literature of medicine. . . . [O]ur preparers of compilations and compendiums, big and little, acknowledged or not, are continually increasing the collection, and for the most part with material which has been characterized as 'superlatively middling, the quintessential extract of mediocrity.' "[3]

THE NEED. A primary problem has been the proliferation of publications. The twenty thousand biomedical journals now published are increasing by six to seven per cent a year.[4] To review ten journals in internal medicine, a physician must read about two hundred articles and seventy editorials a month.[5]

Physicians may receive more than five thousand pages of journal material each month, including advertisements and give-away journals. Much of this contains valuable alternatives and advances in medical practice. Diagnosis is continually being refined by such innovations as ultrasound, computed axial tomography, radionucleotide imaging, and radioimmunoassays. New drugs like histamine H^2 receptor antagonists, calcium channel blockers, and cephalosporins provide additional therapeutic options. Newly described diseases, such as Legionnaires' Disease, toxic shock syndrome, and acquired immune deficiency syndrome (AIDS), also demand attention.

Considerable poorly written or otherwise faulty material infiltrates medical publications. Unfortunately, even peer review in the most prestigious medical journals does not preclude publication of premature, questionably valid, or repetitious scientific reports. DeBakey and DeBakey[6-11] have written extensively on the invalid themes, illogical arguments, inadequate or inaccurate data, and unsupportable conclusions, as well as the ungrammatical prose and generally inferior writing in reputable peer-reviewed journals. In a personal communication, John Williamson reported that his extensive study of scientific publications pointed to a "misinformation explosion," in which only 20 per cent of published reports today meet even minimal criteria of scientific validity. Sir Thomas Lewis, writing in 1944, emphasized the need for critical reading: ". . . reform, to be useful, must render the student of medicine discriminating in a world where a disquieting proportion of what is offered him in conversation and in the generality of journals and of books is inaccurate, slovenly, or redundant."[12]

"It is important for us to recognize that the reasons for writing clinical articles and the reasons for reading clinical articles may have very little in common," cautioned David Sackett. "We read them to find out how to manage our patients; often, however, authors may write them to obtain tenure. It is our responsibility to determine the validity and applicability of what we read; and we certainly cannot depend on the give-away magazines that provide advice but no data."

TECHNIQUES. If the busy physician is to avoid unreliable and unintelligible articles, he must read selectively and critically. Observing certain screening techniques can make reading more efficient, whether it is general reading to keep abreast of current medical events or specific reading to solve problems in practice. "Since we recognize that the clinician is never going to have any more time to read than he has now," continued Sackett, "we have formulated specific guides and, perhaps more important to the busy clinician, some screening questions that the physician can apply as he reads scientific articles."

SCREENING FOR RELEVANCE. All physicians begin by looking at the title and determining whether the article is potentially interesting or useful to them. "Next," advised David Sackett, "review the list of authors; with experience, you will know what their professional reputations are and whether their work has withstood the test of time. Consider the site where the work was carried out, and note whether the patients described are similar to those you see. Turn next to the abstract or summary, which will tell you whether the substance of the article, if true, would be useful to you as a clinician."

SCREENING FOR VALIDITY. "Readers need to be much more critical than editors, and certainly more so than authors, in determining what is valid and what is going to help their patients," continued Sackett. "Some of the reasons we read, certainly those most pertinent to individual patients, are to understand the cause of a disease, to determine whether a new diagnostic test is worth using, to distinguish useful from useless forms of therapy, and to find out the clinical prognosis of a disorder." If an article concerns etiology, the reader needs to ask basic questions about the integrity of the study (proper selection and prospective follow-up, or simply case reports and undocumented clinical impressions).

"If you want to find whether a diagnostic test is useful," Sackett explained, "you can quickly scan the methods section to see if there is a valid basis for comparison between the proposed diagnostic test and some established standard. Alpha-fetoprotein, for example, is the diagnostic test that has been suggested for hepatocellular carcinoma in patients with preexisting cirrhosis. In this instance, the established standard would not be just the microscopic examination of the liver. The patients with negative biopsies should be followed until they have done well for at least two to three years, so that you can exclude hepatoma. Thus in many conditions, we increasingly use the subsequent clinical course as the standard."

If you are reading to differentiate useful from useless or harmful therapy, the key question, Sackett pointed out, is: "Was the assignment of patients and treatment randomized? That is the only way to be sure that the groups are sufficiently comparable to draw valid conclusions. If the methods section includes terms like 'a table of random numbers,' or 'a computer program of randomization,' you can be reasonably sure that it was a randomized trial. If, on the other hand, you see statements like 'patients were allocated at random,' then you should be skeptical.

"Randomized clinical trials offer the most convincing evidence available today in the study of both therapeutic effectiveness and side-effects. We need to compare the incidence of skin rashes, photosensitivity, gastrointestinal upset, headaches, weakness, or dizziness, in patients on placebos with those on active drugs. Some side effects occur so infrequently, however, that the usual randomized clinical trial would not be large enough to disclose them. For those, we must rely on a much less powerful design, the case-control study, in which a group of patients with the apparent side-effect is assembled and then matched with a control group without the disorder (and that is where we usually get into trouble). Discrepancies between the two groups in the incidence of prior exposure to the drug or other factor would constitute some evidence, although not very strong, that the factor precipitated the disorder.

"If we are reading about the clinical course and prognosis of a disorder, we should find out if the patient group was identified at an early, uniform stage of the disease. If not, a host of biases may interfere. For example, what exactly is the increased risk of colorectal cancer in patients with ulcerative colitis, and does it justify a prophylactic colectomy? When you search the literature to find an answer to that question, you become frustrated because the most 'authoritative' studies of the risk of cancer in ulcerative colitis patients are based on 'grab' samples of patients, many of whom were included because they already had cancer. As a result, the cancer risk associated with ulcerative colitis is vastly overestimated in these studies. The way to answer the question is to collect a group of ulcerative colitis patients at an early, uniform point in the natural history of the disease, such as when they develop the first unambiguous symptoms or receive the first definitive therapy. That is the only way to determine the natural history and clinical course of a disease.

"Critical screening of articles not only substantially increases the validity of the conclusions the reader draws from them, but also increases his efficiency considerably. By applying these basic screening principles, the reader can expeditiously identify which papers to keep and where to file them."

Note-taking and Mental Summaries

Note-taking is a time-honored method of crystallizing what you read. Osler used it to great advantage. According to Cushing, Osler was "a rapid, methodical reader with an exceptionally retentive memory, but in addition he had formed the habit of jotting down the gist of what he had read so that it could be drawn on when needed, and moreover he would often augment the notes with some reflections of his own. It was due to this habit of writing as he read that he finally acquired the charm of style which characterized his later essays."[13]

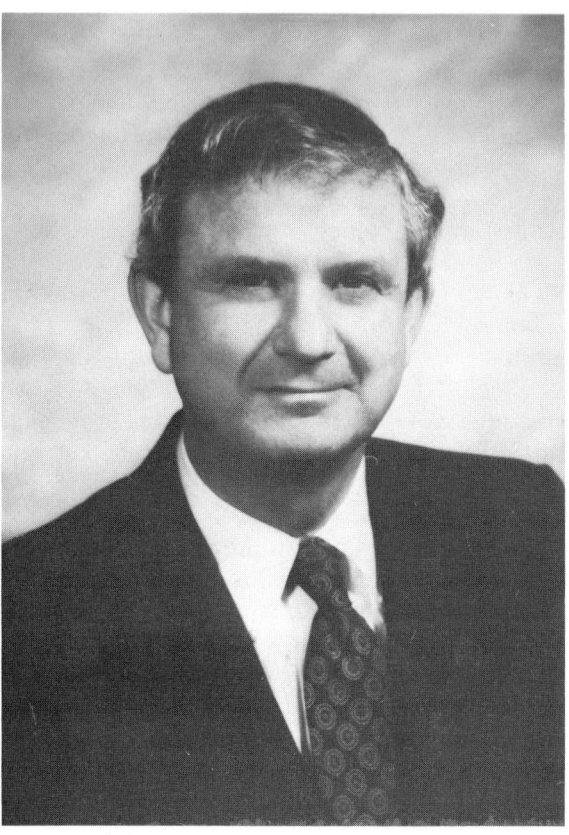

Reading is as important a habit for a physician as brushing his teeth and watching his waistline.

> Robert H. Moser, M.D.
> Executive Vice President Emeritus
> American College of Physicians

2. Reading: Keeping Current

The late Alton Ochsner, Michael DeBakey's mentor, kept a permanent record of his notes. "Just by looking at those notes," he said, "I can recall relatively easily the thousands of references that I have read." Thomas Callister uses cards for note-taking, and reads them when he is having coffee or has nothing else to do, thereafter filing them at home, where they are easily available. "This system works well for me, even though it has been hard on my coat pockets."

Some physicians use a tape recorder rather than cards or paper for note-keeping. Mentally reviewing and summarizing the important points of an article, in a single sentence if possible, helps fix them in your mind. Richard O'Brien enhances his retention by mentally devising experimental approaches to extend the state of knowledge beyond that reported in the papers that he reads.

A Scheduled Time for Reading

Most physicians agree that learning has to be a daily activity, in which you discipline yourself to read several hours every day and construct a reading schedule that accommodates your lifestyle.

To keep unread journals from piling up, designate a special time to read. Daniel Stone gets up at 4:30 a.m. and reads for one and one-half hours every day except Christmas. "When I get home in the evening, I am too tired to read in an active, aggressive way. I may turn the pages, but I am not really absorbing the information. Furthermore, I prefer spending my evenings with my wife. In the morning, on the other hand, there are no distractions. My mind is fresh, and I can really absorb the material." Richard Field reads from 6:00 to 6:30 a.m., when no phones are ringing and there are no intrusions. "In that short time, I cover about four journals a month."

According to Cushing, Osler read during meals: "During this first year in Philadelphia he usually dined alone at the old Colonnade Hotel, diagonally across the street from his rooms, always it is said with books and manuscript on the table, and he was usually to be seen reading and making notes during the course of the meal."[13]

Allan Ebbin keeps a pile of journals beside his bed to read before retiring: "I know of no better way to fall asleep than to read my journals. Since my wife is also a pediatrician, I can put some of them on her pile, and she doesn't know the difference. Seriously, my best learning has always been at home, alone, with a book or journal. There are only a few things that provide more entertainment for me."

Some physicians prefer to read in brief spurts, at intervals throughout the day—5:30 to 6:30 a.m., at work, after work, and before bedtime. Since a set time for reading is not possible for Lawrence Green, he leaves journals on various tables in his office and home, to be picked up when convenient. The late Alton Ochsner also used any brief free time to read. "I try to make every moment of my day count, because there is so little time to do things," he said. "I have on my desk journals of all types, and if I have a few spare minutes, I use that time to read." Norton Greenberger reads on several specific subjects instead of concentrating for an hour on one particular topic, which he finds soporific. "When I read, I decide in advance how much I want to accomplish per unit time. I do not read every word; I read for comprehension, recognizing that I have to get through a certain amount at a given time."

Suzanne Knoebel considers her reading time a reward. "Saturday afternoon or Sunday is my 'R and R' time. If I have problems in patient care that I need to read about, I eagerly anticipate this time. But I caution against trying to 'fit' learning into an already tightly scheduled period; pick a convenient 'R and R' time and use it for that."

Some physicians combine reading with other hobbies. David Covell, for example, can be seen every Wednesday afternoon hiking in the Angeles National Forest above Pasadena reading a current journal, despite the slight risk that engrossing articles can distract attention from tree limbs, snakes, and boulders on the trail.

READING RETREAT. Frederick Ludwig and Gerald Plitman use their vacations to catch up on their reading. Plitman created a two-day "reading retreat" for colleagues, which evolved from the practice he and his wife had of going away for a few days every summer, isolating themselves from their usual routine, to read. For each retreat, they invite two professors, who are asked to select topics and to send copies of the selected publications to all others going on the retreat. Everyone reads the material in advance and comes to the retreat ready to discuss these topics. "It is a restful, relaxing event," said Plitman.

Donald Switz and Dan Mohler have initiated similar reading retreats in Virginia. "The format of dual teachers and many papers has worked well for Plitman; we use a different format," said Switz. "We select three topics per conference and, by rotating the subject, cover all of internal medicine every four years. A single teacher is invited to put together each of the half-day sessions. The teacher selects no more than seven original articles, which he believes are the most important in his field since the last presentations. We ask the registrants to tell us the aspects of each subject they wish to 'catch up' on. We believe physicians learn best when they have a voice in what they will read. Before the reading retreat begins, this information is returned to the teacher, who then has a chance to modify his reading list or to know what to emphasize from his selections. We do not mail the readings in advance, but do distribute a bibliography.

"Like Plitman, we restrict the group to about 25. We retreat to a park-like setting, and families usually come. We make time for walking, loafing, and fishing. The structure of each session is similar to Plitman's. The teacher spends about 30 minutes at the beginning putting the subject of the articles in perspective with respect to current knowledge. We then ask for volunteers to present the pith of each article, after which we retire to read for two hours. When we reassemble, the volunteers present the abstracts, which serve as a basis for discussion by all participants. We spend about 90 minutes discussing the articles in the order the participants desire. There is ample time to ask the teacher for special insights related to clinical cases participants have struggled with.

"Special benefits of the reading retreats are: (1) an opportunity to look critically at original articles, (2) the stimulation of group discussion, and (3) the opportunity to quiz the instructor about clinical matters germane to patients and the articles. We work hard to help participants think about good study design."

Following Specific Investigators

Irvine Page connects facts to people. "I have always been interested in contemporary history; I follow what is going on in the world of medicine largely by associating events with people. History tells me how people make discoveries or observations. My interest in history grows as both the subject and the people grow. A classical example is DNA research. I knew Oswald T. Avery and Colin M. Macleod, both of whom worked on the floor below me at the Rockefeller Institute for Medical Research. I saw the evolution of their work from the beginning, with the accompanying development and skepticism. This is the way I remember things." Donald Seldin also tries to keep abreast of advances by following the work of scientific leaders.

A Historical Perspective

Reading the history of science and medicine provides a good basis for teaching or learning what has happened in the past—how people with keen curiosities were led to important discoveries. Gastone Matioli, however, warns readers: "Validate the historical background upon which the experts base their views. Reviews sometimes distort original intentions or at least phrase them poorly. Americans often ignore history and thus miss the opportunity to identify the source of inherited errors and misunderstanding." Osler advised physicians to "read the original descriptions of the masters who, with crude methods of study, saw so clearly."[14]

General Reading

We use the term "general reading" to refer to that not directed to specific problems in practice or patients under current care. Such reading is enjoyable, useful, and necessary to keep abreast of the general state of medicine. As Paul Wehrle pointed out, "General reading is helpful in following medical progress and disease trends, especially in communicable diseases and new problems." Ian Mackay finds that "General reading provides the opportunity to 'think sideways.' Often, when I have been taxed by a difficult or puzzling clinical problem, or have been startled by an unexpected diagnosis, I am surprised by the number of articles related to that problem that I suddenly encounter; the clinical experience has created an interest in the subject, and I become aware of articles that would otherwise have been overlooked."

Every physician must develop his own method of selection. Most subscribe to several general journals, such as *The Lancet*, the *British Medical Journal*, *The Journal of the American Medical Association*, and *The New England Journal of Medicine*, as well as one or more journals in their subspecialties. They usually review the table of contents, checking off the titles that appear interesting. After scanning the abstracts, and sometimes reading an entire article, they file the most significant papers for future use.

Aids to General Reading

EDITORIALS. A physician who reads the editorials in two or three major journals can keep fairly well informed about new developments. Of Arthur Rubenstein, Professor of Medicine at the University of Chicago and a specialist in diabetes mellitus, Richard Byyny remarked: "When we went on rounds together, I wondered how he kept up with his busy schedule. One day I asked him how he did it, and he said, 'I am absolutely religious about reading the editorials in *The Lancet* because they are succinct and timely.' "

LETTERS TO THE EDITOR. Perusing the letters to the editor in prestigious journals is an enjoyable way to review and gain additional perspective on important medical and related issues of the day. They are not only topical but are often more readable than the more stilted formal articles.

SCREENING AND ABSTRACT SERVICES. The *Medical Letter*, a biweekly publication, and the *Yearbook* publications contain excellent information, with expert commentaries. William Waters has made a habit of keeping the *Yearbook of Medicine* at his bedside and reading two or three articles in it every night. "This is the cream of the literature reviewed by the cream of the experts." Some physicians scan abstract journals such as *Excerpta Medica*, whereas others peruse current awareness newsletters, such as *Medical Alert* and *Infectious Disease Alert*.

Two excellent services summarize publications in surgery. *Selected Readings*, designed by Robert McClelland as a study program for surgical residents, is now used extensively. Each month, subscribers receive a packet of about 50 reprints, along with a thirty-page printed commentary in which each reprint is reviewed. For Richard Kraft, *Selected Readings* is "all any general surgeon needs. I give this service to every member of our resident staff. Twice each month, I meet with the residents for two hours and review this material, to keep them current."

The *Surgical Index* produced by Joseph Ignatius contains abstracts of many of the important surgical articles on 3-by-5-inch cards. These are mailed once a month, saving the physician many hours of screening and abstracting articles.

Self-assessment Programs

Certain specialty societies regularly publish syllabi prepared by experts in the field and containing self-assessment programs, along with objective tests, patient-management problems, and critiques of the questions and answers. Many physicians use the self-assessment programs, such as the Medical Knowledge Self-Assessment Program (MKSAP) or the Surgical Education Self-Assessment Program (SESAP), to keep abreast of new developments or to study for recertification tests. This study combined with the comparison of one's own answers with those of others has proved to be extremely valuable. Between editions, some textbooks offer current awareness volumes, which include self-assessment questions and answers.

Library Visits

Fred Turrill skips lunch to go to the library and look up problems or randomly read. "Most of us have good intentions about looking up certain information," he explains, "but never get around to doing it unless we do it that same day." Visiting the hospital library about once every two weeks allows a physician to scan the journals that he does not subscribe to. For the past thirty years, Thomas Callister has reserved Monday afternoons for such study. "During my first few years of practice," he said, "I would leave the office at noon and go to the library to read. I would eat dinner with Bill Nerlich, and the two of us would spend the evening studying for the Boards. After we passed the Boards, I continued to spend Monday afternoon and evening in the library, and I still spend six or seven hours a week there."

Reading in the General Media

The media often release new information in medicine before it is published in the medical journals. Reporters get *The New England Journal of Medicine*, for example, before many physicians receive it. "A patient reads something in *The Wall Street Journal* and calls his doctor for an opinion about it," said Alan Gordon. "If the physician hasn't heard of it, he appears not to be keeping up." James Moss pointed out that "Many patients were better informed than their physicians about DMSO after it was featured in a story on 'Sixty Minutes.' " David Sabiston pays attention to medical stories in the public press primarily because he may want to look up such topics in medical publications. "You soon recognize that there are recurring themes in the press. This year it may be obesity, and four years later it may be the surgical treatment of obesity. Cancer, like various new concepts in heart disease, is always there. The subjects repeat themselves in cycles, and it is just a matter of keeping each updated." The *Harvard Medical School Health Letter* and the *Mayo Clinic Health Letter* aid physicians in the education of patients about their diseases and general health.

Some physicians post articles on a bulletin board in their offices to convey medical information in the general news to patients. Such a system encourages the physician to assess medical news items as they appear.

Reading to Solve Specific Problems

Full coverage of medical periodicals is not possible, and even if it were, detailed recall is not. If it is true, as most students of adult education believe, that learning is most effective when a specific problem needs to be solved, the overworked physician can spend his available time most efficiently focusing on information that will help him diagnose and treat the patients under his care. Robert Petersdorf considers patients to be the gateway to new knowledge: "If we direct our reading to conditions we see in our practice, we can keep up reasonably well." Practice-related reading can be classified in two categories: reading about recurring conditions seen in practice, such as hypertension or duodenal ulcer, and reading about puzzling problems in individual patients.

Reading on a Topic of Special Interest

Most physicians develop special interests in certain problems, diseases, drugs, or laboratory studies. If the physician has a record of the types of problems seen, the drugs prescribed, and the laboratory studies ordered, he can direct his reading to his personal experience and become expert in specific medical topics. (See also Chapter 10.) Donald Seldin explores certain subjects in great depth as they come up. "I try to organize the material in some way, either in the form of notes or in an oral presentation. I prepare not only a catalogue of items but also a synthesis. If I were studying idiopathic edema of women, for example, I would review the literature on that subject fairly thoroughly, and then try to assimilate the

2. Reading: Keeping Current

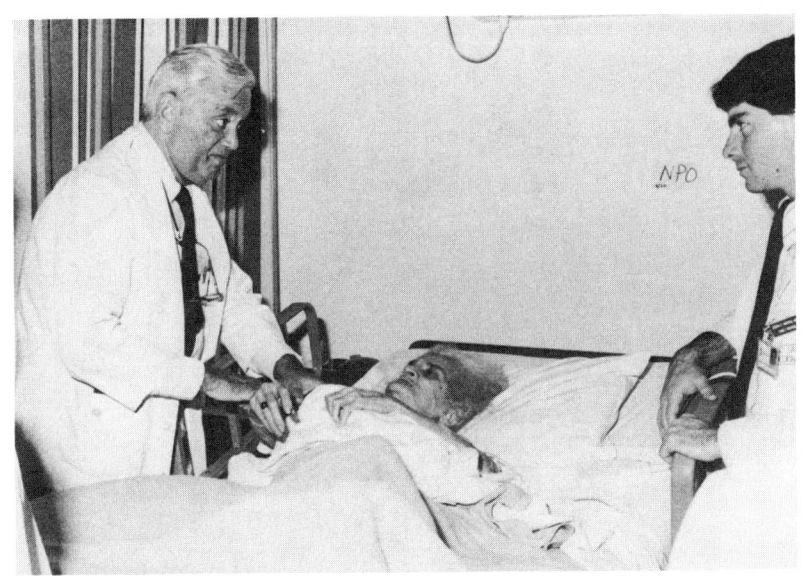

If we direct our reading to conditions we see in our practice, we can keep up reasonably well.

Robert G. Petersdorf, M.D.
President, Association of
American Medical Colleges

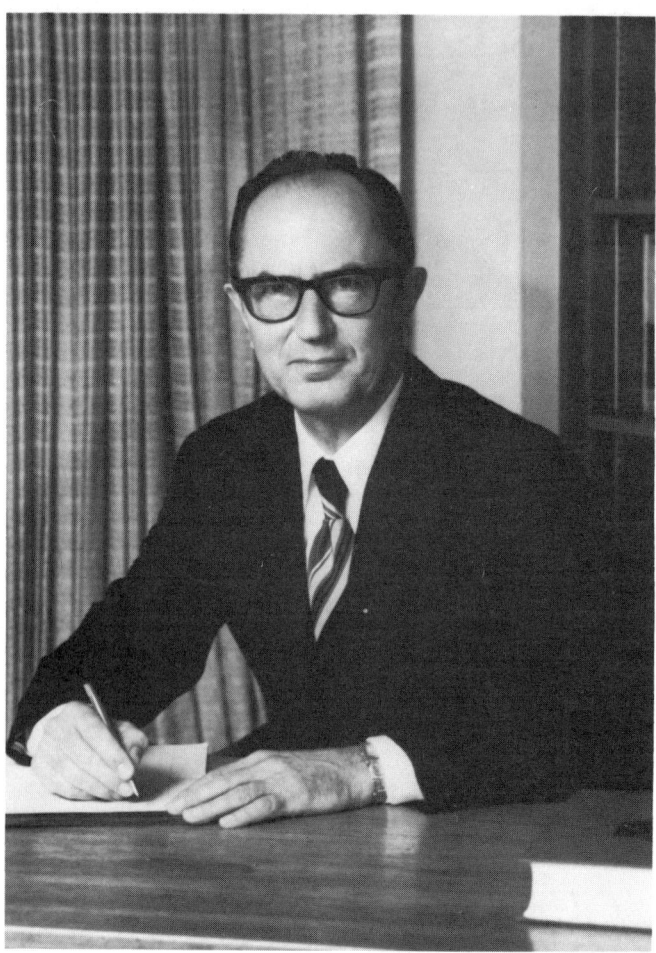

If I were studying idiopathic edema of women, I would review the literature on that subject fairly thoroughly, and then try to assimilate the material for application to my purposes.

Donald W. Seldin, M.D.
Chairman, Department of Internal Medicine
University of Texas Health Science Center, Dallas

material for application to my purposes." Other physicians read on topics they are scheduled to present at medical meetings, in hospital rounds, or informally to colleagues.

Reading on Individual Patients

Eugene Braunwald considers it vital to read about a problem as soon as it arises. "If Mrs. Jones has a mitral valve click and migraine, and you wonder if the two are associated, look the subjects up immediately, not six months later. You will retain the information longer because you will make an association with a specific patient, and this association will help you apply the knowledge you have acquired to similar future problems."

Reading on a particular patient increases retention. "What I remember most," said Edward Shortliffe, "is the information related to specific patients. I may find an interesting article when reading randomly, but it does not stick the same as if I am forced to read because of puzzling questions I have about a patient. Somehow, that becomes better integrated into my memory and helps me deal with similar problems in the future."

Sequence of Study in Solution of Specific Problems

When a clinical problem requires additional information, ask yourself precisely what you know and what you do not know. Framing the right questions helps you to be more efficient in finding specific information. First consult a recent edition of a standard textbook for an accurate sketch of the clinical condition under scrutiny. Then, if necessary, you can read a good review article.

If the information is not available in a standard textbook or in review articles or if you want more detail, you will have to consult appropriate articles in the medical periodicals. Toward this end, you may use a personal reprint file, or you may consult a medical librarian to obtain pertinent references. The personal reprint file, if kept current, is a convenient source of information for solving puzzling problems. (See Chapters 3 and 4.)

*****

Reading is the most common way for physicians to gain new knowledge and review fundamental concepts. Since there is entirely too much medical literature for the physician to read, he must develop methods of screening journal articles for relevance and validity. As George Sarton said, "The art of reading implies the art of non-reading, and more energy is sometimes needed in order to skip rather than continue useless drifting. Many would-be scholars never learn anything not only because they cannot read, but also because they cannot stop reading: they are like asses turning round and round in a mill with blinkers on their eyes."[15] In addition to reading to remain aware of the state of the art, physicians read about their cases, either about individual puzzling patients or about their aggregate experience with various conditions. Scheduling a daily time for reading and developing related activities such as taking notes, following specific investigators, and relating reading to experience will enhance the value and efficiency of reading. Cultivating a historical perspective about the medical literature and disease entities also enriches understanding and provides a basis for coordinating and integrating new knowledge with old. Editorials in leading journals generally keep one alert to new developments.

The physician with limited time can maximize efficiency by emphasizing reading on puzzling individual patients and conditions seen recurrently in practice. All reading and study are enhanced when the physician has a personal study center that includes updated textbooks and reprint files, as discussed in the next chapter.

References

1. Da Costa, Jacob M. Valedictory address to the graduating class of Jefferson Medical College, Philadelphia. Delivered Mar 11, 1874. Philadelphia: P. Madeira, Surgical Instrument Maker, 1874:8.
2. Osler, William. The student life: A farewell address to Canadian and American medical students. *The Medical News* Sep 30, 1905;87(14):630.
3. Billings, John Shaw. Our Medical Literature. In: Rogers, Frank Bradway, ed. *Selected Papers of John Shaw Billings: Compiled, with a Life of Billings.* Baltimore: Waverly Press, 1965:128-129.
4. Price, Derek De Solla. The development and structure of the biomedical literature. In: Warren, Kenneth S., ed. *Coping with the Biomedical Literature: A Primer for the Scientist and the Clinician.* New York: Praeger, 1981:3-16.
5. Warren, Kenneth S. Selective aspects of the biomedical literature. In: Warren, Kenneth S., ed. *Coping with the Biomedical Literature: A Primer for the Scientist and the Clinician.* New York: Praeger, 1981:17-30.
6. DeBakey, Lois: Critical reasoning: A prerequisite for clear scientific writing. *Int J Cardiol* 1984;5:629.
7. DeBakey, Lois; DeBakey, Selma. Muddy medical writing: Is the culprit "bad grammar," technologic terminology, committee authorship, or undisciplined reading? *South Med J* Oct 1976;69(10):1253-1254.
8. DeBakey, Lois. *The Scientific Journal: Editorial Policies and Practices.* St. Louis: The C. V. Mosby Company, 1976.
9. DeBakey, Lois. Releasing literary inhibitions in scientific reporting. *Can Med Assoc J* 24/31 Aug 1968;99(8):360-367.
10. DeBakey, Lois; DeBakey, Selma. Medicant. *Forum on Medicine* Apr 1978; 1(1):38-40, 42-43, 80-81, 83-86.
11. DeBakey, Lois; DeBakey, Selma. The abstract: an abridged scientific report. *Int J Cardiol* 1983;3(4):439-445.

12. Lewis, Thomas. Reflections upon reform in medical education. *Lancet* 13 May 1944;6298(pt 1):619.
13. Cushing, Harvey. *The Life of Sir William Osler.* London: Oxford University Press, 1940:242.
14. Osler, William. In: Bean, William Bennett, ed. *Sir William Osler: Aphorisms from His Bedside Teachings and Writings.* Springfield, Illinois: Charles C. Thomas, 1968:79.
15. Sarton, George. Notes on the reviewing of learned books. *Science* 22 Apr 1960;131(4):1183.

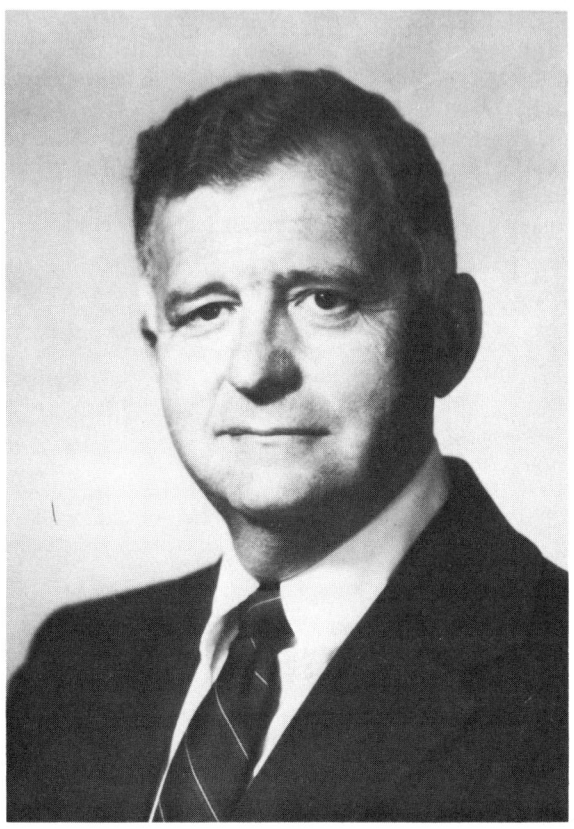

If Mrs. Jones has a mitral valve click and migraine, and you wonder if the two are associated, look the subjects up immediately, not six months later. You will retain the information longer because you will make an association with a specific patient, and this association will help you apply the knowledge you have acquired to similar future problems.

Eugene Braunwald, M.D.

Dr. Braunwald's research, reported in more than 700 publications, has illuminated many aspects of cardiology. He and his colleagues clarified the importance of Starling's Law as a major determinant of ventricular performance in man, and he made critical contributions to the description of idiopathic hypertrophic subaortic stenosis. With colleagues, he conducted some of the earliest studies on beta-adrenergic receptor-blocking drugs and described an important biochemical defect in heart failure— the depletion of norepinephine in the hearts of patients with this condition. Dr. Braunwald's work on limiting the ultimate size of myocardial infarction

Personal Essay

Eugene Braunwald, M.D.
Harvard Medical School
Chairman, Department of Internal Medicine
Brigham and Women's Hospital
and Beth Israel Hospital
Boston, Massachusetts

I lead three professional lives, each with different educational needs. As Chairman of the Department of Internal Medicine, I must have some basic understanding of general internal medicine to make Grand Rounds on the Medical Service, to take morning report with residents, and to deal intelligently with faculty members in the Department who have a variety of skills, specialties, and interests. My second role is that of clinical cardiologist. Several months each year, I function as a physician on our Cardiology Service, where I see both inpatients and outpatients. The third component of my professional life is research in cardiovascular disease and cardiovascular physiology.

I have tried to make my three professional roles support, rather than compete with, one another. As I have observed physicians in academic life whose research is far removed from their clinical work, I have noticed that these two activities are often competitive, not complementary. I am

---

has profoundly influenced clinical cardiology. In a series of brilliant animal experiments, he demonstrated that infarct size after coronary occlusion can be reduced by various interventions, including beta-adrenergic blocking drugs, coronary vasodilators, and anti-inflammatory compounds administered alone and in combination with coronary reperfusion. Recipient of numerous awards, he has been influential in governmental affairs related to cardiovascular research and practice and has served on the editorial boards of several prestigious medical and scientific journals.

Eugene Braunwald is one of the foremost contemporary scholars in the cardiovascular sciences; his contributions are prolific and his influence is profound in both clinical cardiology and basic research on the heart and circulation. Intense intellectual curiosity and extraordinary analytical sensibilities are the foundation of Dr. Braunwald's search for knowledge to treat the countless patients afflicted with heart disease. His example has been an inspiration to his students; more than forty of Dr. Braunwald's former trainees are full professors, department heads, or directors of cardiology divisions in major medical schools throughout the world.

William F. Friedman, M.D.

always skeptical about a person who, for example, is a superb molecular biologist and tells me he wants to practice general internal medicine. These two roles do not support each other. If, on the other hand, he is interested in the fundamental mechanisms of cell division and says that he plans to do cancer research, it makes much more sense.

I have also conducted research primarily on myocardial ischemia for the past thirteen years. In my research, my continuing education is the result of association with my own research fellows and other colleagues in the field. To keep abreast of my research subject, I must read virtually everything published on it, which requires about four hours each week.

If someone asks a question that I cannot answer, I look it up immediately, or I assign the problem to a resident. In our medical center, the information is readily available because we encounter complex problems and hear arguments among talented people on all aspects of medicine. It is almost as if education were forced on me.

I am becoming more and more convinced that the case-study method, which can be done very readily in a hospital setting, is one that we should be pursuing. Instead of giving a lecture on coronary artery bypass grafts, for example, one would select six patients who demonstrate different aspects of the problem. The course based on the case-study methods without any didactic lectures is different from the usual grand rounds in which a lecture is given and a patient with XYZ diseases is presented. The case-study method, in which the discussion is about a patient illustrating something instructive, requires more work because you have to prepare the material and make slides in advance, but it is more effective than simply selecting a patient who happens to be in the hospital and discussing that case.

I have been programmed for the work I am doing; my parents expected me to do exactly what I am doing, and the expectation was made clear to me even before I started school. I sometimes feel that I am acting out a script written by someone else. My parents wanted me to do something that they did not have a chance to do, and they saw that I had the capacity to do it, so they encouraged me. I do not regret that. My professional life gives me joy and considerable satisfaction and rewards.

I intended to practice clinical medicine. Bill Hubbard, then Dean of Students, introduced the elective system in 1951 at New York University. When I went to see him, I thought that I wanted a clinical elective—dermatology or orthopedics, as I recall. He said, "I expected that you would do research," and I said, "No, I do not want to do research. Nothing could be further from my mind." When I sensed that he was starting to become angry, I said to myself, "If I fight this, I will get into serious trouble." I therefore said, "I will be glad to do research." He asked, "What kind of research do you want to do?" I responded, "Oh no. I am doing this to please you, and therefore you must make that decision. I really do not want to do any." He called Ludwig Eichna, who at that time was Chief of Cardiology, and said "I have a man here who would like to work in your laboratory." "Please send him over," was the reply. I joined his laboratory, and within a week my life had changed in that I was exposed to active investigation. Not only did I become enthusiastic about the nature of the work, but I became fascinated by the cardiovascular system.

As one of the editors of *Harrison's Textbook of Medicine*, I must read all the new chapters regardless of the field of my specific responsibility. For two months, I have been reviewing renal disease, a new section of the book.

I also read the cardiac journals in some detail, although not from cover to cover. One of my most rewarding jobs is as Editor of the section on "The Heart and Blood Vessels" in the *Year Book of Medicine*. In that capacity, I receive tearsheets of the world cardiovascular publications every two weeks, and these facilitate keeping up with cardiology. I probably would have resigned from this editorship some years ago, but I did not want to give up a service that is extremely valuable. Virtually every published cardiovascular paper comes to my desk, and I use that material to build a good recent reference file. My own textbook, *Heart Disease*, could not have been written without the reference file I had accumulated for the *Year Book*.

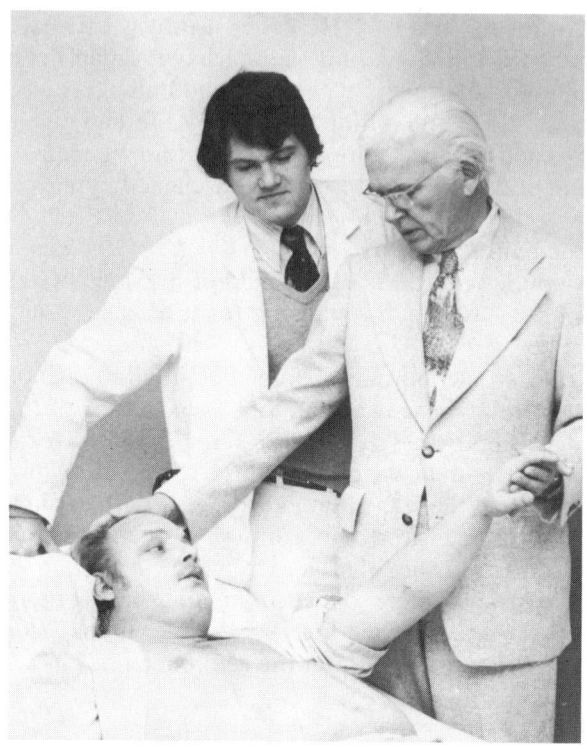

Every physician, whether a specialist or a general internist, should select some clinical condition and begin, at an early date, to develop special knowledge and experience about its natural course and its diagnostic and therapeutic management.

Philip A. Tumulty, M.D.

Dr. Tumulty was twice the recipient of the George J. Stuart Award as Outstanding Clinical Teacher and holds an Honorary Doctor of Science Degree from Georgetown University. He published *The Effective Clinician* and has written extensively on clinical subjects, including the treatment of pneumonia, infectious endocarditis, effects of recurrent malaria, natural history of systemic lupus, scleroderma, giant–cell arteritis and hepatic hypoglycemia, and functional illness.

Dr. Philip A. Tumulty exemplifies what Francis Peabody had in mind when he said, 'The secret of the care of the patient is in caring for the patient.' A gifted, lifelong student of medicine, Dr. Tumulty radiates a compassionate concern for all his patients, whatever their backgrounds, their sorrows, and their fates. His devoted care of his patients, even during the search for a diagnosis, is the kind of therapy each of us would like most to have, and is an unforgettable inspiration to his students and to his colleagues.

Sherman Mellinkoff, M.D.

Personal Essay

Philip A. Tumulty, M.D.
David J. Carver Professor Emeritus of Medicine
The Johns Hopkins University School of Medicine
Baltimore, Maryland

Students and others have asked me: "Why do you find a career in general internal medicine so completely satisfying?" My answer is: Because each day that medicine is practiced properly, I find a full measure of those fulfillments for which we all strive: intellectual enhancement, stimulation, and excitement; an opportunity to increase and expand the best qualities of mind and spirit; a chance to feel the thrill of bringing relief to fellow human beings through the best use of one's intellectual and personal endowments; and finally, the daily experience of seeing and understanding more clearly the depths of human nature, with its intense complexities and eccentricities, its good and bad, its sublimity and depravity, its victories and defeats. A clinician is not merely a bystander looking at life as it flows by him; he is an active participant in it, at some of its most crucial stages, involving his fellow human beings.

To be effective in such a role, one must, of course, have a number of requisites, including a knowledge of medical science and of the nature of man, both based on the broadest possible clinical experience. He must be stimulated not only by scientific facts and intriguing clinical situations, but by the very simple or exceedingly complex problems arising from his patients' human qualities as well. To perform superbly, he must be an eager, persistent, devoted medical scientist, one to whom the joy of living comes largely from experiencing daily the positive effects his knowledge and his talents have on his patients' problems, whatever their source may be.

But how does one prepare for such a totally fulfilling and also demanding career and, once embarked upon it, how does one prevent the practical burdens involved in it from leading to boredom, intellectual and spiritual sterility, and a gradual decline of the stimulus to excellence and of pride in achievement?

Here we come to the significance of the role of continuing education in our clinical careers. While a proper program of continuing education may keep alive the essential qualities of an effective clinician, it cannot create them. It is therefore the role of the medical schools to select those students with the proper gifts, talents, and abilities of mind, spirit, and character and to create a broad curriculum that fertilizes their growth.

Organized lectures and demonstrations are of undisputed value, but they are not the heart of the matter. The key remains in self-education, and, to my way of thinking, clinical self-education has three essential components:

1. Physicians need to have as many and as varied clinical experiences as possible. I see clinical conditions today that I have never seen before, and although they are sometimes insignificant, they may also sometimes be exciting and unusual, as with Takayasu's disease.
2. Having had this new experience, the physician must learn more about it. It is important that the clinical experience come first and the reading after.
3. Discussion with others of one's new clinical experiences is invaluable, not necessarily by formal consultation but perhaps by informal conversations and exchanges.

A major concern of the clinician is involvement in matters springing from the patient's human nature. Surely the greatest study of mankind is man. A superbly trained scientist who is ignorant of the classics of literature and art and who is naive about social, political, and financial factors is not likely to use these factors positively to ameliorate his patient's illness. How can the physician become more sensitive to these matters? A well-organized schedule, permitting reasonable time for hobbies and interests, social and community activities, and reading, is helpful but is not enough. I recommend a program by the local medical group such as that conceived and developed by Dr. George Udvarhelyi of the Johns Hopkins Medical Institutions. In regular informal sessions, often embellished by wine and cheese, those with experiences in widely diverse fields are invited to talk and to answer questions—basic scientists, musicians, actors, clergymen, judges, psychiatrists, social workers, politicians, and others.

Every physician, whether a specialist or a general internist, should select some clinical condition and begin, at an early date, to develop special knowledge and experience about its natural course and its diagnostic and therapeutic management. Such conditions as systemic lupus erythematosus, bacterial endocarditis, and giant-cell arteritis, for example, have intrigued me through the years, always as a result of my having seen a patient with the condition about which I needed more knowledge. Seeing the patient was followed by a gathering of articles, compilation of a filing index, and slow, methodical collections of case material.

The development of subjects of special interest has several advantages. First, it keeps the clinician intellectually stimulated instead of submerged in the purely routine. Second, in examining the natural history of a disease over time, the physician will acquire a richer knowledge of many other disorders that may simulate it. Third, such clinical studies, if carried out well, may lead to a clinical report, and such a report sometimes leads to an important advance in medicine. Finally, and from a purely practical standpoint, such studies help the young clinician become established as a consultant in the community and as a speaker at medical programs.

A clinician, then, should be a permanent, enthusiastic student of disease and of human beings affected by it, so that he may acquire the ability to cure when possible and to bring relief, comfort, and support to his patients. Without a practical and vital program of continued self-education, these priest-like powers of the superior clinician will not be fully realized.

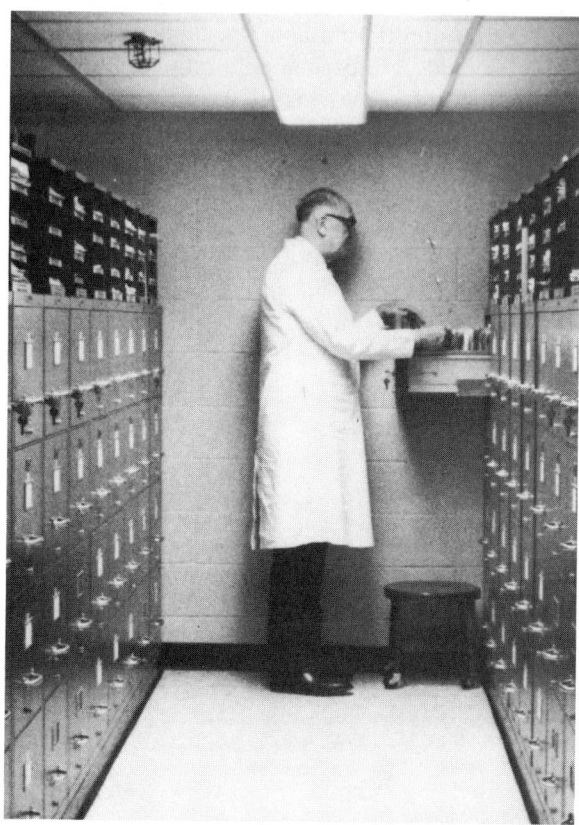

Beyond formal education, a well-developed personal medical library supports continued personal education.

Harold Jeghers, M.D.
Professor of Medical Education
The Northeastern Ohio Universities

3

The Personal Information Center

> [A] man should keep his little brain-attic stocked with all the furniture that he is likely to use, and the rest he can put away in the lumber-room of his library, where he can get it if he wants it.
>
> *Sir Arthur Conan Doyle*[1]

Early in his residency at the Boston City Hospital, Harold Jeghers (co-discoverer of the Peutz-Jeghers syndrome) was prompted by a case on his service to review the publications on herpes zoster. The attending physician, after having heard this young resident's detailed review, asked him to discuss that subject at medical rounds. Jeghers, pleased that his review enabled him to lead an important discussion soon after beginning his residency, was motivated to develop a personal library that would give him quick access to medical information. He subsequently became a pioneer in development of the personal information center. Joseph Van Der Meulen attests to the success of Jegher's methods; the best informed physicians he knows were trained by Jeghers to organize and use a personal reprint file.

The personal medical library is a major tool and convenience in the study of particular patients and subjects. Most important in establishing proper study habits, according to Jeghers, are physical facilities suitable for this purpose. The basic equipment of a "personal study center" includes a desk with drawers, a desk chair, a bookcase near the desk, an "easy chair" and adequate illumination for reading. According to Jeghers, the personal study center is most useful if it is quiet and restricted solely to that purpose. It becomes unique and personal when special items are added and a specialized approach to study is initiated.

Medical Textbooks

Pertinent textbooks, which are a primary information source, are essential, and a personal reprint file is virtually indispensable. "The purpose of a large, multi-authored textbook of medicine," noted Lloyd H. Smith, co-editor of *Cecil's Textbook of Medicine*, "is to furnish a reliable, timely précis of information as an entry point for learning about or refreshing one's knowledge of a certain subject. Annotated references allow the reader easy access to a broader treatment of each topic. A textbook cannot be complete, no matter how massive it may become; each discipline within it has sprouted textbooks of comparable size, and most of the major diseases are the subjects of monographs. No student or physician is expected to read through a compendium of 2,500,000 words. Rather, textbooks are to be consulted periodically and selectively for pertinent information on specific clinical problems. Because patients furnish remarkable memory hooks in our minds concerning their problems, this type of directed reading is generally effective."

The Personal Reprint File

The reprint file is a practical, easily accessible resource of medical knowledge—a unique collection of articles the physician has selected as relevant to his practice. In addition to tear-outs or xerographic copies of journal articles, the reprint file may contain notes on publications related to patients studied, notes and handouts accumulated during conferences, and notes about lessons learned from direct observation of patients. Kenneth Diddie's habit of filing patient notes when the case was a particularly good example of a condition made his retrospective reviews for teaching or publications easier. Such personally collected and annotated material cannot be supplied by any institutional library. Over the years, it will represent a unique record of a physician's personal medical experience and a valuable resource for optimal care of patients. "Whenever I encounter a problem," said Margaret McCarron, "I pull out my file, which includes journal tear-outs, copies of consultation notes, and, in cases of drug overdose (a particular interest of mine), an abstract of the case on forms that I developed. A resident called yesterday, for example, about a patient with a dilantin overdose who had a high dilantin serum level on admission; the level dropped 20% in 24 hours and 10% during the next 24 hours. In my dilantin overdose file, I had three cases with the same kind of dilantin clearance. I could not find this information in books or in the Poisindex microfiche, which I consulted later. However, I had an article in my own file regarding a fatal case of dilantin poisoning in a child, where the half-life of dilantin was 80 hours. This information enabled me to answer his question."

Such information, along with records of personal reading and medical experiences, allows ready access to the material and keeps the physician in tune with medical developments. According to Edward Rosenow, Ted

Howell of the Henry Ford Hospital found that residents having difficulty passing specialty boards improved when they categorized and filed journal articles, a process that helped them organize their thoughts and grasp the material better.

Some methods of filing journal tear-outs and personal notes are relatively simple, whereas others are complex. Each physician must choose the system best suited to his needs and work habits. The important thing is to find a system that you will use.

General Principles

The essential features of a reprint file are (1) simplicity, to ensure ease of storage and speed of retrieval; (2) currency; and (3) manageability through periodic weeding. A personal filing system may have several components: a list of the topic headings under which articles are filed, cross-referencing under several topics, coherent filing organization, and a method of retrieving all reprints on a certain topic.

When journal pages do not contain complete source information, be sure to record on each article the full reference: journal name, volume, issue number, inclusive pages, and date. Or append a photocopy of the table of contents. Otherwise, even though your filing system may permit retrieval of the wanted article, you will not know its source. Other notations may be made at the top of articles, such as a rating of the quality of the article and illustrations.[2]

Methods of Filing

Many physicians choose topic headings for reprint files from the table of contents in a standard textbook.[3-7] Models include *Harrison's Principles of Internal Medicine*,[8] which covers symptoms; *Cecil's Textbook of Medicine*[9] and Davis-Christopher's *Textbook of Surgery*,[10] which cover organ systems; or appropriate subspecialty books. If the table of contents is numbered, those numbers can be used to organize the reprint file. If not, articles can be filed under the major headings and subdivisions of the contents. Telfer Reynolds designed his general internal medicine file somewhat like an index of a general medicine textbook, but created detailed subdivisions that reflect his interests. Still others create new topic headings as new interests develop.

Three popular methods of indexing the files are by alphabetized topic headings, by decimal numbers, and numerically. A fourth method, with edge-punched cards, has been used for filing abstracts and summaries only. Whichever method you choose, keep a central topic index that lists all topic headings and numbers to avoid duplication and to expedite retrieval.

ALPHABETICAL FILES. Reprints and notes are filed in folders arranged alphabetically by broad topic headings, such as gastroenterology. Subheadings, such as peptic ulcer disease, can be delineated by color-coded tabs on the folders. Full capitals can be used to distinguish major categories. The object, of course, is to be able to scan the file quickly to retrieve the desired folder. By using only general headings and subdividing only sections of particular interest and importance to a physician's practice, the files can be kept to a minimum.

DECIMALS. In the decimal system, major topic headings are assigned whole numbers (1.0, 2.0, 3.0,. . .) with decimal subheadings. For example, under category 1.0, subheadings would be numbered 1.1, 1.2, for as many as are needed. Categories can be further divided by adding more decimal points, but the finer the divisions, the more complicated and cumbersome the classification.

NUMERICAL FILES. In the numerical system, each article is numbered consecutively in the upper right corner and filed in a folder by the number, regardless of subject matter. As each new article is filed, the next available number is assigned to it. Each folder holds a certain number of articles, usually between ten and twenty-five. Thus, if the first folder is numbered "1-10," it will hold the first ten articles in serial order. The second folder will be labeled "11-20," and so on.

The numerical system requires an accompanying reference card file arranged by subject, by author's last name, or by both. The card should list the complete reference and the number assigned to the article.

A card file, although not necessary for reprints filed by topics (alphabetically or by decimals), may facilitate retrieval.

Cross-indexing articles may increase the usefulness—but also the complexity—of the reprint file. Articles filed by topic, whether by decimal notation or alphabetically, can be cross-filed by a sheet of paper placed in other pertinent topic folders, referring the user to the file containing the article.

Reprint Indexing Systems

We have described several manual systems for filing reprints to acquaint readers with the specific principles involved. Indexing programs for personal computers are now available and should simplify the use of the personal reprint center. A more complete discussion can be found later in this chapter and in Chapter 17 on computers.

A Detailed System

Baker and Brashear have described a system in which the physician chooses his own topic words to build his categories and cross-index articles.[11] This system contains fewer, but more individually pertinent, categories than those found in textbooks, which may include topics seldom seen by most practitioners and may omit others seen often. The strength of the system is in the personalization, the ease of cross-indexing, and the expansion possible as the user's needs grow or change. The materials needed are file cards (5-by-8-inches), file card box, manila folders (9-by-12-inches), and a manila folder box.

LABELING. Each article is numbered consecutively in the upper right corner of the first page, and topic words are written in the lower right corner of the first page of the reprint.

CENTRAL INDEX. The central index is an alphabetical listing of topic words previously chosen by the user. Baker and Brashear recommend constructing a folded central index sheet by taping together four 5-by-8-inch cards along the 8-inch side, one above the other. Topic words are listed alphabetically on this central index as they come to mind during the initial review of an article. Two columns are made, the A's starting at the top left and the Z's ending at the lower right. Ample space is left between topic words to permit insertion of new ones.

The central index allows the physician to see at a glance what topic words are represented in his reprint file. If the user finds a desired topic already in the central index, he proceeds to record the reference of the new article on that topic word card (see next paragraph). If the topic of the new article is not listed in the central index, the user adds it and then makes a new topic word card for the topic word box.

TOPIC WORD CARD FILE. On cards labeled by topic, pertinent references are listed in ascending order by reprint number. Each card represents a single topic, and the cards are filed alphabetically. The complete reference is recorded for each article: reprint number, author, title, and year published. If necessary, a second card for a topic can be filed behind the first card. Each article is so listed on a topic word card for every topic recorded in the lower right of the first page.

REPRINT FILE. The articles are placed in folders in a file box or drawer, ten to a folder, filed in numerical order.

NUMBER CARD. A "number card" reminds the physician which number to assign to the next reprint. As he assigns a new number to an article, he crosses out the last number on the card and records the next number to be used.

Example of Use

The physician finds an article he wishes to keep. He consults the "number card" to determine the last used number and assigns the next one to this article, writing it in the upper right corner. He records one or more topic words in the lower right corner. He consults the Central Index to see if the topic words are in the file. If they are, he pulls the proper topic card(s) from the topic word box and adds the new number and reference. If they are not, he adds the new topic to the Central Index, makes new topic card(s) for the topic word box file, and records on each the article number and full reference.

When the physician wishes to retrieve articles on a specific subject, he consults the Central Index to find topic words on that subject, consults the topic word cards in the topic word box, finds the numbers of the articles he wants, and retrieves those articles from the proper folders.

Bound articles can also be cross-indexed: type the title of the bound article and the title of the journal, volume number, and page numbers on letter-size paper and then process this sheet as if it were the reprint. In the Baker-Brashear system, the physician writes the topics on the reprint, and at the same time may number the articles. A secretary can be easily trained to do the rest. This system, which also accommodates personal notes, Kodachrome slides, and summaries of patient charts, is simple, fast, personal, flexible, and expandable, and permits cross-filing.

Other Systems

Harold Slocum divides his index key into five major parts: (1) a list of all topics under which he files articles; (2) basic science articles; (3) the 18 major citations of the International Classification of Health Problems in Primary Care (common primary care diagnosis); (4) specific aspects of primary care; and (5) subjects of personal interest, such as office management and patient education.[7]

Ernst solved the space problem by filing abstracts and summaries instead of complete articles.[12] He placed the abstracts or summaries on edge-punched cards, available commercially. To the holes punched around the periphery of each card he assigned specific numbers, representing the topics, and he coded the cards by notching out the space between the topic's assigned hole and the edge of the card. When a needle was inserted through a topic's holes, any cards coded with that number slipped from the deck, and the desired cards were thus retrieved. He was able to retrieve and sort cards rapidly and efficiently. The basic classification was printed directly on each card, and a central index was therefore not needed. Although his was a manual system, automatic card-sorting machines are available.

David Blankenhorn's decimal system does not use cross-referencing: "If I want to do a comprehensive review, I can use the cumulative indexes and computer searches. I confine my reprint file to topics I am particularly interested in. I adopted an open-ended system, and when I have a new category, I simply write it down and enter it. I then assign each file a number. Cardiac physiology is 1, congenital heart disease is 2, rheumatic heart disease is 3, and so on. For rheumatic heart disease, I added 3-1 for

3. The Personal Information Center

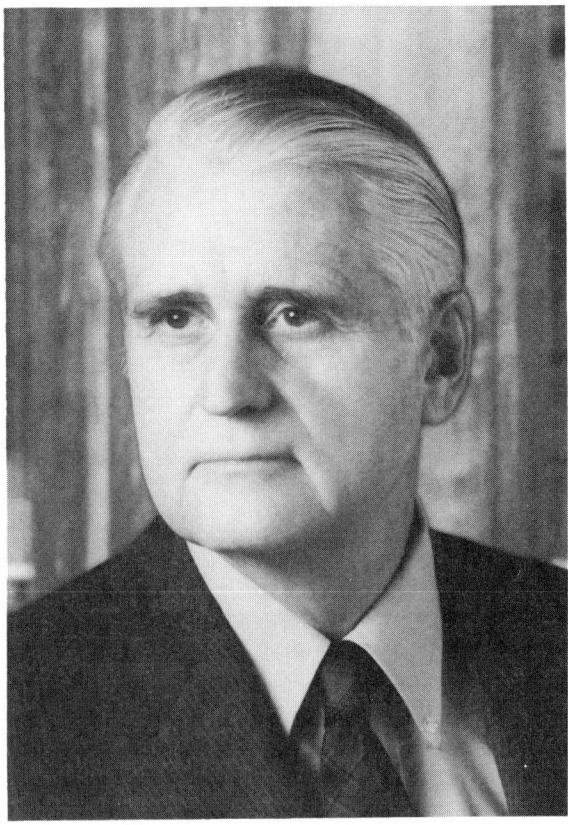

The purpose of a large, multi-authored textbook of medicine is to furnish a reliable, timely précis of information as an entry point for learning about or refreshing one's knowledge of a certain subject.

> *Lloyd H. Smith, Jr., M.D.*
> *Professor of Medicine*
> *Associate Dean, School of Medicine*
> *University of California, San Francisco*

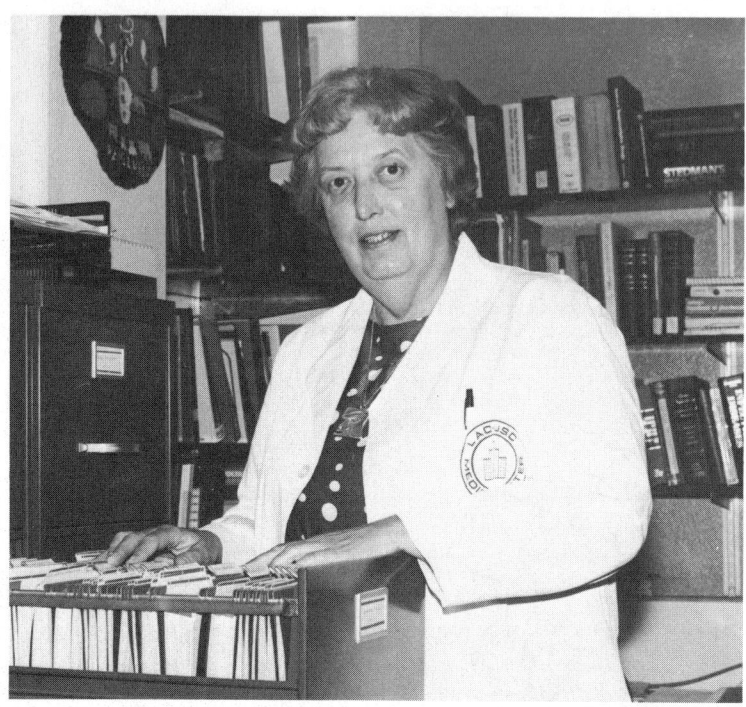

Whenever I encounter a problem, I pull out my file, which includes journal tear-outs, copies of consultation notes, and, in cases of drug overdose (a particular interest of mine), an abstract of the case on forms that I developed.

Margaret M. McCarron, M.D.
Associate Professor of Medicine
University of Southern California

mitral stenosis, 3-2 for mitral insufficiency, and additional subnumbers for other related conditions. I also include an 'unspecified' folder in each major category. I have expanded this system over the years, and when I become interested in some new subject, I find a key word that will remind me of this concept (although it may not be particularly informative to anyone else) and assign a new number to it."

For easy retrieval, Robert Smith files articles according to diagnosis, operation, or surgical complications. "Before doing an extensive review of a topic, I review my personal file. I feel relatively secure that my file will give the information I need to take care of patient problems or to prepare a conference on short notice. For instance, although renal hypertension in children is something that I see relatively infrequently, I have on file published reports on this subject from two or three centers around the country. When, once every year or two, I am called on to treat a child with renal hypertension, I go to that file and see how physicians with extensive experience handle it. I can also go to the library, of course, but it is much more convenient to have the material at my fingertips."

Irvine Page does not systematically file articles he tears out of journals, but writes the subject in the corner of each article. Then he places them in stacks of folders on general subjects. "Looking through these folders jogs my mind about things that I had forgotten," he said. "The literature is so voluminous that no one can keep up with it. I go through the stacks every so often on winter afternoons when I have nothing else to do and discard material that is no longer of interest."

Neil Elgee may have the simplest system of all: placing key articles between relevant pages of his textbook. When the new edition of the textbook comes out, he weeds out his "file."

The Computer

The methods described for indexing a personal reprint file can be enhanced and perhaps simplified by the use of a computer. Software already exists for most common computers that permits cross-indexing of references by topic, subtopic, article title, author, and key words. Thus a physician is able to search, by topic or key word, the references stored in the computer. Only the pertinent references will be displayed on the computer screen, shortening the time spent searching for appropriate articles in the actual files. For example, rather than looking at all the references filed under the topic "hypertension," a computer search can be keyed to display only those references pertaining to drugs in hypertension therapy, that is, filed under the topic "hypertension" and listing drug therapy as a keyword. Duke Baker, who has a home computer, commented that his manual system described above is so quick and simple that he has not yet perceived the need to computerize it. The computer file does not yet take the place of the reprint file; it serves as a quick and easy index to the reprint file (See Chapter 17).

Alternatives to a Reprint File

Eli A. Ramirez prefers simply to shelve his journals. "Over the years, I have tried many types of reprint file systems. Most of them worked well but took too much time to maintain. Several years ago, I began to keep a bookshelf file in chronological order for each of the six journals I subscribe to. Each bookshelf holds about five years of a journal. I file all index issues separately from regular issues so that I can find references rapidly by looking through the index issues together. Then I go back to the bookshelf files to obtain the articles I want in the journals." Others shelve the index issues with the respective journals. Several times a year, Ramirez updates his journal bookshelves and index issues, discarding those older than five years. He favors this method because it requires no additional expense and little time for organization and maintenance.

Keeping the File Manageable

Robert Cheshier, chief librarian at Western Reserve School of Medicine, cautioned against allowing the personal reprint file to become too complex or too massive. "Many physicians put off starting a reprint file because they think a good system has to be complex and time-consuming. As a result, they never start one. Personal files should be limited to articles used frequently, and the physician should select the filing system most practical for him. The redundancy within periodicals is abundant. If you find one good article on a topic, it is not necessary to keep numerous others with essentially the same information. The personal reprint file will assume increasing importance as practitioners organize their files with the aid of computers. Librarians will have a big role in educating physicians and their staffs in the use of the computer."

*****

The personal information center is a must for all physicians. Medical textbooks, the most efficient gateway to knowledge, should be kept current. The personal reprint file helps the physician organize and gain ready access to articles most pertinent to his practice. The process of organization may also enhance the physician's understanding of the materials. The personal library is not, however, a substitute for the services now available in modern medical libraries of all sizes, from a small library in a community hospital to a large society or medical school library.

Most such medical libraries are linked electronically and can provide rapid and detailed access to almost any medical article. The modern medical librarian has access to printed and electronic data bases and, as an information specialist, is prepared to assist the physician. Thus the physician should use both a personal reprint file and a good medical library.

References

1. Doyle, Arthur Conan. The five orange pips. In: *The Complete Sherlock Holmes*. Garden City, New York: Doubleday & Company Inc., 1930:225.
2. St. Clair, Helen D. Teaching residents a personal filing system. *Bull Med Libr Assoc* Jul 1981;69(3):324-326.
3. Fuller, Ellis A. A system for filing medical literature: Based on a method developed by Dr. Maxwell M. Wintrobe. *Ann Intern Med* Mar 1968;68(3):684-693.
4. Singer, Karl. Where did I see that article? *JAMA* 6 Apr 1979; 241(14):1492-1493.
5. Gaeke, Richard F.; Gaeke, Mary Ellen B. Filing medical literature: A textbook-integrated system. *Ann Intern Med* Jun 1973;78(6):985-987.
6. Ambuel, J. Philip. System for filing and retrieving medical knowledge. *Am J Dis Child* Nov 1963;106(5):462-465.
7. Slocum, Harold E. Personal medical reference files for family physicians. *J Fam Pract* Oct 1977;5(4):593-595.
8. Petersdorf, Robert G.; Adams, Raymond D.; Braunwald, Eugene; Isselbacher, Kurt J.; Martin, Joseph B.; Wilson, Jean D., eds. *Harrison's Principles of Internal Medicine*, 10th ed. New York: McGraw-Hill Book Company, 1983.
9. Beeson, Paul B.; McDermott, Walsh, eds. *Textbook of Medicine*, 14th ed. Philadelphia: W. B. Saunders Company, 1975.
10. Sabiston, David C., Jr., ed. *Davis-Christopher Textbook of Surgery: The Biological Basis of Modern Surgical Practice*, 12th ed. Philadelphia: W. B. Saunders Company, 1981.
11. Baker, Duke H.; Brashear, Richard H. Cross-indexed file for medical literature. *Ann Intern Med* Apr 1974;80(4):557-559.
12. Ernst, Richard E. Abstract card classification and retrieval systems for radiologic literature. *Amer J Roentgen* Jul 1965;94(3):741-747.

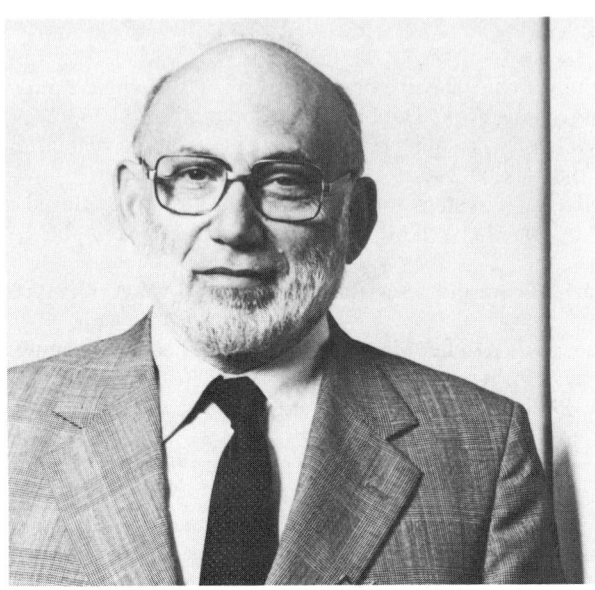

When I approach a problem, I usually immerse myself in it.
Joshua Lederberg, Ph.D.

Dr. Joshua Lederberg, President of The Rockefeller University, received the Nobel Prize in Physiology or Medicine for his work on genetic material in bacteria. His discovery of the mechanism of genetic recombination in bacteria and his career-long work in bacterial genetics were a principal foundation for contemporary research and biotechnology on gene manipulation in bacteria. Working on research in artificial intelligence in the seventies with E. A. Feigenbaum, he spawned one of the first expert systems (DENDRAL), a prototype for practical applications of artificial intelligence. With G. Nossal, he contributed to the conceptual development of monoclonal antibodies by showing that individual immune cells produce single types of antibodies. Dr. Lederberg played an active role in the National Aeronautics and Space Administration Mariner and Viking missions to Mars. His interest in improving communications among scientists, the general public, and government policymakers has led him to write extensively for lay audiences on the social impact of scientific progress.

I have never known anyone who exemplifies lifelong learning more fully than Joshua Lederberg. Throughout his life he has displayed an insatiable curiosity, wide-ranging interests, an extraordinary capacity to integrate information from diverse sources, and unfailing generosity in exchanging information with his colleagues. In addition, he is extremely well organized, highly energetic, and capable of making optimal use of computer technology. One of his trademarks is to send

Personal Essay

Joshua Lederberg, Ph.D.
President, The Rockefeller University
New York, New York

Implicit in my role as teacher and administrator is the need to know more than to do. My present position, as President of The Rockefeller University, requires a broad knowledge of my scientific colleagues' work in many fields. Many of my colleagues go to meetings to listen to presentations, but I prefer to read because I can better direct my attention than if I am at the mercy of the speaker.

Although my main responsibilities are looking for connections between things rather than being a completely informed specialist in any one subject, I use some pretty straightforward techniques of acquiring new knowledge. I scan 50 to 60 articles in *The New England Journal of Medicine, Science,* and *Nature,* and I use a weekly reporting service, the Automatic Subject Citation Alert (ASCA), which includes any article that cites the authors with whom I have been principally engaged in my scientific career. Research that cites any of about three dozen other authors is likely to be among my central interests. In addition, I receive weekly printouts of the titles of published articles by all The Rockefeller University authors. I request reprints or photocopies of 20 to 25 articles a week.

For the past fifteen years, I have been drawn increasingly into national security, international relations, and related political and economic affairs. Much of my reading is in periodicals like *Foreign Affairs, International Security, Foreign Policy,* and innumerable reports from the government, RAND, and other organizations. Most of the books I read are in these fields, as well as in biography and history. The articles in the two dozen series of *Annual Reviews* (whose Board of Directors I chair) are an invaluable grounding across the whole range of natural and social sciences.

I have the titles of useful articles recorded in roughly chronological order, and I keep a computer-searchable file of those I have read. After I look at the articles, they go into a box. Every once in a while, they are organized by date, just to have a systematic way of keeping them some-

---

notes with information and ideas highly pertinent to our own interest based on his monitoring of research literature. He is unfailingly helpful to his students, friends and colleagues. Joshua Lederberg is always keenly aware of moving frontiers and is constantly searching for ways to improve the constructive uses of existing knowledge.

David A. Hamburg, M.D.

where without going to the enormous effort of maintaining a complex system. I keep subject files of reprints on 50 or so topics.

For five years I wrote a newspaper column and needed background material. I now keep paper files and computer entry items—anything from clippings to articles, with my own comments on them—several hundred rubrics.

I do not ordinarily keep both chronologic and subject files on the same material. The material filed chronologically is more diverse, and I am most likely to want something from it if it is within the past year than if it is ten years old. I make a point of discarding paper to avoid being burdened with the idea that I ought to go look for it. It is probably more cost-effective to go back to the library routinely. The only material I make sure I keep is what would not be available at the library or that is for some special personal purpose, like the interconnection of parts of science.

When I approach a problem, I usually immerse myself in it. I find out everything I can that might have some possible bearing on it. I try to identify with whatever phenomenon I am looking at, to put myself in the place of that animal, molecule, bug, organ, or whatever is being described. What does the world look like from that vantage point? A lot of it is subconscious. Without consciously trying to find solutions, I can go to bed at night and wake up in the morning, and there will be some random conjunction or ideas—sometimes elusive and dream-like—that can provide a different angle. I hasten to write it down before it torments me like a lost dream. The most difficult thing is to drop other preoccupations and concentrate on a given issue: the process of preparation may take precious hours.

Curiosity and motivation are essential in continuing education. I've been so curious all my life that I must discipline myself to suppress my curiosity in other directions to accomplish tasks I have agreed to do. Unfortunately, some people were not allowed to express their curiosity early in life, or it was not reinforced.

It is difficult to capture the elements leading to creative development. My own interest in science started at a very early age. My mother saved a piece I had written when I was seven, in which I expressed my determination to be a scientist. My parents responded with partial encouragement and partial dismay; the encouragement was positive and the dismay was challenging. By the time I was eleven or twelve, I was reading college textbooks in chemistry and mathematics. I do not see many youngsters today showing such intensity. I cannot explain my intensity at that age. At a certain point I was reinforced. My parents were proud of me; I did well at school; and my teachers were wise enough to leave me alone. In a classroom in which I was three or five years ahead of the rest, the other students did not pester me, and I did not pester them. I was very much self-taught, working by my own devices.

It was not until I got to college that I found someone willing to provide some kind of structure to my education. That was my mentor, Francis Ryan, at Columbia. It was in his laboratory that I learned about genetics and microbiology, out of which came my early research work. Ryan knew when to be tough and when and how to encourage me. He was a worthy debater, and I had not had many opportunities to argue logically up to that time. He was also a superb teacher—in his communicative skills and in his ability to identify with students—and he was able to draw out my ideas without competing with me. His style was to provide every encouragement for me to deal with a set of problems.

To encourage intellectual interaction here at The Rockefeller University, I organize a luncheon every couple of weeks with some of my colleagues, and I make a point of getting people together who would not ordinarily come together. From time to time, I exchange notes with others about scientific issues. It keeps me alive intellectually. I browse more than anyone else I know—because it is part of my job—and when I see material in an out-of-the-way place that one of my colleagues in a given specialty is unlikely to know about, I send him a copy. If it is helpful one time out of twenty, it is worth it.

Physicians can discuss their cases with their colleagues. Formal, mandatory continuing medical education, on the other hand, may get in the way of one's self-education. Psychiatry, for example, has been advancing relatively slowly: it is hard to distinguish psychiatry decade by decade except for the pharmacological advances. On the other hand, psychiatrists learn from experience and from their patients. So there may be a different need for continuing medical education in that field. The greatest gaps are more likely to be in the broad sphere of medicine than in one's own specialty. Yet the internist does need to know what is going on in surgery, pathology, and other specialties.

4

The Institutional Medical Library

> For the general practitioner a well-used library is one of the few correctives of the premature senility which is so apt to overtake him.
>
> *William Osler*[1]

Although a good personal study center may be the physician's most valuable continuing education tool, and although modern textbooks are useful in answering many clinical questions, the physician's collection at home or the office cannot possibly approach that of the hospital, medical society, or medical school library. Medical libraries have changed and will change even more during the next decade. Librarians have new skills and are acquiring others. Most physicians are not using the library optimally, partly because they are unaware of the ways in which libraries can serve them.

Electronic data bases and cooperation among libraries have largely eliminated library size as a major consideration. The modern medical library can offer special services and has access, beyond its collection, to information at larger regional libraries or even the National Library of Medicine. Ralph Jung has made frequent use of such services: "To learn the most about specific patient problems in my subspecialty, I heavily use an off-line bibliographic citation list generated by MEDLINE to the National Library of Medicine's Interactive Retrieval Service, which is available to me at a moderate cost from the medical library. Not only do I get title citations, but since many articles are now abstracted, I can keep abreast of the worldwide publications on a specific problem. Moreover, should a particular title or abstract intrigue me, I can request and then read this specific article in full. I find this service preferable to using Current Contents or other available systems." (See Chapter 17.)

Modern library services allow physicians to gain prompt access to information pertinent to their special interests. Familiarity with library services and good rapport with the medical librarian are thus invaluable to the physician. The librarian's functions have changed from a custodian of archives to those of a skilled information specialist. The physician has only to define his information needs carefully, and the modern librarian will screen the print and electronic data bases and index systems and will deliver the information requested.

Physicians like Ruth McCormick who regularly use library services are enthusiastic about the results: "One of the most rewarding features of starting private practice is the excellent help I have had from librarians in obtaining information I need to solve patient problems."

The Medical Librarian

The role of the medical librarian is to assist the physician in obtaining pertinent information documents. Robert Braude, Director of the University of Nebraska Medical Center's McGoogan Library, pointed out that as improved management of information reduces the time needed to fill a library request, the physician can spend more time reading and evaluating the information. The physician who does not take advantage of the librarian's expertise may spend unnecessary time searching for information and still miss valuable resources. The more specific the request, the more efficiently can the librarian serve you. Knowing the purpose for which information will be used helps the librarian find appropriate references. For an immediate problem in patient care a few recent review articles may suffice, whereas preparation of a research proposal would require a far more extensive search. Since librarians may be reluctant to appear overly inquisitive about the purpose of the physician's request, it is up to the physician to provide this information.

For example:

> I wish to learn about the current preferred treatment of seasonal allergic rhinitis. I would like a current review article and three or four authoritative articles published within the past year that will address the following questions:
>
> What is the current expert opinion of the efficacy of hyposensitization with specific allergens?
>
> How effective is beclomethasone dipropionate used nasally?
>
> How effective is dexamethasone by nasal-spray inhalation?

"As with any service," explained Nina Matheson, "the best results come from the physician's direct communication with the librarian. When he wants specific information on a medical topic, he should make the request himself unless his secretary can be precise about what he wants. Secretaries are often unable to answer such questions as 'How detailed a search is necessary?' 'How far back in time does the physician wish

4. The Institutional Medical Library

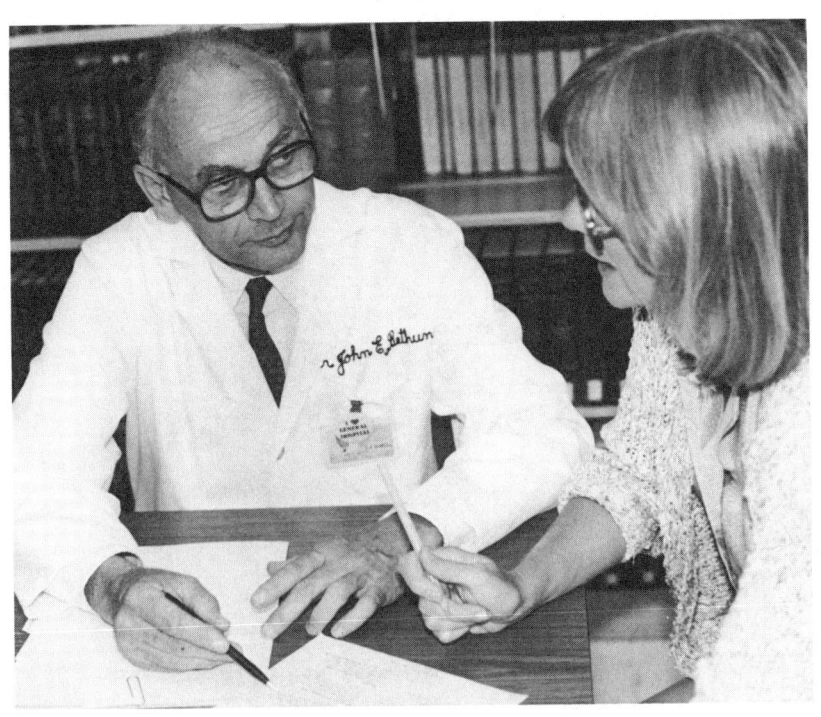

A personal conference with a professional medical librarian is invaluable in circumscribing the precise information to be requested.

John E. Bethune, M.D.
Chairman, Department of Medicine
University of Southern California

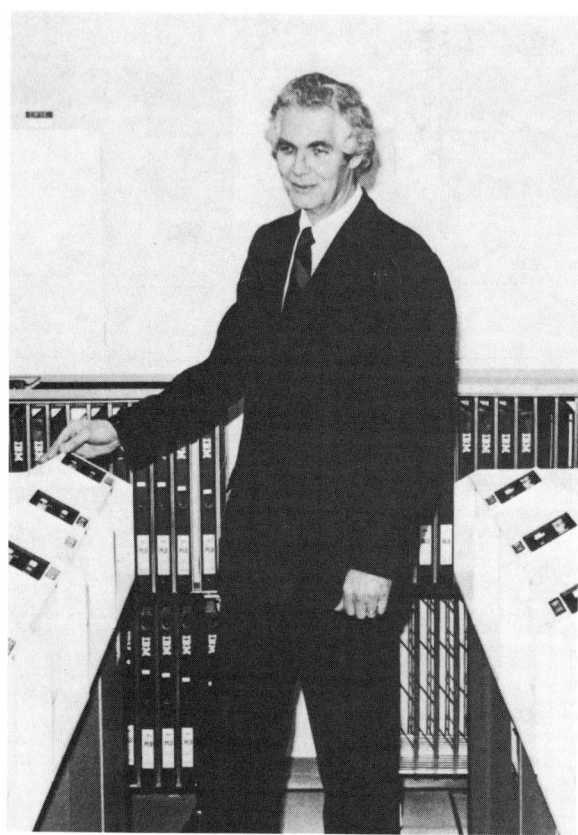

No longer can medical librarians be considered custodians in warehouses for books. Today, with the help of technology, professional information specialists stand ready to retrieve from data banks the specific information requested by clinicians and scientists.

Donald A. B. Lindberg, M.D.
Director, National Library of Medicine

4. The Institutional Medical Library   77

the search to go?' 'Are there other descriptors that narrow the focus of the search?' It is also helpful to have the secretary or other assistant attend orientation programs to learn what services are available and how to use the library, but nothing replaces the personal communication between the physician and the librarian."

Interactive Computer-assisted Searching

A major change in medical librarianship that has revolutionized retrieval of information is the advent of interactive computer-assisted searching. Although manual searches in such sources as the *Index Medicus* continue to be used, librarians and others are increasingly turning to computer searches. On-line data bases are of two types: bibliographic data bases contain citations and sometimes abstracts of documents, whereas non-bibliographic (pragmatic) data bases contain full text or actual data on particular subjects, such as drugs.

MEDLINE

MEDLINE is an on-line computer version of the *Index Medicus* (the index of medical literature published by the National Library of Medicine), the *Index to Dental Literature*, and the *International Nursing Index*, jointly covering more than 3300 biomedical journals and books. In addition to bibliographic citations, MEDLINE contains abstracts for about half the citations entered after January, 1975. The advantages of MEDLINE over its printed counterpart include more access points and speed of identification of relevant articles. The printed index provides subject access only by specific subject headings, whereas MEDLINE allows access also by words in titles or abstracts. This natural-language access-point is particularly useful for current topics such as toxic shock syndrome. In this system an article can be stored under a great many more headings than in the printed index. An article can often be found under twenty or more different headings, but limitation of space in the printed version permits listing of the same article under only three headings. The chances of retrieving an article by computer are therefore greatly increased, even if little is known about it. The computer can also quickly retrieve articles that deal with more than one criterion, such as coronary artery disease in hypertensive male smokers below the age of 35 years. By contrast, finding such articles in the *Index Medicus* requires laborious manual searching.

Other Data Bases

In addition to MEDLINE, the National Library of Medicine produces several other computerized indexes, including TOXLINE, The Registry of Toxic Effects of Chemical Substances (RTECS), CHEMLINE, CANCERLINE, and AVLINE.

TOXLINE covers toxicity of drugs and chemicals, adverse drug interactions, and environmental pollution. It provides abstracts as well as references.

RTECS provides toxicity data and information on threshold limits, lethal doses, and standards for air and water purity.

CHEMLINE enables the user to define chemical substances by preferred chemical names, synonyms, and molecular formulae.

CANCERLINE has three files:
> CANCERLIT provides abstracts of material on cancer from journals, reports, monographs, and conference proceedings.
> CANCERPROJ describes unpublished cancer research in progress.
> CLINPROT is a highly specialized file for clinical oncologists.

AVLINE provides information on audiovisual programs in medicine.

SCISEARCH. One portion of SCISEARCH, available either on-line or as a printed index (Science Citation Index), lists key articles and all subsequent articles citing them. David Blankenhorn uses it to go forward in time from an article of a certain date. "If an article was published in 1978, for example, and I want to know who has quoted the article, I can look under the authors' names and find all their articles that others have cited." The user should be aware, however, that the most frequently cited articles are not necessarily the most valid or authentic, since heavy citation of an author's own publications, failure to cite relevant publications of rivals, and inadequate bibliographic research may all skew the Science Citation Index. Moreover, some articles are cited because they are refuted, not corroborated.

Three other commercial vendors—Bibliographic Retrieval Services (BRS), Lockheed Dialog, and Systems Development Corporation—provide a large variety of additional data bases covering physical and social sciences, humanities, and business. *Excerpta Medica*, a data base available through Dialog, offers particularly good coverage of clinical medicine, with an emphasis on drugs. Its printed counterpart consists of 47 separate sections, each covering a specific medical discipline.

Current-awareness Bibliographies

Through the local medical library, a physician may request periodic updating of references on a particular topic from any of the computerized data bases described here. SDILINE (Selected Dissemination of Information On-Line), for example, covers monthly updates to MEDLINE and produces references four to six weeks in advance of the printed version of each index.

4. The Institutional Medical Library

The physician can, of course, also manually search from the *Index Medicus* and various other reference sources. *Current Contents*, which is published weekly, contains the title pages of more than 1100 journals. Some medical libraries provide selective manual updating services. If a physician does not subscribe to all the journals in his specialty, he can ask the librarian to photocopy the table of contents of certain journals as they arrive. This service is probably most practical for hospital-based physicians with access to small libraries.

Retrieval

Once a bibliography is produced, either manually or by computer, the next step is to obtain the actual documents whose titles or abstracts suggest their usefulness. The availability of documents extends far beyond the materials held by the local libraries. The regional medical library program has an interlibrary loan network that links medical libraries, hospital libraries, and academic libraries. If a physician needs materials not available at his institution, the librarian can request a book loan or photocopy from the nearest library that owns the item.

Audiovisual Sources

Another change in the medical library is the increasing collection of audiovisuals. "Although libraries are identified primarily with books and journals," noted Nancy Lorenzi, "they also contain, or can acquire on interlibrary loan, nonprint media—that is, slides, Audio Digest tapes, videocassettes, l6-mm films, and three-dimensional models of the heart, lungs, and other organs and anatomical regions. Tapes in a media collection may represent an entire conference, and by use of library films, the physician can observe a surgical procedure without leaving his home base." Audiovisuals can also supplement classroom instruction. Librarians can advise physicians about audiovisual programs for particular purposes.

*****

Medical libraries have changed greatly, and medical librarians are now trained to be true information brokers, able to link the physician with the information he needs. The physician's main task is to state specifically what information is needed, how he plans to use the information (for a talk, paper, or patient care), and phrase questions he would like answered. Speaking directly to the librarian, giving the opportunity for questions, is the best approach.

Even more dramatic changes in library services and information management are occurring and will occur in the next decade. (See Chapter 17.)

Reference

1. Osler, William. Books and men. In: *Aequanimitas, with Other Addresses to Medical Students, Nurses and Practitioners of Medicine*, 3rd ed. Philadelphia: The Blakiston Company, 1945:211.

5
The Collegial Network

> To hold him who has taught me this art as equal to my parents and to live my life in partnership with him, and if he is in need of money to give him a share of mine, and to regard his offspring as equal to my brothers in male lineage and to teach them this art— if they desire to learn it—without fee and covenant; to give a share of precepts and oral instruction and all the other learning to my sons and to the sons of him who has instructed me and to pupils who have signed the covenant and have taken an oath according to the medical law, but to no one else.
>
> *Hippocrates*[1]

When one of us (P. M.) visited Timbuktu, Mali, the native physician, upon learning that a visiting physician was in town, went to the hotel. Although he spoke no English, our conversation, through an interpreter, immediately turned to medicine, lasted six hours, and included discussions of patients, practice, and medical education.

A major advantage of being in the medical profession is the warm spirit of fraternity among physicians the world over. After the introductions, it does not take long for two physicians who have never met to become deeply engaged in conversation about the differences and similarities in their practices. This camaraderie is often most dramatic when physicians are visiting foreign lands, but physicians in offices and hospitals have similar educational discussions daily about patients and practice.

Social interaction can promote intellectual stimulation and satisfaction from learning and can enhance memory. "The current avalanche of information threatens to overwhelm me," confessed Irvine Page. "What to do about it? I learn by associating facts with people. For example, in 1935, at a meeting of the Central Society in Chicago, I had lunch in the Cape Cod Room of the Drake Hotel with Dr. W. W. Herrick. Two things I have never forgotten: first, we had red snapper soup with a small cruet of sherry on the side—a new experience for me; second, Dr. Herrick told me that when he first described coronary thrombosis, the presentation fell like a lead balloon. The result: after nearly 50 years, I have forgotten neither red snapper soup with sherry nor Herrick and his experience in introducing a new idea."

Studies have documented the strength of the information network among physicians, which, although informal, provides mutual support for lifelong learning.[2-5] Physicians are constantly providing information to, and receiving it from, their colleagues to help resolve clinical problems. Thomas Wood believes that his greatest source of learning probably comes from interaction with his colleagues, in consultations and informal discussions, as well as in a journal club. "Receiving current medical information from a trusted medical colleague," he finds, "is often as persuasive and useful as the physician's own detailed statistics on a particular subject."

The lifelong student of medicine becomes eligible to join a sophisticated information network by associating with excellent clinicians who are also excellent teachers. You must, of course, uphold your own responsibility in such relations by willingly providing accurate information and contributing your own medical experiences, as well as asking thoughtful questions and listening attentively. It does not pay to be a leech or to try to dominate the relationship. As Francis Moore pointed out, "The more you have to contribute to the education of others, the more welcome you will be in an informal network and the more mutual benefit you and the group will receive."

"As you grow older, it becomes more and more important to associate with young physicians," said Alvin Schultz. "They keep you from withering. They don't accept your answers easily; you have to document what you say. And they have a lot of new ideas." Conversely, young physicians can also profit from the rich experience of older physicians, who are usually anxious to extend a helping hand.

Although you will want to associate with the best informed physicians, you can learn from any colleague. "Even though you may have been the top student at the best medical school and the best resident at the best hospital," counseled James Moss, "every physician you meet will probably know more than you about some aspect of medicine. If you watch him and listen to him, you will discover much that you didn't learn in medical school, and you will then be able to share these new ideas with others."

Learning with Colleagues

"I really don't begin to think until I am in a situation where there is an exchange of ideas, where my opinion is sought, considered, and perhaps challenged, and where some conclusion is reached," said Jack Tetirick.

5. The Collegial Network

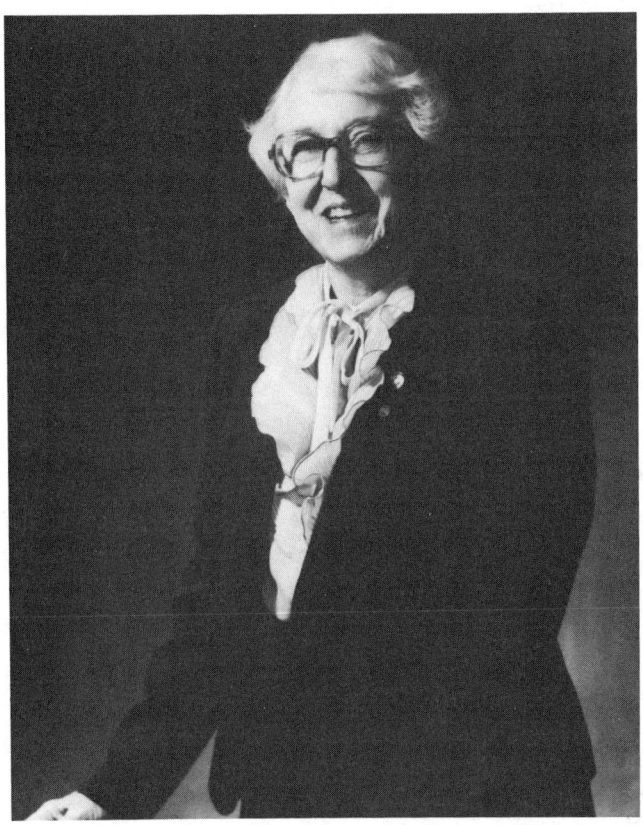

Many young women seem convinced that they will not be accepted or allowed to participate in organized medicine; that simply is not true.

Ruth M. Bain, M. D.
Austin, Texas

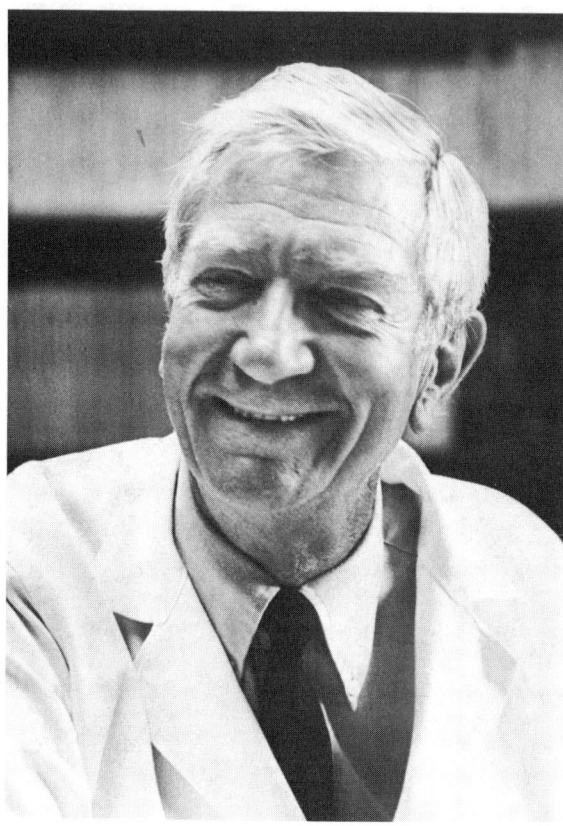

In my professional career, learning from experience, supplemented by reading and discussions with colleagues, has been invaluable.

Thomas H. Brem, M.D.
Emeritus Professor of Medicine
University of Southern California

"The stimulation and the satisfaction of learning come only through social interaction. Maintaining skills in the practice of medicine requires the opportunity to demonstrate those skills to colleagues, with the attendant reinforcement and bolstering of the ego, and then that gentle dangling hook of the fear of losing the circle of approving peers."

Group Practice

Richard Treiman enjoys the advantage of sharing common problems that group practice affords. "It is nice," he finds, "to be able to talk over a clinical problem with an associate who is intimately interested and who will see the patient without a formal consultation or charges. When you run into difficult problems, sharing responsibility relieves the anxiety about whether you are doing the right thing. Every physician should have someone available to share his experiences with." The stimulus of association with a group helps maintain your academic interests and expertise.

Wallace Chambers described the advantages of his group practice thus: "In addition to having discussions almost every hour of the day, we have occasional lunches, and we usually go to breakfast on Fridays, after which we have rounds and see all the group's patients together." Neil Elgee also values the support he receives in group practice: "With fourteen of us practicing together, I have an expert on just about everything at my beck and call. I can reach for the phone and pick my colleagues' brains. It is amazing how that takes care of my needs."

Some groups schedule a specific time weekly or biweekly to discuss specific problems of patients under care, an immediately rewarding practice because the discussion is tied to existing problems. In Robert Volpe's clinic, at the end of the day, several patients are kept—provided they are willing—and their problems are discussed with the staff. "The patients have a chance to speak, and seem to appreciate this. It is one of the highlights of our practice." The late Lorin Stephens belonged to a group of eight orthopedists who closed their offices for two and a half hours Monday mornings to discuss their problem patients. When they felt they needed outside help, they called on an expert, usually a faculty member from a nearby medical school, whom they would pay an honorarium. Sadahiro Yamamoto described a practice in Japan: "Groups of private physicians in Japan organize their practice in a way that allows them to invite specialists from the larger hospitals to speak periodically at their offices."

Desmond Julian considers it crucial to go outside a close-knit group from time to time: "The little conferences among members of group practices are sometimes reinforcements for one another's ignorance. One thinks somebody is a specialist in a certain subject whereas, in fact, he may really be a subspecialist who is considered to have a degree of expertise he doesn't possess. In this kind of contact, the specialists must understand their own limitations."

Some practice groups, such as Jean Creek's, have established sabbatical policies similar to those in universities. The younger members of his group have used the sabbatical to finish subspecialty certification, whereas Creek has used it to expand his knowledge of specific diseases. He spent six months of a sabbatical in rheumatology, for example, at Hammersmith Hospital in London and the other six months in the rheumatology service at the University Center in Indianapolis. Although he does not plan to announce himself as a rheumatologist, he found the experience most helpful because there is no rheumatologist in town.

Solo Practice

Although physicians in group practice may have the edge in developing relations with colleagues, the individual practitioner also has ample opportunities to develop collegial relations through his hospital, local medical society, and even medical centers where he has trained or visited.

Academia

Physicians in academia learn by osmosis—by going to conferences, and seeking out people who have answers to their questions. Richard Byyny, for example, can walk down the hall and find an oncologist, immunologist, or dermatologist with whom to discuss a problem. Manuel Martinez-Maldonado has established a practice in a Veterans Administration hospital that would also work in group practice and even with nonaffiliated physicians. "Every Friday afternoon I hold a session at which anyone on the house staff can present any case he wants. I encourage the staff to bring me cases outside my specialty of nephrology. We develop a working list of no more than four or five possibilities according to the history and physical examination of the patient, and then rearrange the list in the most logical, time-saving, and economical way of determining the diagnosis or excluding the one we have entertained. This technique has been extremely effective because it has helped the house staff think about the tests that are essential for diagnosis."

A Learning Game

Roy Behnke finds the intellectual stimulation of collegial discussions challenging: "Several of my associates on the faculty and I try to stump one another. Every time I meet them, the odds are that they will have a new question for me. If I cannot give them an answer, I have to look it up. A good part of my education comes from talking to my faculty and listening to them. It is surprising what you remember from these exchanges. The exchanges are also recreational."

Curbstone Conferences

Impromptu encounters among colleagues are a useful part of lifelong learning. At such "curbstone" conferences, one physician will question another about a clinical problem he has or about a new drug or diagnostic procedure. Curbstone consultations offer advantages for both parties. The inquiring physician often receives an answer or is directed to a pertinent reference. The consulting physician, through this opportunity to teach, is required to review his experience and thus strengthens his own understanding of the problem. In addition to practical education, the impromptu encounter provides a brief period of relaxation from the physician's busy routine.

A physician should not hesitate to ask colleagues appropriate questions, but neither should he become overly dependent on others. Such dependence is not likely if the physician organizes his thoughts carefully, studies the published information on the subject, and then asks appropriate questions. Kenneth Berge recognizes this problem: "I work hard at solving problems rather than ask for help prematurely; that is a particular temptation in subspecialty and superspecialty institutions. There is always someone around who knows more about a certain subject than I do. I have found that the best way for me to learn is not to call that person immediately, but to bring the problem to a little better state of resolution in my own mind first, and then ask the questions when I am really backed up to the wall. This procedure establishes whether I really do not know the answer—that after having taken the time to search for it, I have been unable to find it myself."

The Telephone

Francis Moore advocates wider use of the telephone for consultation purposes. "One of the advantages of going to a meeting is that you hear someone talk about a difficult case of intestinal obstruction, for example, and later are able to call him up and see how he would handle the patient you now have. Many of us have developed close relations with peers around the country and freely discuss our problems with them by telephone."

Frederick Ludwig, the sole surgeon in a rural institution with eight other physicians, calls various consultants around the country when a problem arises in the operating room. "When I am in a tough situation in the operating room, I simply pick up the phone and call a consultant. Using the telephone freely has greatly enhanced my ability to care for my patients." Don't be bashful about calling a colleague for an opinion; most are flattered by such a call. Medical school faculties are almost always willing to answer questions.

R. J. Williamson belongs to a telephone network: "In the communication system of our hospital, we all have telephone lines in our offices tied into the hospital with a three-digit number. Through my extensions in my office and at home, I can dial any extension in the hospital. I can dictate from any one of those extensions into the hospital, or I can do it by long distance. The cost of the telephone is about twenty dollars a month."

The University of Alabama has established an excellent telephone consultation service for physicians in the state, Medical Information Service via Telephone (MIST). Using a toll-free number to dial the MIST office, the physician states his problem, which is then immediately referred to the proper faculty member for his advice. Although few medical schools have such a formal telephone consultation service, most faculty members, especially those most highly regarded, receive calls regularly from former students, residents, fellows, and other physicians. Thus the telephone provides quick access to information and expert clinical judgment.

Correspondence

Some physicians develop teaching/learning associations through correspondence. Andrew Dale for example, maintains a sizeable correspondence. "When I read an article of special interest about which I have questions, I dictate a letter to ask the author about it or state why I disagree with him. Then he will respond with what he thinks. The exchange is always profitable." Although correspondence is not as popular as it once was, many physicians are enriched by the exchange of letters with respected colleagues and authorities. Correspondence may be especially useful for communicating with fellow physicians in other countries. In the future, correspondence will be expedited by the use of electronic mail (see Chapter 17, p. 259).

Sites of Collegial Conversations

The Lunch Table

Paul Beeson stated the case clearly: "I have always been impressed by the value of the lunch table, where you can sit down and discuss an interesting case. Our profession, after all, deals partly with guess work; we do not deal in absolutes. A solo practitioner is at a terrible disadvantage because he does not have other people to bounce ideas off, and so the lunch table can be a particularly valuable tool for him. Medical students learn a great deal from other students and from informal conversations and contacts. This is the knowledge that sticks; it is study in connection with a case rather than study in isolation, reading in books."

Too often, however, conversation at lunch drifts to automobiles, the stock market, and golf. With just a little effort, physicians can derive greater benefit and enjoyment through discussion of medical topics.

5. The Collegial Network

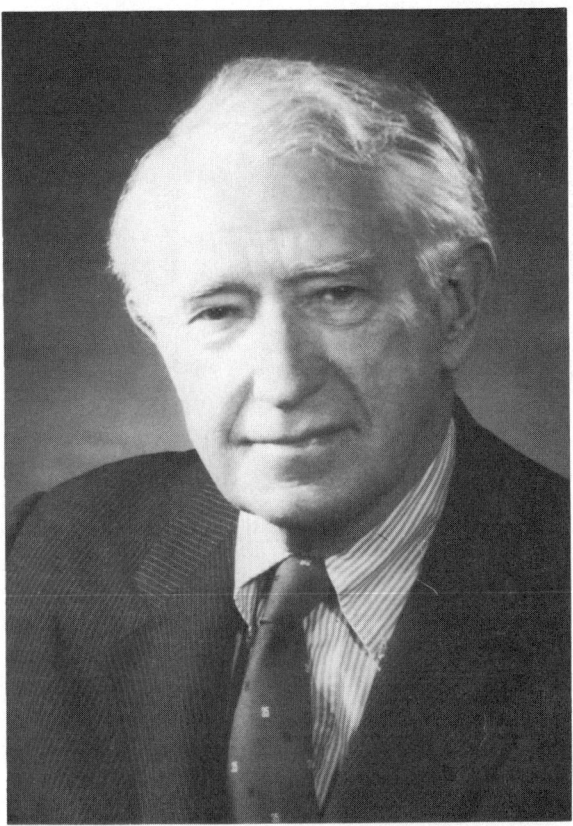

Many of us have developed close relations with peers around the country and freely discuss our problems with them by telephone.

Francis D. Moore, M.D.
Moseley Professor of Surgery, Emeritus
Harvard Medical School

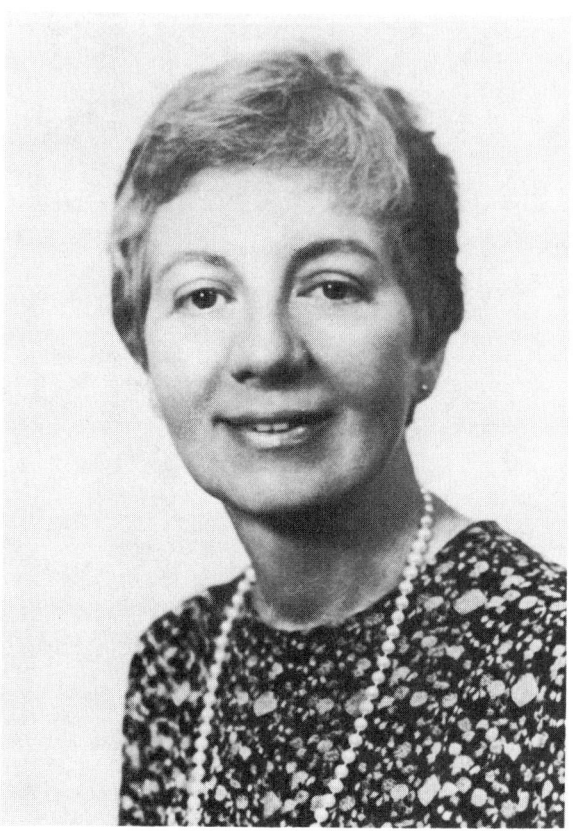

I have good learning experiences from collegial relationships. The "old girl" network, on the other hand, is not yet very effective.

Marjorie Price Wilson, M.D.
Senior Associate Dean, School of Medicine
University of Maryland

H. Ralph Haymond finds that immediately after reviewing a topic is a good time to start conversations on the subject with your colleagues at lunch or elsewhere, "Not only will they be impressed with your knowledge, but they may fill you in on some aspects of the topic that you have overlooked. Even chance encounters can prove valuable."

The Doctors' Lounge

David Covell noted that "The hospital's doctors' lounge is an important forum for doctors of different specialties to learn from one another what is new and important. Recently, for example, a urologist friend described current methods for dealing with renal and ureteral stones by ultrasound techniques, and a pulmonary physician described a recent disastrous case of sleep apnea."

The Bedside of Other Physicians' Patients

Gustavo Kuster described the cooperative spirit among the surgeons at his hospital: "Every week the general surgeons make rounds on all the patients we have in the hospital. We do not fully examine every patient unless one of our colleagues needs an opinion. Instead, we are simply overseeing what is happening within our division. An exchange of opinions ensues. If I do a certain operation, I have to justify it to my colleagues."

Ian Mackay of Australia advocates inviting specialists, like pathologists and radiologists, on hospital rounds and clinical conferences. "They make excellent contributions. Someone on the service should make sure, however, that they are well briefed on the problem to be discussed. It is unfair to throw a strange laboratory result at them and ask them why the laboratory data do not agree with the clinical impression, with the implication that something went wrong in the laboratory."

Bedside rounds with colleagues are most common in teaching hospitals, but all physicians will find the exercise an opportunity for broadening their clinical outlook.

Study and Discussion Groups

> . . . I had form'd most of my ingenious Acquaintances into a Club for mutual Improvement, which we called the Junto. We met on Friday Evening. . . . Our Debates were to be under the Direction of a President, and to be conducted in the sincere Spirit of Enquiry after Truth, without Fondness for Dispute, or Desire of Victory. . . .
>
> *Benjamin Franklin*[6]

In 1911, because Winston Churchill was denied membership in a dining club originally founded by Sir Joshua Reynolds and Samuel Johnson, he established, with Mr. F. E. Smith, a club of his own, called "The Other Club." The membership included such prominent men as Generals Kitchener and Montgomery and H. G. Wells. Churchill invited only those whom he considered both estimable and entertaining. "The Other Club" had such significance for Churchill that he insisted on attending even at the height of the Blitz in 1940 and 1941.[7] For this group, politics was the main topic of conversation, but physicians also can profit from medical discussion groups and, as with Churchill's group, the sessions are most effective when its members are both estimable and entertaining.

Medical colleagues with similar practice problems can profit from discussing individual experiences related to a current clinical problem. For nine years, David Covell has met with eight other internists every Tuesday morning. "We decide what we would like to study, make assignments for each of us to present material, informally discuss the material, and thus learn from one another's experiences. Usually we choose patient-related self-study programs, such as Medical Knowledge Self-Assessment Program (MKSAP) or similar material from major textbooks or medical centers, but the primary value of our group lies in the discussions generated and their relation to our own practice. It is not all serious, however; we enjoy one another's jokes and gripes. Of course, the group would not have lasted so long if we did not all get along. Combining the fun of learning something useful with the fun of a bull session has helped to keep the study group going all this time."

Kunio Okuda of Chiba, Japan, who endorses weekly study sessions to discuss puzzling patients, believes that occasionally inviting young, academically oriented physicians to join the group enhances the discussions.

Visits to Hospital Departments of Pathology and Radiology and the Clinical Laboratory

Pathologists, radiologists, and the clinical laboratory staff are often major teachers in a community hospital. Sir John McMichael, for example, profited greatly from his visits to the pathology department. "Every day I was on duty at Hammersmith, I went to the postmortem room, and never came away without having learned something; often I was a bit humiliated." Ian Mackay confirmed that statement: "Sir John says he visited the postmortem room every day, and he *did*, too. He never missed. Unfortunately, at our postmortem room the presence of a consultant is a rare event."

The radiologist should be consulted personally to help with the choice of radiologic studies needed in difficult cases. Oscar Balchum stressed the value of personal communication: "I learn a great deal from the radiologist. I personally review with him the results for every patient rather than depend on written reports. Often, the radiologist may suggest pertinent articles to read." Edward Shapiro and his partners start their rounds with a visit to the radiology file room. "We go over the files with the radiologists, an experience that has shown the variation in interpretations and opinions among individuals."

"Forming a close relation with the staff of the hospital clinical laboratory, to discuss the indications and outcomes of certain laboratory studies, new tests, and unusual results, is an easy way to acquire surprisingly useful bits of knowledge" in Joseph Lydon's experience. "From my earliest days I sought out peers whose interests were somewhat different from mine. I made it a practice to 'pick them clean.' I would lunch, lounge, loiter, or take advantage of any contact. As a surgical resident, for example, I would lunch with those who were working in the forefront of hypertension. On slow evenings I would go through the x-ray teaching file with radiology residents who were studying for their Boards. I would hang around the pathology laboratory and look at any specimen that came in. I continued this practice with ophthalmologists, orthopedic surgeons, and cardiologists."

Visits to Other Medical Centers

Will and Charles Mayo made a practice of visiting medical centers in the United States and around the world to learn different surgical techniques and policies. One brother would travel while the other maintained the practice. This arrangement was highly successful for the Mayos, who soon developed a leading medical center that attracted, and welcomed, visiting physicians from all over the world.[8]

Today many physicians, especially surgeons, visit medical centers regularly. Occasionally, Frederick Ludwig will visit a medical center with a patient he is referring. Frederick O'Dell, who practices in a small community, takes off a week or two every two years to go to Ann Arbor, to Boston, or to Houston, where he observes in the operating room, talks to the residents, and makes rounds with surgeons. "You can get a lot of useful hints from residents and junior members of the faculty. Not only is the experience enlightening, but it also allows me to form close relationships with many people."

Gustavo Kuster also finds traveling beneficial. "I try to spend one or two weeks every couple of years in centers outside my immediate area—the Midwest or Europe. The instruments and techniques used are considerably different." Additionally, in learning a new surgical technique, he has found it useful to invite a guest surgeon to assist him when he cannot master the technique simply by reading.

A more formal visit may be desired by some physicians. "Unless a physician is in a teaching institution," explained David Sabiston, "he may continue to practice about the same kind of medicine as when he finished his residency. We have mini-residencies at Duke for graduates from outlying areas who can spend two weeks or longer making daily rounds with a particular specialist. These are much better than courses because they allow participation in actual practice, where there is give and take and not just presentations with a stiff question-and-answer period."

Some medical centers are better equipped to receive visitors than others. To avoid inconvenience and disappointment, a prospective physician should have specific goals in mind and make arrangements well in advance of the visit.

Recreational Sites

Fred Turrill likes not only to work with colleagues but to play with them—at golf, tennis, fishing, or hunting—and finds that such relaxation with colleagues is a pleasant way to learn. "Not only do you get to know your colleagues better, but you also learn from the medical discussions."

"Perhaps the greatest learning method of all," according to Desmond Julian, "is to be sharing a ski lift with a distinguished colleague who can pass on his expertise to you. He is trapped with you, he is probably in a very good mood, he is preparing for the onslaughts of the ski slopes, and he is prepared to speak to you very honestly about what he does. One of the problems about many formal presentations is that we speak in generalities and not about specific problems we encounter or about our shortcomings. We miss physical signs; we misinterpret investigations. Until you talk to someone very frankly, as you can on a ski lift, you really don't find the truth."

Learning from Other Health Professionals

A mutually beneficial collegial relationship can also be developed with other members of the health team. Brian Goodell advocates having office staff involved in its own and the physician's continuing education: "If it is a small office staff, you can assign tasks for the collection of relevant information. If someone in our office has read a particularly good article, he will have it copied, distribute it to everyone else who might be interested, and then label and file it for everyone's future reference. Nurses are particularly important resources for this purpose." Desmond Julian thinks he has probably learned more about his patients and practical nursing problems from informal discussions with nurses and other health personnel at coffee and lunch than from the formal sessions.

Joseph Gonnella regrets that physicians do not take full advantage of pharmacists' knowledge: "We still visualize that profession to be the old-time druggist, but in many hospitals there is someone who knows the side effects of drugs better than the doctors, and that is the clinical pharmacist. Some of us, in fact, have graduate students in pharmacy making rounds with us. The director of our pharmacy is a good friend, and since I know he is interested in evaluation of drugs, he and I are always asking each other questions."

*****

This section has highlighted informal learning methods that physicians use each day. These methods may seem self-evident and unsophisticated, but they exemplify the multitude of possibilities available to physicians to profit from the experience of others, to weave education into social and recreational events, and to organize and test thoughts on medical problems. The collegial network in medicine is real and extremely active. It is one of the dividends of being a physician and, if nurtured, will enhance not only the physician's knowledge, but his enjoyment of practice.

References

1. Edelstein, Ludwig. The Hippocratic oath: Text, translation and interpretation. *Bull Hist Med* 1943;(Suppl 1):3.
2. Manning, Phil R.; Denson, Teri A. How cardiologists learn about echocardiography. *Ann Intern Med* Sep 1979;91(3):469-471.
3. Manning, Phil R.; Denson, Teri A. How internists learned about cimetidine. *Ann Intern Med* May 1980;92(5):690-692.
4. Stross, Jeoffrey K.; Harlan, William R. Dissemination of relevant information on hypertension. *JAMA* 24/31 Jul 1981;246(4):360-362.
5. Stross, Jeoffrey K.; Harlan, William R. The dissemination of new medical information. *JAMA* 15 Jun 1979;241(24):2622-2624.
6. Franklin, Benjamin. In: Farrand, Max, ed. *Benjamin Franklin's Memoirs*. Berkeley and Los Angeles: University of California Press, 1949:152.
7. Colville, John. *Winston Churchill and His Inner Circle*. New York: Wyndham Books, 1981.
8. Clapesattle, Helen. *The Doctors Mayo*. Minneapolis: University of Minnesota Press, 1941.

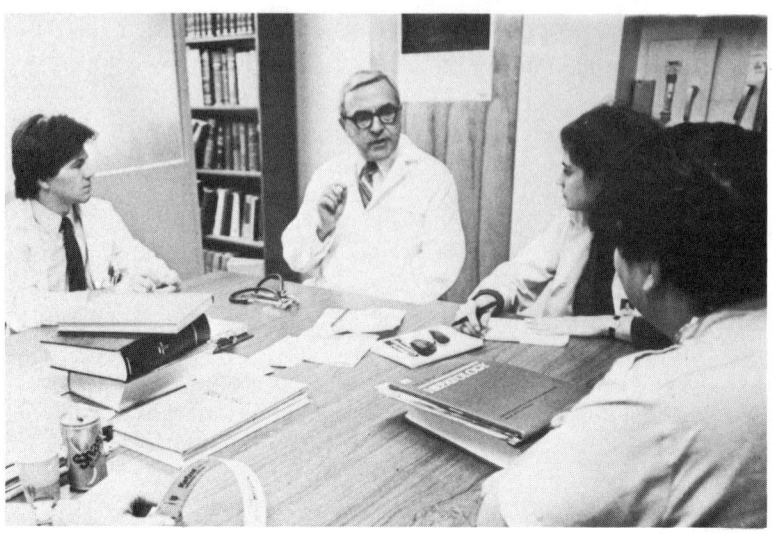

It is useful for doctors to have little groups that provide someone near at hand with whom to exchange ideas and discuss patients or published articles.
Sherman M. Mellinkoff, M.D. (third from right)

The remarkable march toward excellence of the UCLA School of Medicine is in no small measure due to Dr. Mellinkoff's wise and persistent guidance during his deanship since 1962. His outstanding contributions in the fields of medical education and gastroenterology have brought him recognition in the United States and in Europe. Among his awards are an Honorary Doctor of Humane Letters from Bowman Gray School of Medicine; the Ad Astra Award, University of Louisville; Physician of the Year Award, University of California; Abraham Flexner Award, Association of American Medical Colleges; and UCLA Honorary Alumnus Award. Dr. Mellinkoff's contributions to medical literature in gastroenterology and medical education, including publication of several books, have been numerous.

Sherman Mellinkoff is a clinical mentor who never preached. I shall never forget ward rounds as an intern while he was Chief Resident on the Osler Medical Service at Johns Hopkins. Never hurried, Sherm had two important priorities—the patients and the house staff. When a patient question arose, he always examined the patient himself and later shared new clinical insights with us in his gentle, wise way. His manner was invariably good-humored. We especially looked forward to his evening visits, when he became not only an able consultant but a special friend who inspired us to prove worthy of our patients' trust. A caring physician, a wise academic leader, and a trusted friend for many faculty, students, and patients, he gave generously of himself to his family, his profession, and his colleagues. By example, he demonstrated the science and art of medicine as well as the best of personal human qualities.
Carol Johnson Johns, M.D.

Personal Essay

Sherman M. Mellinkoff, M.D.
Former Dean
University of California, Los Angeles
School of Medicine
Los Angeles, California

Continuing learning in medicine is an individual matter. The human mind is so complex that there are many different ways to approach this subject. Most important is the maintenance of curiosity about patients. I like patients and am intrigued by their problems, so medical practice has both an emotional as well as an intellectual attraction for me. I try to look at each patient independently, unprejudiced by other people's opinions. A physician learns more if, when examining a patient, he is unprejudiced by someone else's opinion and takes a history as though this were a fresh, new problem, then seeks information on the basis of questions that arise in his mind from direct observation of the patient. Often, medical students think that they are not going to succeed unless they look at the writeup in the chart by someone else and then determine from it what they should record in the chart or what they should say to the attending physician. If the student can remember that it is much better to be in doubt than to be in error, he will continue to learn.

I have a yearning for knowledge. That desire began before I knew that I wanted to be a physician. It has been traditional in our family to ask questions and to try to get honest answers, but also to admit that we "do not know," the three most difficult consecutive words to traverse the human larynx. That admission, I think, is essential for continued learning. As I remember, this belief was strongly fortified by a teacher to whom I am grateful, the late George DeForest Barnett, who taught physical diagnosis at Stanford. A great man in my view. He did not publish a lot, but he was an inspiring bedside teacher. He somehow inspired everyone who was fortunate enough to be exposed to him.

Another person to whom I am indebted is Dr. Arthur Bloomfield, a profound scholar who always began a discussion of a patient, after the diagnosis was firmly decided, with the history of that disease. That is a good idea, because understanding what people knew about a disease in the past and how the present state of our ignorance or enlightenment was reached is helpful. A great teacher of mine who is also a distinguished medical historian as well as a master of differential diagnosis is A. McGehee Harvey of Johns Hopkins. He inspired one's best effort to be thoughtful and thorough in every clinical problem and to comprehend its historical and physiological implications.

The third person from whom I learned a great deal is one of the greatest bedside physicians I have ever known, Phillip Tumulty, who is also at Johns Hopkins. I have never known anyone who more completely wins a patient's confidence. He inspires confidence because he loves his patients, and they sense it. Confidence is a tremendous asset, not only in caring for the patient, but also in obtaining a history. If a patient is fearful and defensive about his answers, if he thinks he is being cross-examined rather than being given an opportunity to state his complaints and concerns, the history will not be as accurate. That is the recognition that Phil Tumulty brought to me.

I have had a long, close relationship with the gastroenterologists around here, especially the late Mort Grossman. He was a veritable gold mine not only of information, but also of wise interpretations of new developments. In fact, Mort had a little program that I have found immensely helpful. He and some of his staff discussed major topics covered annually at the American Gastroenterological Association meetings. Anyone in Southern California who was interested could attend. The topics were reviewed thoroughly, with opportunities for questions from the floor.

When Mark Ravitch and I were once seeing a patient with jaundice, he told me a story about William Thayer's collar button. Dean Lewis, who was described as the poor man's Halstead, had taken Dr. Halstead's place. Lewis was a good surgeon, but down-to-earth and not particularly eloquent. Dr. Thayer, who had taken Osler's place, was a Boston Brahman, and there was an imperious relation between him and Lewis. One Sunday, Thayer telephoned Lewis to say that he was sending his laundress into the Johns Hopkins Hospital for an appendectomy and asked Lewis to see to it. Dr. Lewis agreed to do so. Some time later, Thayer was in the amphitheater and, to his consternation, he observed Lewis operating in the right upper abdominal quadrant. He asked, "What are you doing?" Lewis answered, "I'm taking out her gallbladder; she has acute cholecystitis." Later, Dr. Thayer asked him, "How did you dare operate in the right upper abdominal quadrant when I told you that the patient had appendicitis?" Dr. Lewis replied: "Well, I asked the patient what she was doing when her pains started. She said 'I was putting a collar button on one of Dr. Thayer's shirts.' " The point is that when a pain is really sudden, as it is with a gallstone getting lodged somewhere, the patient remembers exactly what is going on at that time. But if the pain sneaks up on you, as it does with appendicitis, no such precise answer will be forthcoming.

This is a point I also learned from Phil Tumulty: do not be overly precise. There are times to ask specific questions such as "What were you doing when the pain started?" but there are other times when it is best just to let the patient ramble, and although it may appear that it is a waste of time, it sometimes elicits information that would not come out by direct questioning.

I like biographies of great physicians. I have enjoyed, tremendously, the series that Mac Harvey has been writing about the greats at Johns Hopkins. I have learned more from this kind of reading than from articles on education alone.

I read articles in connection with the patients I have seen or heard about, and that makes what I read come to life for me. Similarly, when I am puzzled (and that is often), I like to discuss individual patients, articles I have read, or ideas with colleagues who are more familiar with the subjects than I am. I test new ideas in the same way.

In consultations, it is best to rely on what Dryden called the "plain style," that is, clear, precise, trenchant English. But we cannot all expect to be Drydens. It is sometimes more helpful, therefore, to obtain the consultation through conversation. One of the worst wastes is to send a patient with lupus erythematosus to the radiology department with the request merely for a chest x-ray or, worse yet, an x-ray of some bone. The radiologist ought to know what the patient's problem is and what question is being asked about that patient.

I have a file at home of landmark reprints to which I refer often. I review my reprint files every once in a while and am amused sometimes that an article that I once thought was important may no longer seem so. At other times I am refreshed and amazed at how classical a particular paper has turned out to be. My file is extremely simple. I use a filing cabinet and manila folders, and classify the material primarily by topic. If I want to look up portal hypertension, for example, I look under "P." Some articles I file by authors' names.

6

Learning from Formal Consultations

> When thou arte callde at anye time,
> A patient to see;
> And doste perceave the cure to greate,
> And ponderous for thee: . . .
> Gette one or two of experte men,
> To helpe thee in that nede;
> And make them partakers wyth thee,
> In that worke to procede.
> *John Halle, 1565*[1]

"Consultation, coupled with a brief review of the literature on the specific subject, benefits the patient, the referring physician, and the consultant," said Paul Wehrle. "Information is always better retained when associated with specific problems." Consultations also promote interaction among colleagues—the basis for much continuing education in medicine. When a consultation is indicated, it is, of course, necessary for the physician to discuss its purpose with the patient beforehand.

Reasons for the Consultation

Conventionally, the referring physician requests a consultation because he needs assistance in diagnosis or treatment or because the patient requires a special procedure, such as liver biopsy. Occasionally, he seeks a second opinion because the patient or the family is unduly anxious or apprehensive. By determining the precise purpose of the consultation before requesting it, the referring physician can expand his own knowledge and save valuable time.

Requesting the Consultation

Seeking Consultation

George Thorn warned against two extremes in consultations: "At one extreme is the physician who balks at a consultation, as though his own knowledge were being challenged. Patients appreciate the physician who seeks another opinion even when he thinks he knows the answer. Every good clinician realizes this, but some, particularly young physicians, may feel that they are expected to know all the answers. At the other extreme is the physician who gives up too easily, hardly ever solving a problem alone and complicating the situation by involving too many others."

Profiting Most from a Consultation

FIRST STUDY THE PROBLEM YOURSELF. When the referring physician and consultant have a common specialty, the referring physician will usually study the case thoroughly before requesting the consultation. When, however, the consultation is outside the referring physician's specialty, as, for example, when an orthopedist seeks advice from an otolaryngologist, the referring physician may not do a comprehensive study of the condition and may not therefore learn as much as he could for application to future patients, especially since the consultant often proceeds with the patient's treatment.

To obtain the most from a consultation in your field of interest, first look up the subject in a standard textbook or in your personal library file. That information will help reduce the scope of the consultation to a few specific questions. Delineation of the problem by one or more explicit questions and a brief review of an authoritative publication on the subject can, in fact, sometimes clarify the problem enough to make a consultation unnecessary.

SUMMARIZE THE RECORDS. All data, including patient records, roentgenograms, and laboratory reports, should be summarized and made accessible to the consultant. While summarizing his data, James Dooley assesses his own performance with the patient, whom he may have observed for ten to twenty years, by carefully reviewing all the clinical material accumulated during this time, including his notes.

When the patient is to be seen in the consultant's office, the referring physician may summarize the clinical information in a letter. For hospitalized patients, the summarizing note is made on the chart. Preparation of either summary, when preceded by a careful review, is educational for the referring physician. Regardless of the type of summary used, it is helpful for the referring physician and consultant to discuss the problem in person or by telephone before the consultation.

6. Learning from Formal Consultations

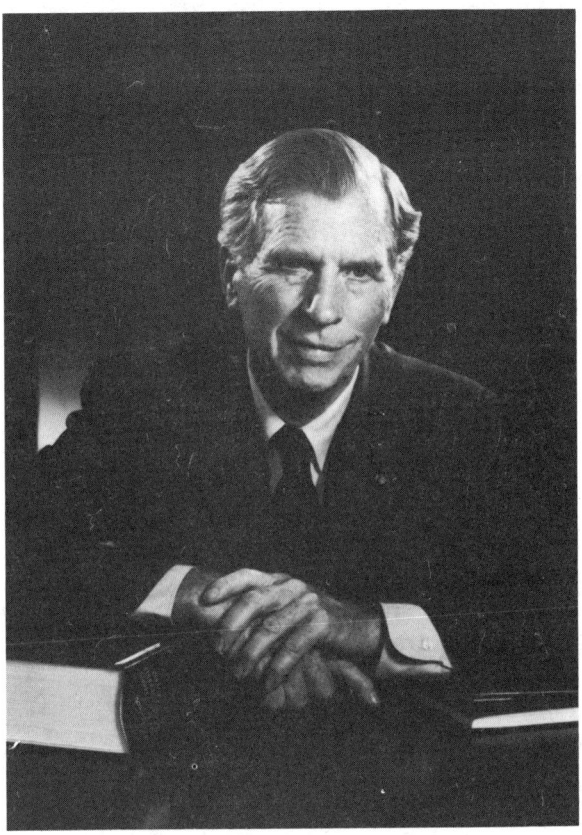

Patients appreciate the physician who seeks another opinion even when he thinks he knows the answer.

George W. Thorn, M.D.
Chairman, Board of Trustees
Howard Hughes Medical Institute

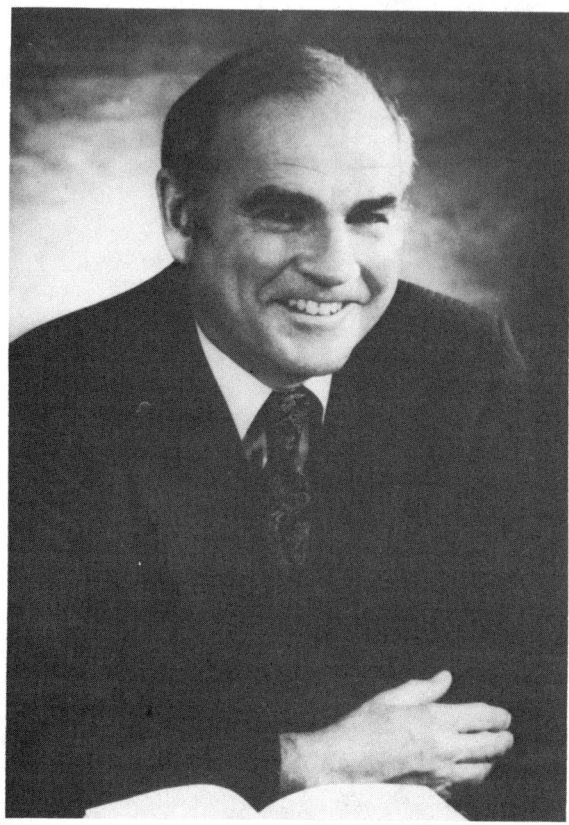

In research, and probably also in practice, maintaining and fostering curiosity— the ability to ask questions each time a new phenomenon occurs —is indispensable.

Baruch S. Blumberg, M.D.
Associate Director for Clinical Research
Fox Chase Cancer Center

6. Learning from Formal Consultations

ASK SPECIFIC QUESTIONS. William Parmley deplores the vagueness of many consultation requests and stresses the importance of informing the consultant of the explicit purpose of the request. The more specific the questions, the more the patient and the referring physician will profit from the consultation.

Example:

This 23-year-old woman with rheumatoid arthritis continues to have significant symptoms while taking 3 aspirin tablets four times a day. A dosage of 14 tablets per day produces tinnitus. Should treatment be changed? Are nonsteroidal anti-inflammatory agents indicated? Should we go directly to gold?

Ask the consultant for a listing of the phenomena that should be monitored.

Example:

What signs, symptoms, and laboratory tests should be monitored and at what intervals? For example, joint symptoms, swelling, fever, and sedimentation rate.

The consultant may also be asked to identify the criteria (signs, symptoms, and laboratory tests) that will require additional consultations.

Warren Williams tests the specificity of his questions by writing his own responses to his consultation requests, outlining diagnostic and therapeutic plans. He then compares his plans with those of the consultant, and they discuss any differences. Consultations thus become a personal and active educational tool.

When R. D. Richards was a young faculty member, he saw a certain patient and decided what he thought should be done. He then asked a senior faculty member to look at the patient and give his recommendation. "To my surprise," said Dr. Richards, "he recommended something quite different from my approach, although I still felt my approach was preferable. At that time, I realized that I had not communicated properly with him, and should have specifically stated what I wished to know. Since then, I have never asked for a consultation unless I really wanted it and have always specified precisely what I wished the consultant to do."

Who Is Present during the Consultation?

Some referring physicians like to be present during the consultation. "I call the consultant," said Edward Shapiro, "outline the problem, and make a date to meet with him at the bedside. I watch him examine the patient, I supply additional information if needed, and I interrogate the consultant. In this way, I learn a great deal. One consultant said I cross-examined him, and I don't deny the accusation." Aaron Feder will not perform a consultation unless the referring physician is there, and will not make such a request himself unless he is present to hear what the consultant has to say.

Most physicians think, however, that the consultant does better without the presence and influence of the referring physician, which may interfere with the consultant's establishing rapport with the patient or may inhibit the patient's responses. Most consultants prefer to have time to organize their thoughts without feeling that they are "on stage."

Providing the Consultation

"A physician conducts a patient consultation under two different circumstances," said Walter Somerville. "In the teaching hospital, he may be attended by junior staff and students eager to learn and imitate, and by hand-picked senior residents and fellows, critical and watchful for a false move or clinical slip. With such continuous audit, the physician is in the ideal environment to bring out the best in himself as teacher and physician.

"The procedure is different when the physician is alone in his office or in a nonteaching hospital face-to-face with his patient. Two techniques are beneficial to the patient and invaluable to the isolated physician. The first is *patient transposition*, in which the patient's thoughts and feelings can be described thus: 'I am sensitive and terrified. I am overawed by the doctor, silent and pompous or unkempt in open sweat-shirt, writing down my anxieties, intimate disclosures, and sexual indiscretions, to be read by goodness knows whom? And that tape recorder? No wonder I feel like running away, screaming, from this horrible experience.' Imagining this scenario from the patient's point of view goes a long way toward creating the proper environment for easy doctor-patient communication.

"The second technique is the *invisible audit*. I surround myself with an imaginary audit-jury, drawn from the most constructive critics in my experience. Closest to me, breathing down my neck is Paul Wood, then Sam Levine, and beside him my most stringent critic, my wife, Jane, whispering emphatically what I'm doing wrong. With my pomposity deflated, affectations minimized, and extempore guesswork challenged, I'm ever aware of my watchful friends. And the patient gets the best service I can give," concludes Somerville.

The Consultant as a Learner

Paul Harvey cited another advantage of consultations: "The consultant has the chance to examine a patient and think over a clinical problem without doing the basic work and with most of the tests completed. This

6. Learning from Formal Consultations

review of the work of others is a unique opportunity to see how others approach problems."

The questions asked by the referring physician may offer a useful perspective. The request may stimulate the consultant to review a recent specialty textbook or personal library file or even do medical library research. If the specific reason for the consultation is not clear, the consultant should ask the referring physician for further information.

Teaching What Not to Order

To promote cost-containment, the consultant should point out unnecessary studies that were ordered before he came on the scene, even though such disclosures may be ticklish. In Desmond Julian's opinion, "Consultants don't do enough teaching about when certain tests are *not* needed. Every time you order a test, even an electrocardiogram or roentgenogram, let alone an invasive procedure, you should ask yourself if the information will improve the care of that particular patient. The consultant can often diplomatically point out the limitations of some laboratory work that is ordered."

The Consultant's Report

On completion of his evaluation, the consultant will write a letter from his office or make a consultation report on the hospital chart. Restricting the length of the report forces the consultant to summarize and communicate better. Writing succinctly also reinforces retention. Within twenty-four hours of the consultation, the consultant should call the referring physician.

Daniel Stone pointed to the instructional value of consultations: "The teaching in my consultation is largely through the letters I write afterwards, in which I review my thinking with the referring physician. I also cite references, and if the physician does not have access to a good medical library, I photocopy relevant articles and append them to the letter."

The inclusion of references must be handled delicately, since some referring physicians may consider such citations to be condescending. On the other hand, many physicians turn to consultants who are known to be outstanding teachers and who often provide useful references in diagnostic workups and treatment.

"The report sent from the consultant to the referring physician upon discharge of the patient," in Desmond Julian's opinion, "doesn't convey much to the referring physician if the diagnosis or treatment is buried among a mass of data representing the results of tests that he does not understand. I recommend a brief letter, which outlines the diagnosis, the basis for the diagnosis, the treatment selected and its rationale, or, in a complicated case, a more detailed letter further explaining these points." Even the most effective letter does not eliminate the need for a personal discussion after the consultation, whether face-to-face or by telephone.

Discussing the Consultation

Almost all referring physicians arrange for a personal meeting or a telephone conversation with the consultant afterwards to discuss details or to ask further questions. Sherman Mellinkoff cautioned: "Physicians sometimes forget the value of conversation. We habitually write notes to consultants in the chart, which is fine—it was prescribed by Hippocrates and remains a good idea today—but I don't think you learn as much or help the patient as much if you rely exclusively on notes in the chart by the attending physician, consultant, or others caring for the patient. If something important develops regarding the patient, it is a good idea to discuss it directly with the consultant. Then both the consultant and referring physician will understand the problem better."

Reporting to the Patient

"The patient often has high expectations of the consultation, and although the consultant may try to withdraw and say he will discuss the case with the patient's doctor, the patient usually wants to hear the consultant's opinion directly," as Ian Mackay pointed out. "Consultants should be given an opportunity to express an opinion and perhaps offer a little reassurance to the patient, but this is a delicate issue in the referring physician-consultant relationship."

Desmond Julian added: "The consultant and referring physician should see the patient together after the consultation. It's remarkable how often patients see as major discrepancies the minimal differences in what two physicians tell them. If, for example, I recommend a 1,000-calorie diet and another physician recommends 800 calories, the patient may think, 'These doctors can't agree.' Joint decisions are desirable regarding matters that may seem inconsequential to us but very important to the patient."

The Follow-up

The formal consultation should not end with the consultant's written or verbal communication. When the referring physician remains responsible for the patient's primary care, he should keep the consulting physician posted on the patient's progress. Follow-up telephone calls to review the case or clarify points benefit the patient as well as the referring physician and consultant.

"Whether the consultant should see the patient *again* is," in Ian Mackay's words, "often a touchy matter in hospital practice when a good relationship develops between the consultant and the patient." If the consultant considers it advisable for him to see the patient again, he should so indicate and thus avoid disturbing the referring physician-consultant relationship.

The Ideal Consultation

To learn the most and ensure the best advice for the patient, the referring physician should delineate the precise reasons for requesting a consultation. Unless the problem is in a totally different specialty, he should read about the subject in a current textbook, collect all existing data on the patient, summarize the records in a letter or a note on the hospital chart, and formulate specific questions for the consultant.

"In the ideal consultation, the referring physician is present on my arrival, describes the problem he wishes to consult me about, and introduces me to the patient," said Desmond Julian. "That's important because it shows a collaboration of colleagues rather than a physician giving up and having to pass the problem to someone else. After he introduces me to the patient, he leaves while I talk to the patient privately. In this way, the patient is not fearful of telling a different story to one physician from that told to another or of contradicting himself. I take the history and do the physical examination myself. Then I meet the referring physician again and discuss the problem with him. Sometimes something emerges that requires action or further elucidation, or some contradiction in the story may need to be resolved. I like to go back to the patient with the referring physician and explain our joint opinion about diagnosis or treatment."

Even when the patient's problem is discussed in person or by telephone, it is still necessary to write a letter or consultation report. The consultant's report should be clear and concise, providing specific advice on diagnostic and therapeutic plans, along with the rationale on which that advice is based. If the consultant is not to follow the patient himself, he should be notified when significant changes occur. Each of these steps offers opportunites for active participation and enlightenment.

Reference

1. Halle, John: *An Historiall Expostulation: Against the beastlye Abusers, bothe of Chyrurgerie, and Physyke, in oure tyme: with a goodlye Doctrine and Instruction, necessarye to be marked and folowed, of all true Chirurgiens.* London: Thomas Marshe, 1565. Edited by TJ Pettigrew. London: The Percy Society, 1844:31, 32.

7

Formal Courses and Conferences

> [Lectures] are a temptation to the more contemplative mind to learn diseases by the study of models, rather than of the things themselves. They tend to divorce him from the workshop and the chips and fragments and rude designs that lie about within it, and introduce him into a room swept and garnished and hung round with masterpieces for his contemplation. This may be all very well for gentlemen who patronise the arts; but this is not the way to make the artist.
>
> *Peter Mere Latham*[1]

Formal courses and conferences are the second most popular method of continuing medical education, after reading.[2-4] Numerous studies have shown that physicians learn facts from such formal instruction.[5,6] Courses that focus on physician performance in specific clinical situations, however, can not only transfer facts but can also alter that performance, even though such changes are difficult to measure.

Critics have focused on the limitations of courses and conferences. Since they are memory-based, knowledge so acquired may not be used for weeks or months in the care of patients and may therefore be forgotten. The educational needs of physicians may also vary widely, and yet courses and conferences, which are group enterprises, emphasize common needs, not individual needs. Jesse Rising, who spent decades organizing courses, said: "After retiring as the Associate Dean of Continuing Education, I became a volunteer in the Department of Family Practice at the University of Kansas Medical School, where I have been learning general medicine again for the past two years. From that experience I am convinced that the critical factor in CME is to take care of patients. Courses are interesting, but learning comes from studying patients."

To Claude Organ conferences are often simply dull. "To inspire the participants, the course director must create a spirit of learning. This sounds trite, I know, and it is easier said than done."

Despite their limitations, formal courses and conferences can keep physicians aware of current knowledge and new developments, can broaden understanding, and can put the practicing physician in touch with experts and peers. Physicians who gain the most from courses are able to relate course material to their own clinical experience. The fact that these gains are difficult to measure after standard courses or conferences does not vitiate such instruction in a comprehensive lifelong educational program.

Reasons for Attending Formal Courses and Conferences

Physicians are motivated to attend formal courses and conferences by both inner standards and extrinsic forces, such as peer pressure and licensing regulations.[7-12] The motivations varied slightly in different studies conducted, depending on the phrasing of questions, but can be grouped into several broad categories. Physicians frequently cited as motivating factors the opportunity to review and increase medical knowledge by becoming more aware of the general state-of-the-art (with the assumption that the knowledge will make the physician more competent), and by acquiring information pertinent to specific patient problems. Physicians also use courses for self-assessment, to compare their knowledge to that of experts in the field and to compare their work to accepted standards of practice. Continuing medical education is also seen as an integral part of professionalism by society and the medical community. Professionals are expected to sharpen their knowledge and skills continually. A change of pace from practice and contact with colleagues and faculty are also cited as motivations to attend courses.

Expected Benefits

For Patrick Storey the single most important benefit of attending a conference or CME short-course is a recognition of what the registrant does not know and what he cannot do. As Oliver Wendell Holmes bluntly stated, "The best part of our knowledge is that which teaches us where knowledge leaves off and ignorance begins. Nothing more clearly separates a vulgar from a superior mind, than the confusion in the first between the little that it truly knows, on the one hand, and what it half knows and what it thinks it knows on the other."[13]

Reinforcement of the physician's past knowledge is more valuable to Richard Caplan than the slight new information he may acquire. "Nor must we forget the attitudinal advantages—the re-ignition of lagging fires, the recharging of batteries, the renewal of excitement. Further, a course or conference allows us to place ourselves in the fertile mode of an active learner, free from daily professional responsibilities and interruptions."

7. Formal Courses and Conferences

Even if a physician's knowledge is up-to-date, as Jack Lein said, "attending a course will reinforce the assurance that he is doing his best."

For George Race, the ripple effect is the primary benefit from formal courses. "When the physician hears something new, his interest is piqued, and he will then consult journals, books, or experts on the subject to learn more about it. Furthermore, the contacts that participants make with a course faculty often allow them to identify consultants with whom they can establish ready communication."

"A continuing education course is a wonderful, legitimate excuse to leave the responsibilities for children, spouse, and patient care behind," said Karin Jamison. "The setting is usually some lovely hotel in a different environment. It is fun to meet people from all over the country and share experiences, joys, and problems, and to discover that what is difficult for one may be difficult for all. Such recognition gives a sense of relief. Even though the meetings are intense, they are still a restful experience. It is an unusual opportunity to laugh at oneself with trusted others who understand. Lastly, for the women, it is a wonderful opportunity to shop without having to get back home or to the office. On a more serious note, it is very gratifying to take back home some information that is helpful to one or more patients."

Registrants in courses given by the University of Southern California voiced views of expected benefits similar to those in published studies. Several of those views cited here illustrate the expectations physicians surveyed place on postgraduate courses and the benefits they derive from them:

"It is regenerating to be away from any distractions at home and thus be able to concentrate on the course. I expect to feel more stimulation from the renewal of academic knowledge and to gain more clinical confidence." (Peter Best)

"I want to update my concept of patient care and reassure myself that I am maintaining a high standard of medical practice." (Gerard Farinola)

"Courses give me an opportunity to coordinate the material I read in the literature, and to hear directly from the people in the forefront of their specialties." (Unsigned)

"I expect to get the most advanced knowledge in the field from the course, since I can find the day-to-day knowledge and information in textbooks." (Ragheb Sawires)

"Courses make reading more meaningful, placing the importance of the material in better perspective. Often the writer of an article has spent much of his life doing research on a particular subject and is therefore somewhat biased about the significance of his work." (Wenzel A. Leff)

"I compare what I hear at the course with what is currently in the literature. I expect to come away with a summary of what is new on a subject that will be clinically useful to me." (Daniel Hoffman)

"I want to learn how medicine is practiced in different places and review important developments that I may have missed or do not have in proper perspective." (Unsigned)

"I get the opportunity to compare my method of practice to what is taught in the university hospitals." (Rokay Kamyar)

"I want to increase my medical knowledge and demonstrate to myself how much I don't know, as a stimulus to read." (G.E. Wiebe)

"Courses offer a more provocative approach than sitting at home and reading." (P. B. Jorgensen)

"Attending courses permits me to dilute parochialism a bit—to get views on medical subjects other than those prevalent in my locale." (Donald Jacobs)

Selecting a Course or Conference

Content

In deciding whether to take a particular course, Donald Petit suggested that physicians ask themselves: "Do I want a board review? Do I want to find out what's new on a given subject? Do I want to learn something because I think it might be good for me, for example, basic science for clinicians? Courses or conferences for physicians should have a clear statement of content so that the physician will know in advance what he can expect." More specifically, Edward Rubenstein advised that "The scale and the level should be explicitly stated. For instance, does the program deal in depth with a subject, or does it consist of a number of compressed sessions highlighting the most important or most timely points? Does it emphasize basic science or does it focus on practical clinical matters? Is it intended for specialists or subspecialists or physicians with other primary interests?"

Lawrence Highman chooses courses that provide current information on problems that arise in practice at his small rural hospital. "I want to find out what changes I can make or what equipment is needed to improve my care of my patients." It is, of course, the physician's responsibility to determine whether the content will make a difference in his practice. Richard Caplan suspects that most physicians "respond with a somewhat more visceral than intellectual awareness of what they need. Furthermore, the present methods used by educators to demonstrate needs leave much to be desired. Who is to say that 'visceral wisdom' is not a reasonably good measure of what we need to learn?"

Faculty and Sponsor

The reputation of the sponsoring institution/organization is a fairly reliable index of the competence of the faculty and the value of a medical education conference. "An outstanding course," in Donald Petit's opinion, "depends first on the quality of the faculty—its ability to impart knowledge, its enthusiasm, and its style. Does the faculty stimulate me to learn? Is the experience really enjoyable?"

Course Design

A program that promotes active participation is most beneficial, with ample opportunity for questions or concerns of the participating physicians through direct question-and-answer periods or discussion forums. Programs are enriched by multiple formats such as lectures, panel discussions, and problem-solving sessions. Informal periods at lunch and coffee breaks are useful for discussion among participants.

Facilities and Site

Are the chairs comfortable, and are the tables convenient for writing? Is the lighting good? Are the audiovisual facilities adequate? Is the temperature comfortable? These may seem like minor factors before one attends a conference, but once the sessions are under way, their absence can become a major detriment.

National or regional courses or conferences are held at medical schools, hospitals, hotels, convention centers, or at vacation sites, where programs are popular but controversial. "With tuition of $75 to $125 per day, air travel, and the trend of conducting courses in posh resort areas, not to mention the cost of maintaining the office and staff while the physician is away, cost is becoming a tremendous factor," noted Wenzel A. Leff.

On the other hand, a relaxed setting is important because it removes physicians from the tensions and distractions of practice and thus allows better concentration. A relaxed setting may also lower the barriers between faculty and participants and permit interaction to continue at the beach, poolside, or dinner table. Because a vacation setting is also pleasant for the faculty, it may attract superior teachers. In our view, a combined course and vacation will enhance educational activities rather than detract from them, provided that the sponsor plans a superior course that leaves no question that the prime purpose is learning. Recreational activities should be scheduled outside of course hours. Courses that appear to be simple tax dodges, with little or no educational value, are deplorable. That such courses exist does not argue against the superior programs set in vacation surroundings. Participants must be particularly alert in assessing the quality of the faculty and suitability of topics to ensure the legitimacy of the program and the applicability to their needs.

Fruitful and Worthless Courses

Some interviewees gave examples of fruitful as well as worthless courses. Cited most often as worthwhile were courses with information for practical clinical application, with opportunity for interaction with an outstanding faculty, and with emphasis on new information and skills rather than overviews. The most useful courses, in Robert Palmer's view, are those that apply directly to the physician's own practice, whereas the most worthless are those that suggest that the only proper care of patients is given in a large medical center or "Ivory Tower" setting. In J. Young's opinion, controversy and discussion are crucial components of a good course. "Passive didactic instruction does not really encourage intellectual growth. A great number of panel discussions are worthless, the 'professors' merely scratching one another's backs."

Ensuring Optimal Benefit

Preparing for a Course or Conference

When Frederick Ludwig goes to a meeting, he has a specific goal in mind. "A day or two in advance of the meeting, I will study what I am going to be dealing with. Then at the meeting, I take notes, and when I get home, I organize my thoughts and dictate a summary for my secretary to transcribe so that I have a record of it. Later I can go back and consult those notes." Donald Feinstein also reads the abstracts the night before. "I feel that it is extremely inefficient if I do not prepare." Trying to think in advance of something worthwhile to contribute makes Kenneth Berge much more attentive to the content.

Being Active during the Course

Most interviewees said that they take notes during the sessions, and some rewrite them the same evening to reinforce the concepts. Summarizing your notes while the presentation is still fresh in your mind gives "double-exposure" to important ideas. Some physicians try to corral the speaker after the presentation for further questions not answered during the sessions, or to discuss particular cases with other participants. A good course syllabus is a great help but, unfortunately, is rare.

Follow-up Study

After a course, some physicians summarize their notes or the provided syllabus and file the material under the appropriate heading in their files. New information can be condensed into a few basic statements, written on one sheet of paper, and reviewed periodically over the next few days. To disseminate new information, as well as help to retain it, the physician can dictate and distribute to interested colleagues a summary of the meeting. Also, a presentation based on the subject can be given to the hospital staff. Many physicians probe further into subjects that engage their interest or that they do not fully understand, looking for articles to compare, refute, or reinforce what was covered at a conference.

Daniel Bird uses his active learning participation in courses to improve patient understanding. "As an aid in patient education, I have typed short summaries of lectures I've attended and have placed them in a special corner of my waiting room or occasionally mailed them to certain patients. This has ensured the wide dissemination of accurate and timely medical information and strongly underlines the concern of the physician for the welfare of his patient. Patients take these sheets of information home, discuss them with family and friends, and thus introduce the doctor to many persons as one who both knows and cares."

Conferences Offered by Hospitals and Specialty Societies

The general principles discussed under formal courses and conferences are applicable to all such programs, although hospital conferences and annual sessions sponsored by specialty groups may present a different orientation than courses offered by medical schools.

Hospital Conferences

All hospitals have staff meetings, many have section or departmental meetings, and some have general educational meetings. Hospital conferences are convenient for physicians and can be designed to solve specific medical problems in the hospital. They also promote interaction with one's peers and may enhance the physician's visibility while improving cooperation among physicians, nurses, pharmacists, and other health professionals.

In place of medical grand rounds consisting only of a clinical lecture, Samuel Rapaport prefers a patient presentation to serve as the springboard for more generalized comments on mechanisms or treatment. Paul Beeson favors morbidity and mortality rounds, along with case reviews and medical pathology reviews. "These sessions permit physicians to review frankly what happened and where the treatment went wrong. Nothing sticks with you like a mistake. Having someone looking over your shoulder and saying 'No, it is not what you think it is, but it is this,' gives you a healthy humility. I have had just enough experience in private practice to know that no matter what you do, 90 per cent of your patients are going to get well, and unless someone points this out to you, you may begin to feel that what you are doing is responsible."

Hugh Lawrence also lauded the review of morbidity data, with open discussion of cases, followed by an audit. "The audit report suggests a plan of action, and a later audit indicates if there has been any progress.

I found, for example, when I came here about seven years ago, that several different bowel preparations were used by the twenty surgeons. We discussed this and found the infection rate in intestinal surgery to be about 18 per cent. We narrowed the protocols to four, and the infection rate dropped to 5.8 per cent. The new practice was presented at a morbidity and mortality conference, which led other surgeons to refine the protocol, with a further reduction in infection rate to 1.8 per cent. We found, however, that some surgeons were having a higher infection rate than this. At first we thought that the nurses were not carrying out the procedures, but an audit showed that certain doctors had not been writing orders satisfactorily."

Analysis of hospital patient care data can be used beyond conference planning, extending into direct conversation about quality assurance. If a physician is having a high complication rate for a given disorder, Hugh Lawrence will approach the physician privately. "I will not communicate with him by memorandum or letter, but will go to him personally, solicit his help with the problem, and ask him how he would approach it. I will pick the physician with the next worse complication rate and say, 'You are one of two people here who are having a problem, and I just wonder how we can eliminate it.' In this way, I encourage him to produce the action himself."

Death conferences and clinicopathologic conferences, which have been important educational tools in the past, have declined in popularity because they focus on exotic diseases and rare diagnoses. James Moss would like to see these conferences directed toward patients with avoidable deaths. Unfortunately, the litigious atmosphere today makes discussions of this kind very difficult.

Morbidity and mortality rounds can be inordinately dull, "a slow unfolding of the inevitable, ending with a pathology demonstration," according to Ian Mackay. "In addition, although an outcome may be unfavorable and the criticism severe, there may have been, in retrospect, no other course to follow or the course followed may not have been at all unreasonable at the time."

Francis Moore encourages the staffs of small hospitals to review their own experiences. "The average surgeon or internist or pediatrician probably does not analyze his practice data. The purpose of staff committees and staff review groups in small hospitals should be to encourage that kind of review of one's own work."

Desmond Julian advocates a switch from mortality to morbidity. "Whereas the postmortem room used to be the main learning area, with all the tests we have today on living patients, the biopsies and the radiologic investigations, we learn more from morbidity conferences than mortality conferences, that is, from what goes wrong in patients who survive."

Discussions of medical care in which the physician should have acted differently is essential, but some physicians may have a tendency to cover up their actions, as Paul Wehrle explained: "Facilitating discussions with

7. Formal Courses and Conferences

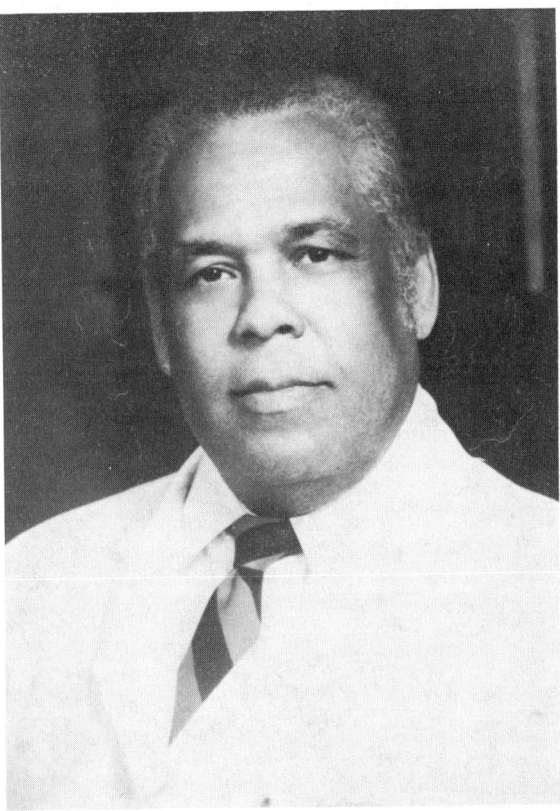

The half-life of a scientific knowledge is five to seven years, which makes learning a dynamic and perpetual process.

Claude H. Organ, Jr., M.D.
Professor of Surgery
The University of Oklahoma

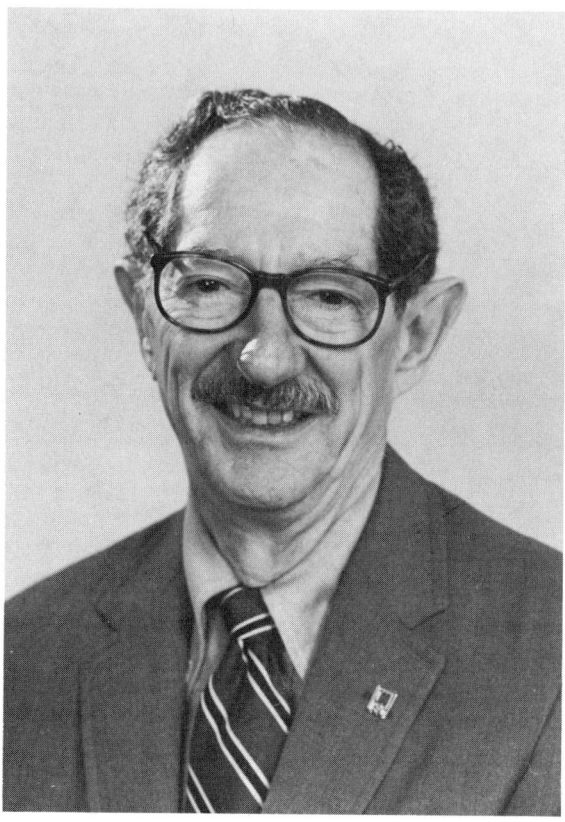

Formal education is too ritualistic. Self-directed learning is likely to be more flexible, more active, and more pragmatic.

Stephen Abrahamson, Ph.D.
Chairman, Department of Medical Education
University of Southern California

medical colleagues is an interesting art and requires a certain amount of understanding. Some practicing physicians in small rural private hospitals are unwilling to discuss candidly patients who have been mismanaged. Each staff member knows precisely which physician treated which patient and must use special tact to make constructive criticisms and suggest alternate diagnostic or therapeutic approaches. Unless the discussion leader is experienced and diplomatic, the atmosphere can become tense and painful for those responsible for the medical decisions under scrutiny." It is best to relate these meetings to educational activities, lest overly harsh punitive measures drive the staff underground.

Claude Organ considers the best hospital meetings to be those directed at deficiencies disclosed by a properly designed audit. He advises physicians to resist wasting time at hospital staff meetings on administrative and statistical reports that lead to no conclusions. The primary purpose, after all, is to improve patient care through education.

Annual Sessions

Annual sessions of specialty and state societies and associations can provide excellent opportunities for learning and reviewing the state of knowledge. As in any other educational event, preparation and participation make attendance more productive.

ADVANTAGES. Programs sponsored by a subspecialty society, which usually give an in-depth view of the latest research and clinical information, differ from the formal course given by a medical school, which is often a review of a topic. The formal course or conference generally entails broad coverage, whereas annual sessions often spotlight recognized authorities on given subjects.

Because of its many concurrent sessions, an annual meeting may have a wider appeal than a three- or four-day postgraduate course, and may provide better opportunities for division of groups by special interest. Unlike most postgraduate courses, it usually also has commercial and scientific exhibits, which may include teaching media, such as computer-based or audiovisual programs. The commercial exhibits usually orient the practitioner to new drugs and devices.

Discussions with fellow physicians from different areas of the country are enlightening. As William Davis has found, "You learn as much or more in the halls between papers as you do from listening to the presentations." The "Meet the Professor" sessions with informal discussion of clinical problems provide divergent views.

LIMITATIONS. Not only do annual out-of-town sessions require a protracted absence from one's practice, but large meetings do not always offer the best opportunities for fellowship and may be dominated by political rather than professional issues. The large audience can also be an obstacle to learning, with less opportunity for face-to-face interchanges.

There may also be housing problems, and less choice of scheduling. On the other hand, the physician can choose the month and general location he wishes for a postgraduate course.

Of little value are prolonged discussions of rare diseases and syndromes that few physicians will ever see, as well as presentations of new diagnostic procedures or therapeutic measures that have not been studied adequately and that may subsequently prove to be of no benefit. For Marsha Wallace, it is a mistake to design information for everyone from country doctors to those in urban centers, each with vastly different needs. "By the time basics are rehashed, there is often little time left for what is new."

Sabbatical Leaves

Lilia F. Nikolaeva of Moscow described a program that has been successful in the Soviet Union and that is obviously more detailed than the short refresher courses and annual sessions in the United States: "Every three to five years, physicians may attend various institutes for several weeks. During this time participants are granted leave from their practice and are provided lodging in addition to their regular salaries. Located in the larger cities, the institutes have become especially attractive to rural practitioners as an opportunity to keep up with new developments in medicine and to obtain cultural enrichment."

*****

Courses and conferences are traditional and remain popular. When most physicians think of continuing education, they think of a classroom presentation. Courses and conferences may define to the physician directions for further study, reinforce past knowledge, acquaint the physician with experts in the field, provide opportunities for informal discussions with peers, as well as teach new facts and developments. Such group teaching and learning help keep the profession aware of the current state of knowledge and of contemporary standards, but cannot provide all the detail a physician needs to conduct his daily practice. Courses are therefore no substitute for reading or for colleague consultations on specific problems. Physicians who have developed methods for reviewing their practice according to problems seen, drugs prescribed, and studies ordered may profit most from courses and conferences because they can compare their experience and performance with those of the instructors.

References

1. Latham, Peter Mere. A Word or Two on Medical Education. In: Martin, Robert, ed. *The Collected Works of Dr. P. M. Latham.* London: The New Sydenham Society, 1878:562.

7. Formal Courses and Conferences

2. Manning, Phil R.; Denson, Teri A. How cardiologists learn about echocardiography. *Ann Intern Med* Sep 1979;91(3):469-471.
3. Manning, Phil R.; Denson, Teri A. How internists learned about cimetidine. *Ann Intern Med* May 1980;92(5):690-692.
4. Vollan, Douglas D. Scope and extent of postgraduate medical education in the United States. *JAMA* 26 Feb 1955;157(9):703-708.
5. Manning, Phil R.; Abrahamson, Stephen; Dennis, Donald A. Comparison of four teaching techniques: Programmed text, textbook, lecture-demonstration, and lecture workshop. *J Med Educ* Mar 1968; 43(3):356-359.
6. Manning, Phil R. Pre- and post-course testing as a teaching aid. *The Mayo Alumnus* Jan 1966;2:18-20.
7. Stein, Leonard S. The effectiveness of continuing medical education: Eight research reports. *J Med Educ* Feb 1981;56(2):103-110.
8. Richards, Robert K.; Cohen, Rita M. The value and limitations of physician participation in traditional forms of continuing medical education, Part II. Kalamazoo, Michigan: Educational Services Department, The Upjohn Company, 1983.
9. Houle, Cyril O. *Continuing Learning in the Professions*. San Francisco: Jossey-Bass, Inc., 1980.
10. Schuknecht, Harold F. The risks and limitations of the course as providing competent training. *Trans Am Acad Ophthal Otolaryngol* Nov-Dec 1976;82(6):640-641.
11. Meighan, S. Spence. Continuing medical education: Philosophy in search of a plan. *Northwest Med* Nov 1966;65(11):925-929.
12. Cervero, Ronald M. A factor analytic study of physicians' reasons for participating in continuing education. *J Med Educ* Jan 1981;56(1):29-34.
13. Holmes, Oliver Wendell. Border Lines of Knowledge in Some Provinces of Medical Science. In: *Medical Essays: 1842-1882*. Chapter IV. Boston and New York: Houghton Mifflin Company, 1911:211.

8

Technology in Traditional Continuing Education

> One of the chief ways in which traditional methods [in education] have been adapted or replaced has been through the application of new technological developments.
>
> Cyril O. Houle[1]

Despite numerous attempts and projects, television, videotapes, and even film have not drastically changed the traditional methods physicians have used for the past thirty years for continuing education.[2] Reading, lectures, and discussions with colleagues remain the most popular forms of lifelong learning. In a 1968 survey of Utah physicians designed to assist with educational needs, C. Hilmon Castle found that television, radio, audiotapes, and records occupied less than 15 per cent of the hours spent by physicians in continuing education.[3] For the most part, these media have been used to bring lectures and panel discussions to the physician's home or office. Technology to date has thus used traditional classroom approaches.

New methods of continuing education are being developed through the use of videodiscs, microcomputers, and on–line data bases. These techniques offer a chance to link education, both in time and subject matter, to the physician's practice. The use of technology in practice-linked continuing education is discussed in Chapters 17 and 18.

Audiotapes

Of all the electronic approaches to continuing medical education, audiotapes are the most popular. The pioneer in the field, Audio Digest, was founded in 1953 by the late Jerry L. Pettis and Claron L. Oakley, who still serves as Executive Editor and Senior Vice-President of the California firm.

"The purpose of Audio Digest," according to Mr. Oakley, "is to bring the best medical lectures and panel discussions directly to the physician in his home, office, or automobile. We record presentations of the most prominent speakers at the most popular conferences and courses, and carefully edit and condense the best in them for our international subscription audience. Physicians attest to the value of the biweekly tapes for learning new developments in medicine and reviewing fundamental concepts. Subscribers like being able to hear famous teachers."

A major advantage of audiotapes is that they can be played while the physician is driving or during other waiting periods. Some listen to tapes during lulls in office activity, while commuting by train, while shaving and dressing, while using an exercycle, and even while sunbathing. Even more unusual methods have been reported: "My tape recorder is equipped with an oscillator, and I can pick up the sound on my transistor-broadcast-portable receiver anywhere in the house or nearby vicinity." "I can work in my garden and listen at the same time." "While jogging three miles a day, I listen to Audio Digest on a Walkman strapped to my back." "I row every morning before breakfast. I can go through one tape a week." "I listen while I'm at the barber shop every Friday."

Other tape services are offered by various societies. American College of Cardiology Extended Learning (ACCEL) is produced for cardiologists, and the American College of Physicians produces the ACP Audio Cassette Program for internists.

The Telephone

In 1966, in an experiment to permit physicians immediate access to current, pertinent, and authoritative information on a 24-hour basis, the University of Wisconsin Department of Continuing Medical Education, headed by Thomas C. Meyer, instituted a Medical Dial-Access Library. The library comprised about 400 audiotapes of 4 to 6 minutes, each containing core information on a wide variety of topics. The topics were mainly on emergencies or recent discoveries, or were subjects that were difficult to find in the usual references, titles such as "Management of Bee Stings," "Prevention of Knee Injury in Athletes," and "Marriage on the Rocks."

The service, initially provided without charge, had 15 to 20 calls daily, but did not prove to be self-supporting. It was phased out in 1977. The technology, however, proved useful and popular for consumer health education, and the University of Wisconsin has continued to provide five-minute consumer-oriented audiotapes on a dial-access system (HEALTH-LINE). At present, the system contains more than 600 tapes. The two major problems are financial support and updating.

The Teleconference

In 1965, Thomas Meyer inaugurated a program of conferences transmitted by telephone to community hospitals. Outlines and printed visual materials or slides were mailed to each conference station two weeks in advance of the scheduled program. An outline was given to each participant, and the 35-mm slides were projected as called for by the speaker. From 10 to 15 questions were discussed after each 30-minute talk. Dr. Meyer likened the system to a large "party line" over which everything that the lecturer said could be heard from the speaker phone by the health professionals seated in conference rooms at their community hospitals. The questions and answers could also be heard by everyone on the circuit. In 1966, Meyer and associates compared physicians who had participated in a telephone course in electrocardiography with medical students who were taught the same course in a traditional lecture format. The acquisition and retention of knowledge, as measured by pre-tests and post-tests, were similar in both groups. In 1980, 185 program sessions of one to two hours each were presented for 4,874 health professionals in 55 hospitals located throughout Wisconsin. The total cost per student contact hour that year were estimated at $5.33.[4]

One-way Radio

The Physician's Radio Network (PRN), a one-way radio program, broadcasts medical information to more than 90,000 physicians. The programs reach virtually every city in the United States through 38 stations throughout the country. A special radio capable of receiving signals from an FM sideband is provided free of charge to physicians. A one-hour program is repeated hourly over a 24-hour period, with a new program each day. Because this is a commercial endeavor, however, the programs are interrupted by advertisements.

Two-way Radio

Dr. Frank Woolsey pioneered a radio network in 1955 at Albany Medical College. Like teleconferencing, two-way radio conferencing is interactive and convenient for both the lecturer and the audience. According to Woolsey, this technique in no way resembles one-way radio broadcasting. Those in remote regions, who are able to listen only to broadcasts of the two-way conferences, receive more pertinent instruction than they would from listening to a typical one-way radio broadcast. They hear the questions posed by their peers, and they hear the answers. Radio and teleconferencing eliminate time-consuming travel for lecturers and participants. The interactive communication is all-important, since student and professor can exchange ideas promptly and spontaneously.[5]

Films and Videotapes

Films sponsored by medical societies and pharmaceutical companies have been available for many years. The Network for Continuing Medical Education (NCME), for example, distributes videotaped programs to hospitals and medical schools. Videoclinics are sponsored by the AMA, and Video Digest is available through Audio Digest. According to Janis Brown, Associate Director, Educational Resources Division, at the University of Southern California's Norris Medical Library, use of videotapes by medical students is high. Perhaps this early exposure will alter traditional methods of study as current students become physicians.

Television Satellite

Although television has been used in CME for years, this type of instruction almost disappeared. Most programs have not used the video adequately and feature only a lecturer or panel, so the effect does not differ from instruction by telephone, radio, or audiotape. The production costs, however, are far greater. In the opinion of Brayton and Caldwell, the early optimism of educators, producers, and hardware purveyors of medical television was unjustified. Predictions of a multimillion dollar medical audiovisual enterprise, pressed to fill daily requests and threatening the existence of medical journals, conventions, and postgraduate divisions of medical schools, have not materialized.[6]

The development of television satellites has regenerated interest in television for continuing medical education. Since 1974, the Washington, Alaska, Montana, and Idaho (WAMI) Program has used television satellites to deliver educational programs to isolated rural areas.[7] Consultations with faculty at the University of Washington School of Medicine (the only medical school in the WAMI area), as well as independent learning programs, were thus made available to individual practitioners. M. Roy Schwarz noted that: "In some circumstances, physicians in remote sites participated in grand rounds via television. Patients were presented from television studios in the remote sites."

In the independent learning programs, participants who received continuing medical education instruction by television satellite were compared, by use of pre- and post-study test performances, with physicians who received independent study programs through the mail. Materials included outlines of the study programs with goals and objectives, audio– and video–cassettes, slides, films, reprints, and textbooks.

In some areas, local physicians developed community discussion groups to review the study programs, while other physicians, after studying the material, had the opportunity to react by television with faculty at the University of Washington. On the basis of pre- and post-study testing, the group that interacted with the faculty learned the most. Physicians participating in community discussion groups were next, followed by those physicians who studied independently. Interaction, either through television satellite or in small groups, enhanced learning.

The Veterans Administration has tested video seminars, teleconsultations, grand rounds, and outpatient clinics designed for patients. The American Dietetic Association (ADA) began experimenting with satellite delivery of continuing education in 1976. The programs are two to three hours long and feature a live panel of dietitians and physicians, sometimes with taped segments of case studies or clinical demonstrations. Participants, who see the program at designated sites around the country, receive study materials in advance. An audience of 1,500 to 1,700 registrants is typical, and toll-free telephone numbers are available for questions and answers.

The American Hospital Association (AHA) uses satellites to broadcast six to eight educational and informational programs per year to members at viewing sites around the country. Increasingly, hospitals are being equipped as viewing sites. "Video teleconferencing is now a routine activity for the AHA," said Vice President James D. Houy. "Audiences, which range from 2,000 to 4,000, are usually linked by telephone lines to the lecturers for live question-and-answer sessions."

The Hospital Satellite Network is using satellite technology to develop educational services for health professionals across the country. Most of their programs, however, will be directed to patients and the general public. "Satellite telecommunications is a cost-effective way for creative educators to enhance the speed and accuracy of information transfer, which is critical to the current practice of medicine," said Ronald J. Pion, Executive Vice President and Director of Medical Affairs for the Hospital Satellite Network.

Computer-assisted Instruction

In computer-assisted instruction (CAI), the new information is communicated to a learner by a computer. It enables the learner to interact directly with information programmed to meet specified educational objectives and thus promotes inquiry, information manipulation, feedback on learning progress, and self-assessment of performance.

William Millard, Associate Professor of Medical Education at the University of Southern California, noted that "The ability to connect the computer with audiotape, videotape, projectors, or microfiche permits developers to design multisensory learning programs. Such programs enable learners to participate in simulations and problem-solving and thus more closely approach realistic situations. A number of studies have demonstrated a considerable reduction in student learning time and favorable cost-benefits with CAI over other instructional methods.

"Among barriers to the effective use of CAI is the lack of high-quality software designed to meet specific CME needs," said Millard. "Health professionals are also apprehensive about using computer learning resources because of a lack of knowledge and experience."

Videodisc

The videodisc permits the storage and presentation of sound and of still and motion pictures, which can be used with a computer-managed learning system. A personal or institutional library of videodiscs, when linked with a microcomputer, can offer problem-solving, self-instructional case studies, and patient management simulations. The learner is required to select answers to specific questions during the audiovisual presentation, and is immediately advised whether the selections are right or wrong, and why.

The American Medical Association (AMA), using optical videodisc systems with computer-assisted instruction, has created several pilot programs in tutorial formats or as patient management problems. Leo Leveridge, formerly of the AMA, considers the videodisc to be unique in directly accessing any still picture, motion picture frame, scene, or sequence quickly and precisely, unlike reel-to-reel motion picture film or videotape. "Each learner can go at his own pace, skipping the familiar while dwelling on the new or complicated. The videodisc also permits active learning at times and places convenient to the physician.

"Microprocessors with the videodisc player allow interaction between the learner and the teacher. By being tailored to what participants, by their responses to multiple-choice questions, show they do not know, such interactive systems save time and prevent boredom. On videodiscs, the expert can present patients with medical problems that are often overlooked, misdiagnosed, or mismanaged by physicians lacking special knowledge or skills."

In one patient-management program developed by the AMA, after presentation of a patient with a pulmonary problem, the learner is asked to choose among several therapeutic options. If the wrong choice is made, the program explains why it is incorrect and automatically shows the recommended procedure. This approach is repeated as laboratory reports, roentgenograms, and fluoroscopic and bronchoscopic views are displayed, after which the learner is asked to venture a diagnosis and recommend treatment. The author of the program substantiates the correct diagnosis and shows how the patient was treated.

A tutorial format on the treatment of facial lacerations showed an actual emergency repair. According to Leveridge, "The learner is asked to identify which of the steps shown was performed correctly. If an incorrect choice is made, the learner is so informed and is given the reasons. The recommended procedure is shown to all who have made the wrong selection and is an option for those who responded correctly.

"Learning reinforcement is immediate, at which time it is most effective. The program can also be designed so that the learner cannot proceed without complete mastery of each step. Video design and production are not, in themselves, extraordinarily difficult. The major task is designing and producing effective interactive audiovisual programs in any medium."

The videodisc can store more information than any other existing medium—ten billion bits of information per side. With such capacity and convenience for retrieval, videodiscs should have a broad application for reference, archival use, and education.

Learning Resource Centers

Learning Resource Centers (LRC), which are usually housed in health profession schools and libraries, contain audiovisual and telecommunications devices for individual and small-group use. Through linkages to national information networks, LRCs allow users to reach resources beyond local holdings. Both print and nonprint educational materials are directly accessible for independent study. Services are customarily provided to help users select and procure educational programs tailored to individual needs. Some LRCs lend materials for home study.

William Millard believes that future LRCs will provide expanded learning resources and services accessible from remote-site computer-based telecommunication systems in the home or office. The continued refinement of microstorage and display systems will also encourage personal instructional libraries.

*****

Until recently, most continuing medical education methods have involved traditional programming. The "knowledge explosion," however, has accelerated the growth of technical methods of teaching that permit considerable flexibility in time and place of instruction. Their ultimate value will be decided by their substance and their effectiveness in fostering learning as determined by the marketplace.

References

1. Houle, Cyril O. *Continuing Learning in the Professions*. San Francisco: Jossey-Bass, Inc., 1980:203.
2. Vollan, Douglas D. Educational methods in postgraduate teaching. *JAMA* 9 Apr 1955;157(15):1302-1309.

3. Castle, C. Hilmon; Storey, Patrick B. Physicians' needs and interests in continuing medical education. *JAMA* 14 Oct 1968;206(3):611-614.
4. Meyer, Thomas C. Teleconferencing as a medium for continuing education of health professionals: A fifteen year perspective. *Mobius* Apr 1983;3(2):73-79.
5. Woolsey, Frank M. The Albany Medical College two-way radio conferences. Presented at the Symposium on Continuing Medical Education Methods and Goals, Georgetown University Medical Center, Washington DC, May 15, 1968. Sponsored by the Regional Medical Program of Metropolitan Washington.
6. Caldwell, Kathryn S.; Brayton, Donald. Use of television and film in continuing education in the health sciences. *J Biocomm* Jun 1974;1(1):7-16.
7. Schwarz, M. Roy; Schaad, Douglas C.; Evans, Franklin W.; Dohner, Charles W. Communications satellites in health education and health care provision: The WAMI experience. *JAMA* 5 Aug 1983;250(5):636-639.

9

Learning from Teaching

> Men learn while they teach.
> [H]omines, dum docent, discunt.
>
> Seneca, *Letters to Lucilius,*
> Volume 1, Book 1, Letter 7,
> Section 8, 64 A.D.[1]

The word "doctor" is from the Latin *docere*, meaning to teach. The title of "doctor" became associated with the medical profession after the fifteenth century, probably because only the medical doctors, of all the members of faculties, went out among the people. "Doctor," by common usage, thus became associated with medicine. Physicians often find themselves teaching patients, colleagues, other associates, and the general public. Academic physicians have primary responsibilities for teaching, but all practicing physicians have such opportunities. In our interviews, we have explored teaching as a method of learning for the physician, have elicited ways of ensuring self-education as a by-product of teaching, have reviewed the attributes of master teachers, and have discovered how practicing physicians create opportunities to teach clinical medicine.

Benefits of Teaching

"The safest thing for a patient," Charles Mayo was quoted as saying, "was to be in the hands of a man engaged in teaching medicine. In order to be a teacher of medicine the doctor must always be a student."[2] Leigh Thompson identified three ways teaching helps him to learn: "First, it stimulates me to search published material, learn new facts, and update my knowledge. Second, it forces me to organize my knowledge for my presentation. Third, it provides the opportunity for feedback from the audience."

Attributes of Effective Teachers

In addition to knowledge of one's discipline, Joseph Van Der Meulen listed the following attributes of outstanding teachers. "They must be able to abstract the essentials from a subject and present them in an organized and interesting way. They should be able to accommodate their pacing to the complexity of the subject. They should be receptive to constructive criticism, be adaptable to change, and remain current. They must be sensitive to the needs of the audience and to its receptivity. Sensitivity is probably innate; I doubt that it can be acquired, but the other attributes can be acquired by experience and constructive feedback."

"An outstanding clinical teacher," said Clifton Cleaveland, "shows a profound regard and empathy for each patient seen on teaching rounds. A second attribute is a dedication to upgrading and renewing one's own fund of clinical information. Thirdly, the outstanding teacher will stimulate open, frank, nonthreatening channels of communication with house staff and students."

For William Waters, the compulsion to share new learning, insights, and revelations is the competent teacher's primary attribute. "Other qualifications include verbalism, enthusiasm, intellectualism, warm feelings for students, and—not by any means least—brains. Most of these can be developed by example and experience."

C. S. Lewis had a similar view. "The primary attribute for teaching is interest in a subject and in young people, coupled with a willingness to impart information. A continual striving for excellence is one of the most important of these attitudes, along with the urge to help one's fellow man, particularly when in need."

Edwin Overholt emphasized "intellectual honesty, high intelligence, enthusiasm, attention to detail, and a joy in interacting with one's colleagues. A teacher must respect his colleagues. The help that an outstanding teacher can give his colleagues and his house staff is the ultimate reward. Teachers should encourage young physicians with a potential for teaching to pursue such a career. Exposure to an outstanding teacher is a great motivator." The opportunity to give case presentations and literature reviews, with constructive comments from their teachers, is extremely valuable to house officers.

A good teacher should possess enthusiasm, self-discipline, and the ability to transmit ideas with clarity, humor, and intelligence. The teacher must show respect and sympathy for his students without pandering to sloppiness of thought or performance.

Teachers must know the subject from all standpoints, according to Leigh Thompson, including personal involvement in research and practice. "They must present the right amount of information in the right sequence with the right timing and the right graphics."

One phenomenon that is clearly a handicap, according to Thomas Burns, is a large information differential between teacher and audience. "We all

9. Learning from Teaching

know people with a great fund of knowledge who are barely able to impart any of it to their peers, let alone to house staff or medical students. On the other hand, information seems to flow readily from house officers to medical students and from senior students to their juniors. A common characteristic among great teachers in medicine is an ability to uncover the learning receptors of students so as not to impede the flow of information down the gradient."

Early in his career, Antonio Gotto learned a valuable lesson about the importance of sympathy and understanding in teachers. "During my initial year as a Rhodes Scholar at Worcester College, Oxford," he said, "I completed the equivalent of the first year of medical school except for biochemistry because my tutor, Hans Kornberg, (now Sir Hans, Biochemistry Professor at Cambridge and Master of Christ College, Cambridge) had been in America. Dr. Kornberg was then a young investigator in the Medical Research Council Unit under the direction of Sir Hans Krebs, Professor of Biochemistry at Oxford. Dr. Kornberg invited me into his laboratory during the summer after my first year. I was to assist an eminent American scientist who was on sabbatical with Hans at Oxford. The first project was to purify an enzyme from yeast, which we would then use in the assay of a bacterial enzyme. The purification and preparation of the enzyme went well. At the end of each day's work, we stored the preparation in the refrigerator. At the end of the fourth day, the American biochemist had to leave early and so asked me to store the enzyme. I decided to return after dinner to try to carry the purification an additional step. Before I left for dinner, I placed a beaker containing the enzyme in an ice bucket, covered all of it, and put it in the refrigerator. When I returned two or three hours later, I found to my dismay that the container had been moved to one side by another researcher. As a result of this and partial melting of the ice, the beaker was now submerged and the enzyme preparation was mixed with the water in the container. I filtered the liquid from the ice and tried unsuccessfully to re-precipitate the protein by adding ammonium sulfate to the saturation. The preparation was lost beyond recovery.

"The next morning it was my embarrassing duty to explain all of this to the American visitor. His face turned a deeper and deeper shade of purple as I detailed the mishap. When I finished, he immediately called for a private conference with my tutor, during which (I was subsequently told) he had strongly urged that my career as a biochemist be terminated posthaste and I be returned to medical school. Fortunately for me, my tutor was somewhat more sympathetic and allowed me to pursue another project with him. This project turned out very favorably, and Hans Kornberg and Professor Krebs invited me to go with them to the International Congress of Biochemistry. There they invited me to drop the medical degree temporarily and pursue a doctorate in Biochemistry under Kornberg. The lessons I learned from this experience were not only to be more careful, particularly with other people's projects and materials, but also

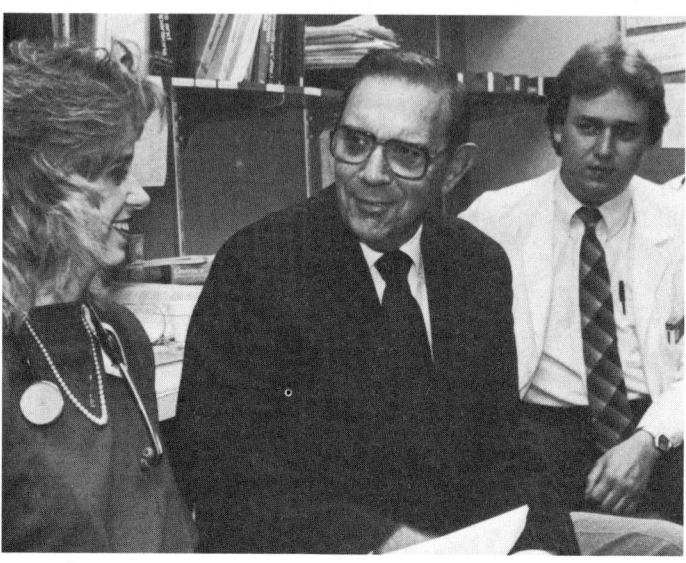

The primary attribute for teaching is interest in a subject and in young people, coupled with a willingness to impart information.

Ceylon S. Lewis, Jr., M.D. (center)
Clinical Professor of Medicine
The University of Oklahoma Tulsa Medical College

9. Learning from Teaching

to lend a sympathetic ear to a young student or scientist who finds himself in a jam."

"A common mistake made by those in medical education," said Thorpe Ray, "is assuming that events such as graduation from medical school and completion of residency or fellowship mark the end of something. In reality, they mark the beginning of a career of perpetual study. The recent graduate should be prepared for his clinical training program, and the finishing resident should be prepared for his lifelong study. By this time, the habit of critical reading should have been established, as well as the self-evaluation and honest self-criticism that are essential for continued intellectual growth and maintenance of clinical skills. The source of useful knowledge and information for the physician is often self-instruction. Teachers help most by establishing sound reasoning and a disciplined approach to clinical problems. A good teacher should clearly demonstrate an approach that identifies the patient as an important and interesting person. The best teachers demonstrate that medicine is fun and learning is fun. They stimulate and attract students of medicine at all stages. Sometimes the manner of doing or saying something determines whether it will be remembered by students.

"I am intrigued by the common statement that half of what one learns is wrong. I wonder if those making the statement can list ten or twenty examples to validate it. The list usually falls short of ten. Our 'new' knowledge usually extends in depth and usually helps us to understand what we already know."

Bobby Alford recalled an incident from his student days touching upon Michael E. DeBakey's insistence on preciseness of evaluation and statement of fact. "Dr. DeBakey had operated on Dr. Mims Gage of New Orleans for an abdominal aorta. It was the custom in those days for the students assigned to Dr. DeBakey's patients to make the presentation to Dr. DeBakey on rounds at the bedside with regard to the status of the patient. In this particular instance, one of my classmates began by saying, 'Dr. DeBakey, Dr. Gage is doing well. . .' and gave the required laboratory results, after which he said that Dr. Gage was 'a little bit distended.' Whereupon Dr. DeBakey turned to Dr. Gage and said, 'Mims, are you distended?' and he replied to Dr. DeBakey, 'No, Mike, I am not distended.' Dr. DeBakey then turned to the student and said, 'A patient is distended or not distended, but he is not a little bit distended.' Dr. DeBakey's emphasis on precision made a lifelong impression on me."

"Not all teaching experiences are pleasant or funny," according to Linda Clever. "I remember two nameless professors. They 'led' by bad example—and no one emulated them. The first asked the patient in a rheumatology clinic if she 'had any trouble with your temperomandibular joint.' Her puzzled look spoke volumes and reminded us to use lay language. The other professor asked an endocrine patient at grand rounds, 'How long have you looked like a frog?' Humiliation is never humorous, nor does it put anyone at ease."

John Martin Askey recalled the words of a mentor during his resident days at the University of Pennsylvania. O. H. Perry Pepper, Clinical Professor at Penn, advised him one day as they rode to Pepper's home for an afternoon of tennis, "John, always have an 'arbeit.' " Askey remembers Pepper as a great stimulator who considered the main qualities of an investigator to be "the simplicity to wonder, the ability to question, the power to generalize, and the capacity to apply." At 86, Askey's continuing education arises primarily from trips to the medical library, he says, but, "the virus for keeping me in contact with medicine still continues."

Full-time Faculty

The teaching principles described by physicians in academia are equally applicable to the practicing physician.

"To me, teaching is essential for learning," said Saul Farber. "Throughout my adult life I have learned mainly through teaching. You learn a great deal from your students while trying to impart knowledge to them. I never go into a teaching session without being prepared. No matter how many times I present lobar pneumonia to medical students, I always read something about that subject the night before, and I never fail to learn something that I had not known before or to gain a new insight that had not occurred to me before, as, for example, about pathophysiology. When I return from a teaching session or rounds, I look up things that I think I should have known or try to find the answer to a question that has arisen. Preparation before and catch-up after the sessions have been very useful and extremely enjoyable."

The importance of preparation was impressed on Ralph Wallerstein during his training under William Castle, whose work on intrinsic and extrinsic factors in pernicious anemia led to the fundamental understanding of that disease. Late one night, Wallerstein noticed a light in Castle's office and, entering to say hello, found him busy studying and writing a presentation on pernicious anemia to be given to medical students. The fact that Castle, an international expert on pernicious anemia, felt it necessary to prepare for a lecture to students left a strong impression on Wallerstein.

As Lloyd H. Smith noted, "The subject matter of medicine is so vast that no one can master more than a part of it. Moreover what we learn is eroded by new insights from basic and clinical research. One's most cherished aphorisms are continually being disproved by indisputable facts. Teaching requires a reappraisal of one's beliefs, a 'loosening of certainties,' as Will Durant said. You must defend your ideas once more both to yourself and, more important, to those being taught. Most of my teaching is done on ward rounds rather than as formal lectures. Fortunately, young people are remarkably forgiving of one's knowledge lacunae and are willing

9. Learning from Teaching

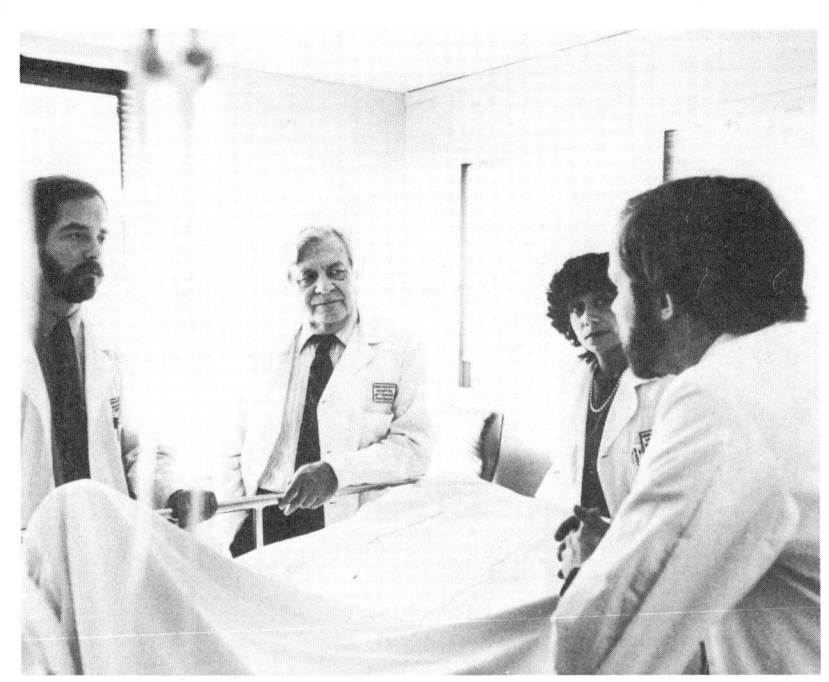

Throughout my adult life I have learned mainly through teaching.

Saul J. Farber, M.D. (second from left)
Chairman, Department of Medicine
New York University Medical Center

to play to one's strengths, if they can be found. This assumes that the teacher has a genuine interest in medicine (it cannot be feigned), is humble before the facts, and is a reasonable and secure master of ceremonies who brings out the best in all who participate in the complex sociology of ward rounds.

"When one is caught off base, which happens to all clinical teachers, it is imperative (a) to admit it, (b) to praise those who are better informed, and (c) to return the next day better prepared on the subject. Even when the clinical teacher is not well informed about a specific problem, he must remember that education is what is left when he has forgotten the facts. His personal interaction with the patient or general approach to the problem may be of more permanent value to those being taught than his instant recall of statistics and references."

Physicians should never be reluctant to acknowledge their limitations of knowledge, as one student learned from Dr. Julius Bauer. According to Samuel Rapaport, the student was presenting a case on rounds. He was doing very well, even as the questions got harder and harder. Finally, Dr. Bauer asked a question to which the student replied: "I am sorry, Dr. Bauer, I knew the answer to that question but I have forgotten it." Dr. Bauer countered: "I am sorry too, for you were the only person in the world who knew the answer to that question."

"The best self-education for clinical teachers is to remain conversant within a broad sweep of medical problems by being on the firing line frequently," said Lloyd H. Smith. "Preferably, they should teach in a way that encourages questions and alternative approaches. Unless their intellectual epiphyses have already closed, this approach will inevitably lead to their growth as teachers, physicians, and human beings."

"Multiple heads are far more important and productive than one head," in Saul Farber's experience. "No matter how uninformed a medical student or house officer is about a particular subject, his insight and curiosity often disclose an aspect of the situation that the teacher was unaware of." Arthur Fox pointed to yet another advantage of teaching: "Teaching demands knowledge of facts and communication skills. If one does not communicate ideas clearly, the loss of interest, or the confusion, of students and house staff is quickly apparent. If they are bright and aggressive, they will tell you when they do not understand or when they disagree. I learn from the bright young people who prove to me that I have not martialed my facts. Then I go back and read further to prove points."

Preparing papers for speaking commitments at postgraduate courses keeps Dame Sheila Sherlock up-to-date in her field. Preparing outlines and handouts to accompany lectures is a useful learning tool. The one who gets the most out of a talk is the one who has to prepare it.

The most important point, for William Waters, is never to give the same lecture twice. "Throw away your notes and start from scratch; reread, rethink, reorganize. The result is relearning, new learning, better information, new insights, and, of course, a much more spontaneous, enthusiastic lecture, seminar, or rounds." The technique that works for Marvin Turck is to "think of the two particular points that are clinically most relevant after I have read something, listened to a seminar, or interacted in a consultation. I then try to use those two points in teaching."

Ralph Haymond advised physicians "to associate with students with inquisitive minds for they will stimulate you to keep current, even if only to avoid embarrassment. And if you never teach, you can assemble all the information you would need for a lecture, as a method of reviewing your own knowledge of a topic." Robert Manning's words summarized the consensus: "The old rule that you don't know something until you can teach it has a lot of validity."

Full-time Practitioner

For those near medical schools, a teaching appointment is invaluable in keeping up with new knowledge. Serving on the voluntary clinical faculty of a medical school may be an economic hardship, but it prevents obsolescence. "After World War II," related Rodney Rodgers, "I returned to three years of residency in medicine at Philadelphia General Hospital. I found myself shockingly ignorant, but was obliged to teach interns and medical students. The training was largely clinical and intensely correlated with patient care. I spent all my spare time answering specific questions that arose while in house staff teaching. It took six months of hard work before I caught up from my two years away from education. I resolved then to practice in a town with a medical school, to which I would volunteer my teaching services so as never to allow myself to decay again."

Physicians who practice at some distance from medical schools can still teach in local hospitals, as Alan Gordon does by conducting morbidity and mortality conferences. Although Richard Field has literally had to go to great lengths to maintain his ties with medical schools, it has allowed him to bring to his community up-to-date general surgery. As an associate professor at Tulane University and at the University of Mississippi School of Medicine, both of which are 100 miles away, he attends grand rounds and teaches students one day a month.

"The most important aspect of teaching," according to Saul Farber, "is the security of knowledge of the teacher. People in practice can feel secure by preparing in advance, and they can become as outstanding teachers as full-time academicians."

"Questions from students often point to inadequacy in your own knowledge," noted Sidney Howard. "Then my pride forces me to update my information."

"The practitioner, perhaps without giving himself full credit, does a great deal of teaching and learning every day," said James Wyngaarden, Director of the National Institutes of Health. "The kind of learning that

142 Medicine: Preserving the Passion

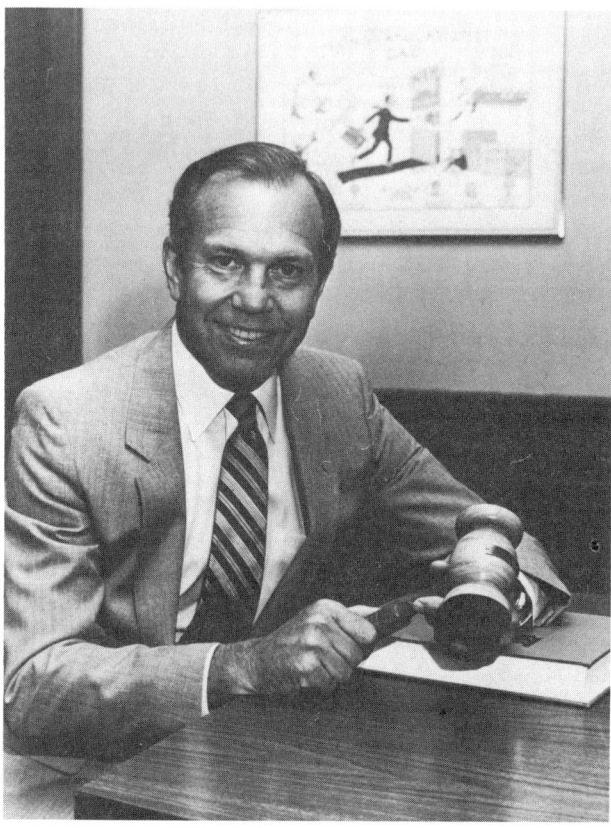

The kind of learning that appeals to me is that in which the roles of student and teacher are mixed, each learning from the other while working toward a shared objective. This is the kind that takes place on the wards with patients and in the laboratory with fellows.

James B. Wyngaarden, M.D.
Director, National Institutes of Health

9. Learning from Teaching

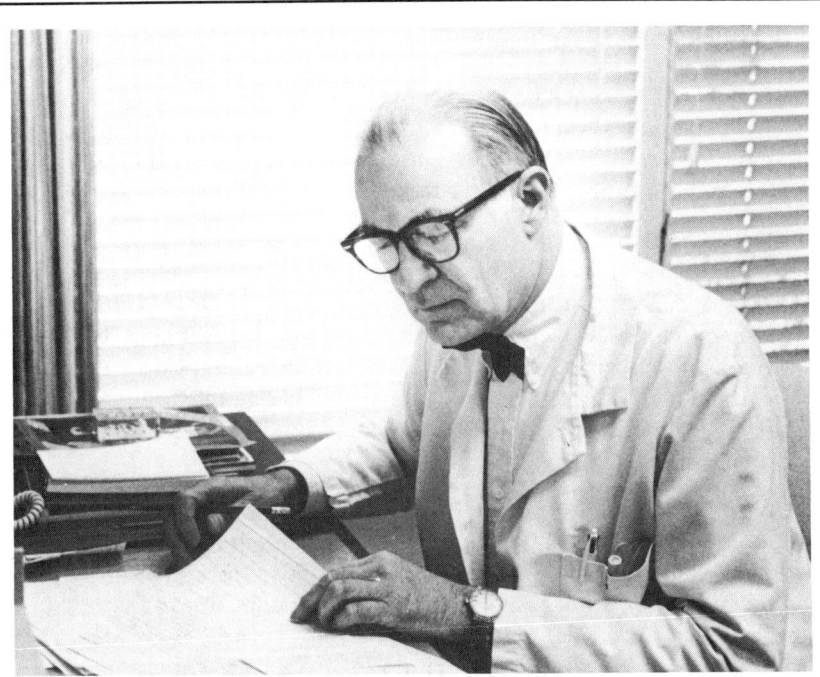

Educationally, the practicing physician should advance from passive recipient to active participant—from partaker of information to questioner to discussant to imparter.

> *George E. Miller, M.D.*
> *Founding Director, Center for Educational Development*
> *University of Illinois at Chicago*

appeals to me is that in which the roles of student and teacher are mixed, each learning from the other while working toward a shared objective. This is the kind that takes place on the wards with patients and in the laboratory with fellows. The mere transfer of information is certainly necessary to establish a joint knowledge base, but the kind of learning that is the most fun and the kind of teaching that is the most fun involve participatory collaboration."

WRITING AND SPEAKING. Richard Field tries to prepare at least one paper each year. "I usually invite one of the people on the staff to be a co-author. We try to stimulate our mutual thinking and share anything that we might consider useful by writing it up and publishing it. The writing is a wonderful learning experience, as is the presentation of exhibits at state medical meetings and at the American College of Surgeons' clinical congresses." Meeting interesting people and the pleasure of traveling are added benefits from such presentations.

TEACHING THE OFFICE STAFF. As James Wyngaarden noted, "The practitioner must do a great deal of teaching when interacting with patients, the nursing staff, physical therapists, or other hospital staff. The physician must not be unduly impressed by rank; the concept of rank is one of the greatest deterrents to learning."

Brian Goodell, who has participated in in-service training sessions in community hospitals in his area, pointed to the reduction in turnover rate and the improved communication such sessions provide. "We make sure that the nurses have access to their literature in the library. I encourage them to give me articles from the nursing journals because they are often very practical."

One of the provisions of employment for nurses in Richard Parkinson's office is participation in a continuing education program. "I devote about one-half hour three days a week to continuing education. The program, which consists of a review of basic science and clinical medicine, forced me to review all the subject material. The first nurse that came to work for me was an LVN, whom I assisted in obtaining her RN license, and then later trained so that she was able to pass the physician's assistant examination with a high mark. Another medical assistant who handled the business end of my practice was so fascinated by that nurse's progress that she entered the field of nursing. She is currently working on her nursing degree, and I try to keep ahead of her and to discuss with her the clinical significance of our cases."

*****

The very nature of medicine requires that physicians be teachers. Teaching is an impetus for study; it requires the teacher to acquire, review, and organize the knowledge to be taught. In good teaching, teachers are also learners, and exchanges of ideas, challenges, and feedback make learning a lively affair.

9. Learning from Teaching

The distinguished teachers we interviewed all stressed the importance of preparation. None was willing to rely totally on memory. The practicing physician who has the opportunity of teaching will profit immeasurably from the experience. Those without access to medical school teaching services will benefit from participating in hospital staff meetings and from teaching nurses and office staff. Informal discussions are also an excellent way to gain knowledge. The physician who devotes time to teaching his patients will be amply rewarded by their improved cooperation.

References

1. Sénèque, *Lettres à Lucilius*, Tome I, text established by François Préchac and translated by Henri Noblot. Paris: Société d'Édition "Les Belles Lettres," 1945:21.
2. Mayo, Charles H. Quoted in: *Proceedings of the Staff Meetings of the Mayo Clinic*, 28 Sep 1927;2(39):233.

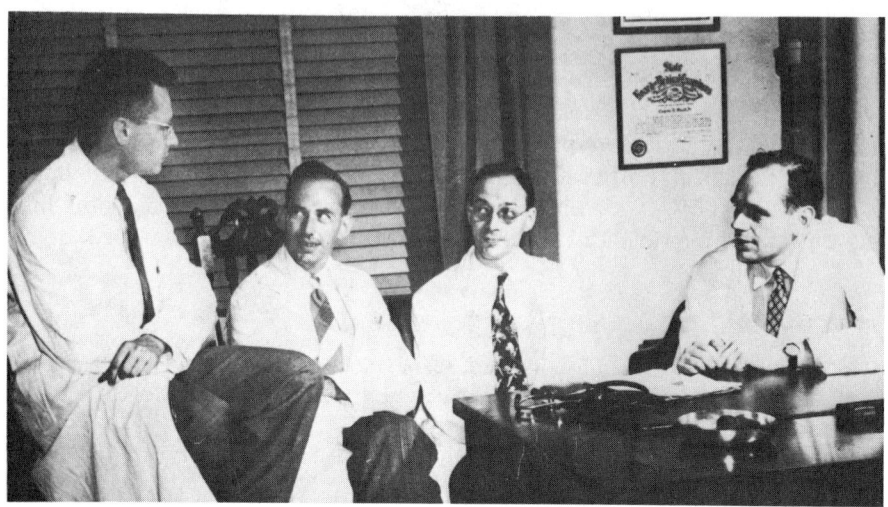

The method a physician selects for lifelong learning must give pleasure or other rewards, because human beings will not continue a program that does not have tangible dividends.

Eugene A. Stead, Jr., M.D. (extreme right)

As Willis Hurst said, "Dr. Stead is one of the greatest in medicine of this century." Dr. Stead has distinguished himself by his contributions in diverse fields of medicine, including a better understanding of the role of forward failure and kidney function in congestive heart failure. He organized the first program for physician assistants in the United States and has been active in the development of information sciences, clinical epidemiology, and bioengineering in academic institutions. Dr. Stead's magnetic qualities have contributed to the development of many leaders in medicine throughout the world.

The most remarkable thing about Dr. Eugene Stead is that he seemed to take a genuine interest in the goals and aspirations of the individual physicians he was training. He never confused administrative decisions with personal decisions. He could be extremely critical and point out a flaw, but it clearly was related to performance and not personality. He could tell you that you were the biggest jackass in the world and an hour later meet you at a cocktail party and treat you in a civil manner, with no sense that there was any hurt intended earlier. In his teaching, one never felt that there was any hierarchy in the room.

Morton Bogdonoff, M.D.

Personal Essay

Eugene A. Stead, Jr., M.D.
Florence McAllister Professor of Medicine, Emeritus
Duke University School of Medicine
Durham, North Carolina

Lifetime learners organize their practice to allow time for study, and because they enjoy using their brains, they continue to learn. During medical school and residency training, the mentors ask the questions and offer praise when the answers are correct. The physician is ready to leave the fold when he asks himself searching questions about his patients and vigorously pursues the answers. The rewards include satisfaction from exercising his brain and improving the quality of his medical practice, as well as the opportunity to hone his knowledge by teaching others.

My first professor of medicine was James Edgar Paullin, an Atlanta internist who served as a President of the American College of Physicians as well as of the American Medical Association. Two mornings a week he saw patients at Grady Hospital, taught students and residents, asked questions, and used the library. He received no money for his teaching services, but allowed his private practice fees to increase as his reputation grew throughout north Georgia and the entire South. His patients never resented his unavailability on those two mornings because, as he explained, "If I'm going to give you first-rate medical care over the years, I must have continuing medical education. I'll do two things: I'll be certain that your needs are covered by someone else when I'm not available, and I'll charge you for my educational time because you are getting the kind of service nobody else in this community can give you." The old gentleman did extraordinarily well. He was the outstanding practitioner in the state; he gave first-rate care; and he died with an estate I wouldn't mind having.

In Boston, Sam Levine, a distinguished cardiologist, followed a similar pattern, spending every morning in the Peter Bent Brigham Hospital. At one time he was paid a salary of $500, but it took him roughly 24 years to rise to that level. Then Dr. Soma Weiss came along and said, "You know, I don't have much free money to pay my young people." Since I was one of the young people, I was interested in that. Soma said, "Sam, you don't really need $500, do you?" Sam said, "No, I don't need $500." So, Sam lost his $500, but he still came to the Brigham Hospital

---

Some of the ideas in this essay appeared in the *AMA Continuing Medical Education Newsletter*, Volume 10, Number 9, pp. 2-7, September 1981, and are included here by permission. Copyright American Medical Association.

every morning. He saw patients, asked questions, and tried to get answers. Louis Hammond of Johns Hopkins and Paul White of Massachusetts General Hospital had similar arrangements.

Those educational days were not designed to pay the overhead of practice. They were set up as educational time required by patients' needs. Patients were asking questions the doctors were unable to answer. This was an extraordinarily efficient way to learn. I had always been surprised that people took the last year of residency training because, if you can multiply, you can see that a year distributed over seven years of practice can be used to greater advantage. There are 52 weeks in a year, and that's a lot of time. A young person can go into practice in the community a year earlier than he would if he took that last year of residency, and he can say to the people, "I'm going to give you the best services over the years, but that requires that I continue my education." He can then set aside one day a week to see patients without remuneration, as a part of his continuing education for seven years. I don't care how much you teach him in the last year of residency, he will be licked by the forgetting curve. No matter what he knows at the end of the residency, he won't retain much of it seven years from then. But if he learns every week, he will lick the forgetting curve.

Not only that; he will have built in a way to control his practice. Instead of the practice running him, he will run it. Unfortunately, there are not many people who have the discipline to carry out this program. The ones who do will be the outstanding doctors in their regions, states, and communities. They will be learning from their patients. And they will profit from what has been discovered and rediscovered by educational experts: when you are active, it helps you lick the forgetting curve, and when you are passive, the forgetting curve always licks you.

The reason we tie learning to patients is simple. Two kinds of knowledge are stored in the nervous system. There is knowledge that requires effort to extract. For example, if I keep poking at a student who knows a certain number of things, I can finally get him to put out the information. It may take a half-hour or three-quarters of an hour to get it out because he had never before used or manipulated that material. The training and education directly tied to patients is designed to take that stored information and mobilize it for use in a variety of contexts.

Education is added to practice when the doctor says, "I'm going to look at this problem outside my usual practice pattern. I'm going to take time to ask a series of questions that I cannot ask about every patient. I'm going to find out some of the things I don't know."

It is easier to start with the patient than it is to go to a meeting and pick up information and then take it back to the patient. I know some physicians in North Carolina who rarely go to meetings, but there's not very much you can ask them that they don't know. They have an extraordinarily simple system; they practice medicine. They learned as residents to ask relevant questions. They read *The Journal of the American Medical Association*, *The New England Journal of Medicine*, *The Lancet*, and the *British Medical Journal*. They ask, "What new knowledge will be useful in my practice?" Then they use the new material in their practice. It is an effective way to learn.

The educator should cultivate in the student primarily an attitude. I have been accused of never teaching anybody anything. In general, the accusation is correct. I never lecture at Duke. I teach attitudes because everybody else is teaching facts. I ask questions like: How can you have a good time practicing medicine and taking care of difficult patients? Those are very fundamental questions that are not asked often enough. I spend a fair amount of time trying to answer them. I am not, however, against facts; you cannot function without them.

The formation of the correct habits and an efficient style in caring for patients is the best and most economical way to practice medicine. It is when the patient does not fit the pattern that you have to refer the difficult problems to someone else or take the more time-consuming thinking and learning route. Patterns are set up not only in the way you practice medicine, but in the way you finance and organize your office.

If you were to say to me, "But I don't know how best to use the time that I set aside for learning from patients," I would reply "See some patients for education and not for production. Look at the patient's problems as if you were reading a book. During that time, ask yourself questions and, because memory is finite, write down some of them. Spend the rest of the time searching for answers to those questions. That takes discipline, but it also pays financial dividends."

Sometimes I am asked, "Are case reports a useful device for continuing medical education?" I always reply that they have great educational value. Their preparation requires discipline. An unfinished case report is worthless. If you have ten case reports in that many subjects, you will be fun to see patients with.

I want to continue my own education for three reasons: (l) learning is fun, (2) I am competitive and would like to give the best care in the community, and (3) I would like to be paid well for it. A simple, consistent program is superior to periodic elaborate programs. My own educational program differs because I have a lot of peculiarities. People are always wanting to know what Board certified me. The Board of Internal Medicine used to call me and request that I serve as an examiner. I couldn't do it because it would not be fair, since I have never taken the examination of the Board of Internal Medicine, or of any other board.

I don't know how many program brochures for continuing education I throw away every week. With the best of intentions, we may have created a monster. Continuing education courses are becoming a major source of income to the educational establishment, but there is little evidence that they change the behavior of doctors.

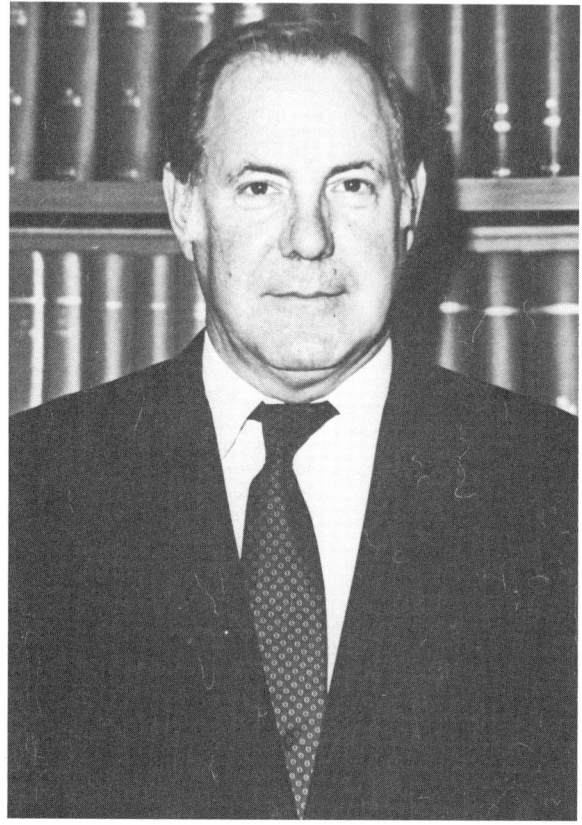

One of the reasons we academicians like our work is that we learn a lot by osmosis. We go to conferences, and we seek out people who have the answers to our questions. So my advice to young physicians is to surround yourself with people who can educate you.

Norton J. Greenberger, M.D.

Dr. Greenberger has been extremely active in prestigious medical organizations. He has served as President of the Central Society for Clinical Research, the American Gastroenterological Association, and the Association of Professors of Medicine, as Secretary-Treasurer of the American Board of Internal Medicine, and as a Regent of the American College of Physicians. He has also served as Editor of the *Journal of Laboratory and Clinical Medicine* and of the *Year Book of Medicine*.

Norton Greenberger is the best organized person I know. He is a warm, compassionate, dedicated teacher who has spent much of his career trying to make learning fun.

Willis C. Maddrey, M.D.

Personal Essay

Norton J. Greenberger, M.D.
Professor and Chairman
Department of Medicine
Kansas University School of Medicine
Kansas City, Kansas

Reading

As editor of the Gastroenterology Section of the *Year Book of Medicine*, I receive 10,000 articles a year to review, from which I select about sixty-five for abstracting in the *Year Book*. The first cut will come by title and summary, the second by the reputation of the authors and journals, and the third by whether the articles will be of interest to a practicing physician. Most of these articles come from journals I have already read, so I am getting a second look at them, and that is a form of reinforcement.

I distribute my reading rather than concentrate it. With a list of the disorders that I want to read about and a list of the reading materials to provide the answers, I will sit down not only with a textbook of medicine, but with selected references from my reprint file or other primary resource material. I have an extensive reprint collection of more than 40,000 articles, organized by disease system. The file is constantly updated, and not a day goes by that I do not use it. I also have about twenty-five years of bound journals that cover three walls of a very large office.

The average student's attention span in the library is about two minutes. I read in my den, where I know I will not be distracted. I read titles; scan abstracts, tables, graphs, and diagrams; and read the introduction and first and last paragraphs of the discussion. Then I ask myself what the message is in one sentence. If an article is written poorly and I cannot understand it, I am not going to waste my time with it; it impairs my efficiency.

When I finish reading an article, I construct mnemonics and try to reproduce the material that I want to remember. I also force myself periodically to see if I can recall that information. So when I am with students or house staff on rounds, I go through the lists for teaching purposes to reinforce my retention. Another trick is to talk about what you have read. At the end of morning reports, I will ask if anyone has read anything interesting the night before.

If we are on rounds and a question comes up that I can't answer, I will assign someone to look up the answer and give a five-minute report with references. When we have coffee during rounds, we make a list on the board as a reminder to me to give a short, off-the-cuff talk on specific subjects when I finish rounds. That forces me to try to recall information I may not have used for some time.

10

Analysis of Practice

> We physicians had need be a self-confronting and a self-reproving race; for we must be ready, without fear or favour, to call in question our own Experience and to judge it justly; to confirm it, to repeal it, to reverse it. . . .
>
> *Peter Mere Latham*[1]

To profit most from experience, the physician needs some objective means of examining his practice. Practice analysis shows what you are actually doing and provides evidence of deficiencies that need correction. Beverly Payne has found that when clinicians view their practice in the aggregate, as in research participation, "There are compelling observations that lead to significant changes in behavior."

William Budd's duties as a country doctor permitted him to make observations and collect evidence that typhoid fever was a communicable disease.[2] William N. Pickles tried to stimulate other country doctors to keep records of epidemic diseases: "We country practitioners are in a position to supply facts from our observation of nature, and it is, I feel most strongly, our plain duty to make use of this unique opportunity."[3] Sir James Mackenzie believed that research in the physician's office was a necessity, for the general practitioner "has opportunities which no other worker possesses—opportunities which are necessary to the solution of problems essential to the advance of medicine."[4]

In 1879, following an undistinguished career as a medical student, Mackenzie entered general practice in a small English town. "About 1883 or 1884," he wrote, "I resolved to begin a series of careful observations entirely for my own improvement, never dreaming of research, for I was under the prevalent belief that medical research could only be undertaken in a laboratory or, at least, in an hospital with all the appurtenances. I merely sought to find out something about the nature of my patients' complaints. . . . I had thus placed before me two definite objects, at which aim: (1) understanding of the mechanism of symptoms, and (2) understanding of their prognostic significance. When. . . I look back upon my work, I can recognize that it was this simple resolution and these definite aims which guided me to such success as I have achieved. . . . I may point out that the necessity for such an investigation, with these aims, could only be found necessary by one who had, in his daily work, found the need for them."[5] Mackenzie's detailed records of patients with heart disease enabled him to become one of the leading heart specialists of his time, and a pioneer in symptomatology.

The study and analysis of practice give the physician a good perspective and a formal record of his own work, thus permitting him to profit maximally from lessons learned. This, we think, is the most rewarding kind of continuing education.

The practice of medicine can and should be a scholarly and intellectual process. "The only way I have found to do that," said Warren Williams, "is through the study of the practice itself. I tried to develop my practice by emulating my medical school professors, who seemed to know exactly what they were doing. When I first started my practice, it seemed to be one sore throat after another, getting people in and getting people out. It was not intellectually stimulating until I started my practice study and analysis." John Fry found that simple, inexpensive methods of recording, reviewing, and analyzing everyday work not only yield better services, but add immeasurably to his enjoyment of medicine. Thus, practice analysis, while delivering the most benefit to the physician from his experience, enhances his zest for his work through greater immersion and gives direction to his future study. These advantages increase the likelihood of improving his patient services and enriching his professional life.

The physician may organize his practice for study by:
1. indexing patient charts by clinical problem, to permit a critique of aggregate experience in specific conditions;
2. keeping statistics on the problems seen, drugs prescribed, and laboratory studies ordered by the physician;
3. compiling and classifying salient clinical features observed in specific problems, diseases, and procedures, recording mistakes, and lessons learned;
4. performing audit of patient records; and
5. tracing, and reacting to, patient outcome.

Indexing Patient Charts by Problem

John Fry keeps a card index of all patients diagnosed with certain diseases, which permits him to calculate incidence/prevalence rates and facilitates follow-up reviews on patients with particular diseases. He also collects the following sets of data: (1) day sheets that record all physician-patient contacts by patient's name, age, sex, diagnostic group, and referrals for studies or consultation, and (2) an age-sex register that provides an up-to-date population at risk. His studies have enabled him to reduce his volume of work per patient and therefore to treat more patients, to lower his prescribing costs, and to minimize his referrals to consultants. It takes him a few seconds per consultation to record the data, and a secretary enters the data weekly into a ledger. Fry's analyses of these data led him to be more conservative in the use of antibiotics,[6] and his studies of emotional disorders, acute back pain, hay fever, and hypertension in his practice prompted changes in treatment of these patients.[7] This recording system allowed him to set down his long-term experience in following patients in family practice, and the disease index provided information that led to his book *Common Diseases*.[8]

William Cooper keeps an index of all his patients categorized by disease. "If I read an article that does not quite agree with my recollection of my clinical experience, I can use the index to review my patients and compare my experience with the author's view."

Warren Williams lists patients' names on cards under diagnoses so that he can pull those cards to study specific conditions. "Simply recording this information made me pay attention to details and ask certain questions that I had never before considered, such as: What is a 'problem?' What is worthy of being indexed? It was an intellectual process that had not been alive in me before. I use a simple indexing system that has worked very well, although it has limitations. I have about 600 5-by-8-inch filing cards in a box, each labeled with the name and code number of a disease, according to the *International Classification of Diseases, 9th Revision, Clinical Modification* (ICD 9CM). When I diagnose a patient's problem, I write it on a problem sheet. When the secretary transcribes my dictated notes, she looks at the problem sheet, and if the diagnosis does not have a check beside it, it means that the patient's name has not been entered in the cross-index file. She will then add that patient's name, address, and date of visit to the appropriate 5-by-8-inch diagnosis card, and put a check by the diagnosis on the problem sheet.

"Initially, the hardest part of this system was having to refer to the index book for code numbers. I kept a 'cheat sheet' on my desk, listing the code numbers of common problems, and after a few weeks, I had memorized most of those numbers. At one point, the receptionists decided, without consulting me, that they would no longer use code numbers, but would file alphabetically by diagnosis. That did not work, however, because of the multiple terms we use to mean the same thing. With my manual system, it is difficult to identify patients with certain multiple problems, such as hypertensive diabetics or depressed hypertensives. A computer could do it in a second, and this will probably push me into the computer world soon.

TABLE 1. Listing of patients by diagnosis. (Courtesy of Warren Williams, M.D.)

Patients with Depression*

311

Name	Phone	Name	Phone
Theresa White	(H) 740-3280	Mary Jones	(H) 841-3335
	(W) 740-0811		(W) 388-4000
Ted Carpenter	(H) 771-0651	Jane McKay	(H) 790-6611
	(W) 841-0101		(W) 850-8765
Kay Moore	(H) 388-3077	James Warren	(H) 773-3141
	(W) 771-8220		(W) 790-1188
Edward Clancy	(H) 773-9988	Melinda James	(H) 388-9674
	(W) 790-0001		(W) 771-2222
Helen Thomas	(H) 740-3292	David Hardy	(H) 850-3626
	(W) 771-5502		(W) 388-9191
Gloria Byrne	(H) 790-9871		
	(W) 388-6666		

*Fictitious names and numbers

"Indexing by problem and diagnosis is one way to get a practice profile. When I go to a meeting, I assign office tasks to my receptionists, such as counting the number of patients with a particular problem and listing them in tabular form (Table 1). In 1973 I returned from a cardiology meeting and found a completed practice profile on my desk. Aside from smoking and obesity, the most frequent diagnosis was depression. I then searched for cardiology, and found it to represent less than 1% of my patients. It dawned on me that this was a beautiful tool to define the postgraduate education I required. I had not attended a single psychiatric meeting or read a psychiatric journal, and yet depression was the most common problem I encountered. I realized that if I wanted to do the most for my patients, I had better enroll in some psychiatric programs. Until then, I had been concentrating on subjects I liked, and now I had a tool to point out a practical approach.

"Indexing by problem also helps identify patients taking specific drugs. For example, when tolbutamide was under scrutiny, I could determine which of my patients with diabetes mellitus were taking tolbutamide. Each Fall I call all my patients with chronic obstructive pulmonary disease and diabetes mellitus to come in for their flu shots. Every time I have called a patient unsolicited, I have received positive feedback.

"Once a month we close the office and call in a consultant for our own grand rounds. Using the diagnosis index, we assemble the records of patients with a specific problem and go through them with the consultant. We ask certain patients to be present for these sessions, and they love it. The whole staff participates, and as a result we have all changed our ways of doing things. I have learned, for example, how to use certain drugs more effectively. We also learned that we were not doing a satisfactory job in patient education, so we changed our methods.

"We always ask the consultant for a composite written report on the grand rounds, and we ask that it be constructively critical. Since we close the office for a half day and pay the consultant about $300, we lose income on that day, but this intellectual part of practice is both enjoyable and instructive. There should be time to make a living and a time to enjoy practice and learn. Anyway, it is far cheaper than going to a meeting that is not pertinent to your practice. The information gained in our grand rounds is 100% applicable to our practice, and the patients ultimately gain."

Keeping Statistics on Clinical Problems, Medications, and Laboratory Studies

The Need

Through extensive work in identifying educational needs in physicians' offices, S. E. Sivertson and Thomas Meyer found that the average physician really did not know what his practice constituted. Said Sivertson, "Early in our work, we asked some physicians to predict their practice profile. They were unable to do it accurately. They were so far off, in fact, that we could not use their predictions to help plan their continuing education. The physician frequently told the consultant 'This is the first time I have understood my practice and how my continuing education should be related to it.' In addition, older physicians would say, 'My practice and I are growing old together. I need to focus more on geriatrics.' "

Studies done in the past ten years by Robert C. Mendenhall, Director of the Medical Activities and Manpower Project at the University of Southern California, have focused on what happens in the physician's office with the different types of patients seen. "We did not specifically ask the physicians to estimate the prevalence of particular problems in their practice, but we have had considerable feedback indicating that they were surprised by the clinical mix," said Mendenhall. "For example, cardiologists and gastroenterologists have consistently been surprised by the large number of nonspecialty problems seen in their practices." In an experiment to see if feedback about ambulatory practice would influence the behavior of an internal medicine house staff, Reid and Lantz found that only 50 per cent of resident physicians could correctly guess the relative frequency of types of patients they saw.[9]

Jeremiah Barondes kept a detailed record of patient visits in his practice. "For three months I kept track of the reason for each patient's visit along with the diagnosis. In nearly a thousand office visits over three months there were only two instances of nephrologic disease and five of hematologic disease, whereas nearly 350 patients had cardiovascular disease.

There were relatively few gastrointestinal or infectious problems of major consequence." Every physician can profit from this type of study.

Aggregate data that permit analysis of the problems seen, drugs prescribed, and laboratory studies ordered facilitate the study of practice. If the physician also knows the costs he generates, the time he spends with patients, and the reasons for his consultation requests and hospital admissions, he can improve his practice management.

Recording the Data

One popular method of recording patient data is the E-book, a diagnostic index suitable for primary care morbidity enumeration. Named for Dr. T. S. Eimerl, who first devised this method of record-keeping, the E-book is a looseleaf notebook with overlapping 3-by-5-inch sheets.[10] After a patient visit, the physician records the patient's name, date of visit, date of birth, diagnostic code number, and referral information. He follows the same procedure for each episode of illness except for a chronic illness such as diabetes, which is entered only once. This information is then transferred onto index sheets corresponding to the diagnostic code numbers. Data may be entered manually or by computer.[11] Hiram Cury encourages his residents to use the E-book to classify their work and to use the classification to direct their continuing education. Other systems based on this principle have been described elsewhere.[12]

Using a recording system based on the E-book, Robert Moorhead, a general practitioner in New South Wales, devoted 20 minutes a day to collecting data on each patient visit for one year. He then compared his data with published studies of the practices of general practitioners and found striking similarities. He discovered many facts about his general workload, its geographic characteristics, patient age groups, and diseases commonly seen that were useful in teaching and formulating questions for further research. As a result, he was able to improve his practice management.[13]

For every patient visit, Thomas Inui uses a general medical encounter-form, which consists of two sheets to be completed by the physician. Pressure-sensitive paper attached to each sheet provides a duplicate page, for entry of the information in the computerized data base. The first page, on which is recorded patient-identifying information (age, sex, date of visit), problem seen, and visit notes, is placed in the medical record. The second page is a prescription, which the patient takes directly to the pharmacy. This page is kept by the pharmacy staff and is used to record refills issued. Drug information entered into the computer identifies the clinician by a number.

Amos Arnon has devised a hardbound notebook, *My Practice in My Pocket*, which fits into the resident's white-coat pocket.[14] It contains clinical information about the resident's patients and their families. Data can be arranged under demographics, problems and diagnoses, clinic visits, referrals, hospital admissions, pregnancies, well-baby care, contraceptive use, follow-up appointments, and chronic diseases.

Cumulative data such as this permit a description of practice activities, identification of patients with particular conditions for further study, description of patterns of laboratory test-ordering, and drug prescribing. From such cumulative data, the physician can analyze his practice and compare it to findings from similar practices, published reports, and local and national standards. He may find, perhaps with the help of a consultant, that he is diagnosing certain conditions more often, or less often, than other physicians are. Such a finding would not necessarily mean that the physician was at fault, but that he should re-evaluate the implicit or explicit diagnostic criteria he is using. If he finds that he is using certain drugs more, or less, than his peers, he may wish to learn more about these drugs, their indications, efficacy, side effects, and contraindications.

One must, of course, be careful not to overestimate the significance of small numbers. As Jeffrey Latts said, 125 patients with pneumonia treated with chloramphenicol without adverse effect may give the physician a false sense of security unless he realizes that serious marrow toxicity occurs with chloramphenicol only once in every 60,000 to 100,000 courses of therapy. The compilation of outcome figures, however, allows the physician to compare his results with larger series. We recommend this approach mainly to enhance understanding in practice and to give direction for future study.

Notation of Salient Clinical Problems

To facilitate learning from experience, some physicians keep cards on patients with certain problems, on which they make notations about unusual manifestations, the value of certain laboratory studies, the effect of treatments, and lessons learned, so their cumulative experience can be coordinated and reviewed. From an analysis of the patient data Paul Dudley White recorded on 4-by-6-inch cards, he was able to determine the frequency of rheumatic heart disease and hypertension, among other conditions, and this information formed the basis of his first book. (See essay by Willis Hurst, pp. 28–29.)

Norton Greenberger's note cards contain the patient's name, hospital number, and major diagnosis or problems. The diagnosis is also entered into a log book, so that if he wants to review the last two hundred patients he has seen with regional enteritis, he can do so. "If a patient has an interesting set of diagnoses that I need to read about, I will make a note to do that. About two or three days a week, I review my note cards and read on those selected subjects. I make the same kind of note cards when

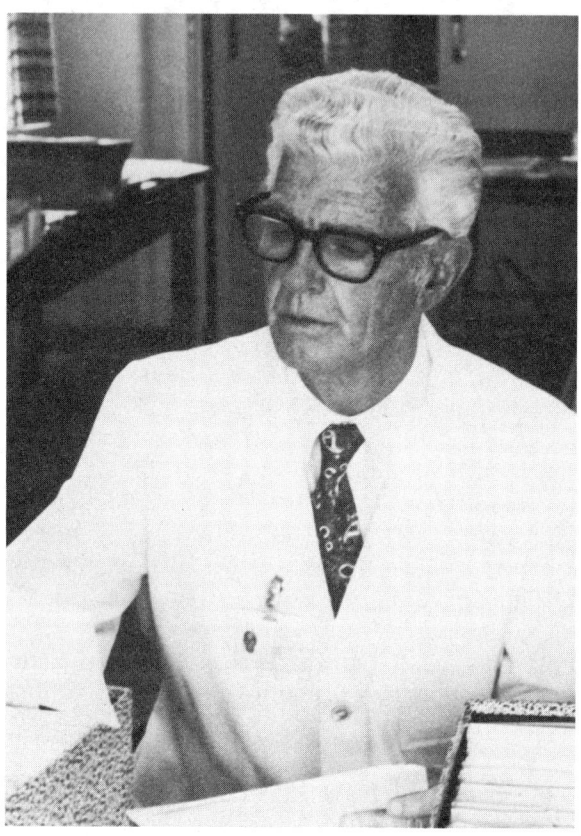

Any time a question comes up on a particular disease, we can pull out forty or fifty cards . . . they often answer a question quickly on the basis of our past few years' experience.

Telfer B. Reynolds, M.D.
Professor of Medicine
University of Southern California

10. Analysis of Practice

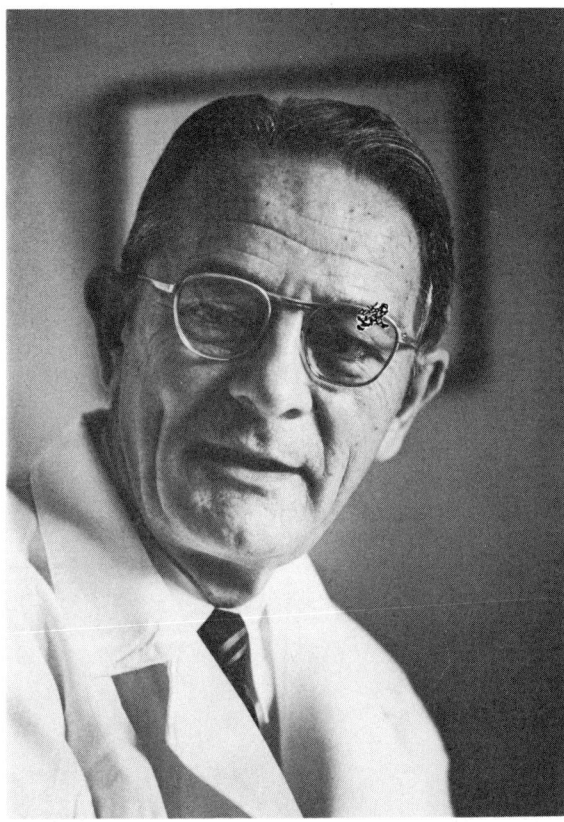

The most important function of a medical school is to make the student a self-educator.

Clarence J. Berne, M.D.
Emeritus Professor of Surgery
University of Southern California

I am in morning report. I also record in my book the name, hospital number, diagnosis, major problem, unusual clinical features, and medication. By surveying all my patients with acid peptic disease or pancreatic insufficiencies, I can see what medications I have prescribed."

Telfer Reynolds categorizes his cards by disease. "We have thousands of cards in the file, divided into two sets: one comprising the consultations made by residents on my service and the other the cases I have seen personally. Any time a question comes up on a particular disease, we can pull out forty or fifty cards and spend a half hour sorting them. It is not real research—you would have to go to the charts to get the full data—but they often answer a question quickly on the basis of our past few years' experience" (Figure 1).

John Romano has developed a similar system for psychiatric patients. "I keep index cards on hospital patients studied on teaching rounds. On a card is the name and age of the patient, the date of the meeting, diagnosis, and so on. I also dictate detailed summaries on patients studied on teaching rounds, recording the patient's story, my observations, interviews with the patient and family, conclusions, therapeutic programs, and so on. One copy is sent to the state hospital for the patient's record, and one is kept in my personal file. I use these files to identify a patient that I have seen before and to cluster diagnostic groups. If you want to study a population of patients, this is a good way to do it."

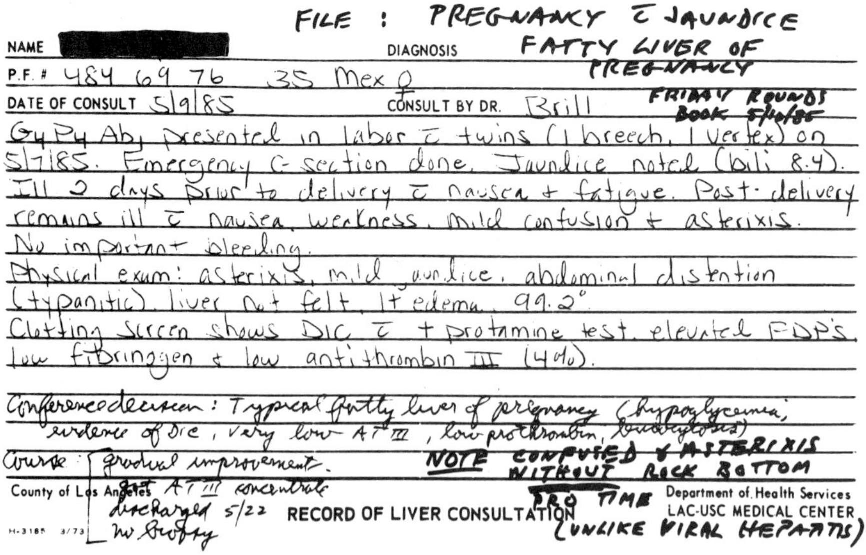

FIGURE 1. Patient card with significant clinical data, filed by diagnosis. (Courtesy of Telfer B. Reynolds, M.D.)

10. Analysis of Practice

A valuable asset in clinical practice, in the opinion of Walter Somerville, is a memory aid to assemble the physician's personal experience in specific diseases or procedures. "The data cards originated by Paul Wood (Figure 2) are designed to tabulate the main features of selected conditions or procedures. A comparison of this information in the aggregate with the reported experience of others leads to logical decision-making. For example, salient features of each candidate of percutaneous transluminal coronary angioplasty (PTCA) are annotated by hand. Time-consuming minutiae are left to the detailed case record. Within weeks, impressions emerge, eventually to be confirmed or discarded. Keeping records like this helps the physician draw on his entire experience rather than only the past few cases."

Notes on Experience

Since her medical student days, Celia Oakley has kept notes on what she learned during the day. "As a student, this was a considerable amount,

NO.	NAME	S. AGE	PLACE	AP	MI	EX	L Main	AD	CX	RC			E.C.G.	X RAY	PTCA Result
1	—	M/60	P	2	+	+	—	+	+	+			Ant M1	+	+
2	—	M/50	H	3	0	+	—	0	+	+			Inf MI	0	+
3	—	F/65	H	3	+	+	+	0	0	+			N	0	—
4															
5															
6															
7															
8															
9															
10															

Form No. M59B. PTCA

FIGURE 2. Card used by Walter Sommerville to tabulate clinical data on patients having percutaneous transluminal coronary angioplasty. Clinical data can be similarly tabulated for patients with clinical conditions of particular interest. AP, Angina pectoris; MI, Myocardial infarction; EX Test, Exercise test; L Main, Left main coronary artery; AD, Left anterior descending coronary artery; CX, Left circumflex coronary artery; RC, Right coronary artery.

but I had the time and the inclination to review what I had written. Now I am busier, but I still jot down the things that I learn each day."

Bruce Zawacki notes in his diary any problem that arises in the course of practice or during presentations, after which he looks up material for reading on the subject. Robert Smith carries with him a record of each patient he has operated on and notes if the operation was unusual in any way. "In this little book I also record my contacts with the referring physicians, to make sure that we keep a good exchange and that I dictate letters. I can get about six months' use out of one book. I carry the book with me everywhere except to the shower. With the pressure of all the administrative and patient-care duties I have, if I don't make notes and outline each day's schedule the evening before, I am apt to forget something. The diary has become my auxiliary brain. I really couldn't function without it. For our grand rounds or our weekly vascular conferences at Emory, it is also useful to look back through the book and select quickly a half-dozen interesting and unusual cases."

Learning from Mistakes

Osler advised physicians to record their mistakes: "Begin early to make a threefold category—clear cases, doubtful cases, mistakes. And learn to play the game fair, no self-deception, no shrinking from the truth; mercy and consideration for the other man, but none for yourself, upon whom you have to keep an incessant watch. . . . It is only by getting your cases grouped in this way that you can make any real progress in your post-collegiate education; only in this way can you gain wisdom with experience. It is a common error to think that the more a doctor sees the greater his experience and the more he knows."[15]

Jane Somerville considers her study of mistakes to be the single most useful exercise she has undertaken. John Fry also keeps a "black book" of mistakes in his drawer, adding to it periodically.

Auditing Patient Records

Audit of medical records is a major method of determining what goes on in the care of patients. Adversaries of the use of chart audit point out that medical records are often incomplete, that changes as a result of medical audit are due only to improved documentation, and that the actual care given patients does not change significantly. This is a weak argument. Documentation of care is necessary, since no one can remember all the details of a patient's history, physical examination, laboratory studies, and progress without proper notes. Since medical care without complete documentation is based on faulty data and guesswork, inadequate records cannot be justified.

Lawrence Weed identified four characteristics of chart audit: thoroughness, reliability, sound analytic sense, and efficiency. A former student of Lawrence Weed, Harold D. Cross, and his partner, Charles S. Burger, and associate, Ann Holland of Hampden, Maine, use three types of chart audits to study their practice for these characteristics: (1) patient audit, (2) technical or procedural audit, and (3) analytical audit.

Patient Audit

After the examination, patients receive a copy of their medical record, which is a problem-oriented narrative statement of each of their problems. They are asked to read this carefully for completeness, accuracy, and understanding and then to return the audit sheet with their comments, additions, and other corrections. About 35 per cent of patients comply. Dr. Cross believes that making patients partners in their health care by including them in the audit improves accuracy of patient data and patient cooperation and may reduce the threat of malpractice.

Technical or Procedural Audit

The procedural audit is a check on the completeness of the record. The typist who transcribes the physician's notes also reviews the medical record for completeness by comparing the data assembled with the information defined in advance as a minimal data base for a comprehensive health evaluation. The physician is informed in writing of any omissions. A nurse or staff member then reviews the record to verify that the physician has responded appropriately to any omission noted by the clinical staff.

Analytical Audit

Once a month five charts of each physician are pulled in random fashion and audited by one of the other physicians for analytic sense and efficiency. After a twenty-four-hour "cooling-off period," the physician being audited responds to the audit point by point, either justifying the medical action or indicating how he will correct any deficiency. If differences between the physicians continue, both will consult publications to validate or update their knowledge and views.

Tracing and Reacting to Outcomes

Without a specific mechanism for follow-up, physicians are often unaware of the therapeutic results in their patients. In this sense, they know less about their practice and their performance than a football coach knows about the performance of his players and their opponents. "Without statistics, we would be unable to maintain a high level of performance," said Tom Landry, Head Coach of the Dallas Cowboys. "We use a quality control system to monitor our football team, that is, we set guidelines for our individual player's performance as well as for our team performance. Our quality-control coach accumulates all the data and alerts the staff when performance levels are below guidelines. We are then able to make adjustments to prevent possible losses in future games. Our most vivid results come when we fall into a slump late in the season. We then concentrate on weaknesses and apply proper adjustments. This usually corrects the weaknesses and returns us to the winning path. Without statistics, however, we would not be able to identify the problems."

Coach Joseph Paterno of Pennsylvania State University also finds that recording and analyzing data are invaluable. "We do not practice without a doctor on the field. He records in a diary everything that happens at each practice. We keep a record of the temperature, the type of drills, the number of injuries, and so on. We can tell if more injuries occur when we scrimmage two days in a row or when we have a one- or two-day break between scrimmages. If we are having more sprained ankles than usual, we can review our records and compare the current year with past seasons. Statistics help us keep our team healthy. I use medical statistics to make determinations about equipment, style of practice, type of drills, and when not to practice.

"We also use statistics on the performance of other teams to determine their tendencies and therefore our best strategy in certain field positions and at certain downs. We are constantly reviewing our computer kick-out for a better evaluation of the other team."

Medicine is admittedly more complicated than athletic enterprises, but the analogy points up the value of analyzing one's performance. Once problems are identified, solutions can be sought. A study of results requires a routine method of tracing patient outcomes.

E. A. Codman was a strong advocate of the "End Result System." "In brief," he wrote in 1918, "it is this: That the Trustees of Hospitals should see to it that an effort is made to follow up each patient [the staff treats], long enough to determine whether the treatment given has permanently relieved the condition or symptoms complained of. That they should give the members of the Staff credit for taking the responsibility of successful treatment and promote them accordingly. Likewise they should see that

10. Analysis of Practice

all cases in which the treatment is found to have been unsuccessful or unsatisfactory are carefully analyzed, in order to fix the responsibility for failure on:
1. The physician or surgeon responsible for the treatment.
2. The organization carrying out the detail of the treatment.
3. The disease or condition of the patient.
4. The personal or social conditions preventing the cooperation of the patient.

This will give a definite basis on which to make effort at improvement. . . .

"The Idea is so simple as to seem childlike. . . . It is simply to follow the natural series of questions which any one asks in an individual case:
What was the matter?
Did they find it out beforehand?
Did the patient get entirely well?
If not—why not?
Was it the fault of the surgeon, the disease, or the patient?
What can we do to prevent similar failures in the future?

"We believe that the general acceptance of a system of hospital organization based on the truthful record of the answers to these questions means the beginning of True Clinical Science."[16]

Many surgeons send questionnaires to their patients at intervals of three, six, or twelve months to determine the success or limitations of their procedures. Michael DeBakey writes his patients or the referring physicians at regular intervals to inquire about their progress. From his analysis of results so obtained, he has been able not only to monitor his clinical experience continually, but to recognize certain patterns of disease that have led him to devise new surgical treatments, such as excision of aneurysms, coronary artery bypass, and others.

Richard Treiman follows every patient with use of a large accountant's sheet with about twenty items across the page. "In the first seven columns I record the date of the operation; the patient's name, sex, and age; the indication; the operation; and the graft and suture material used. I record the patient's cardiac history and note the presence or absence of hypertension, diabetes, or chronic obstructive pulmonary disease. I also record any postoperative complications, the result of the operation, and, when the patient returns, follow-up observations. I have coded some of the cases according to whether the patient had angiograms or carotid surgery. In addition, I keep track of every operation I do by recording in my little operative book the date and patient's name, as well as the names of my interesting nonsurgical patients. A surgeon has to know the results he gets, and his records are therefore important."

Bruce Zawacki maintains an alphabetized file of operative notes, supplemented with review articles on new techniques. "Before performing a procedure not done regularly, I use this file to review my experience and the articles I have collected. I also often present a particularly difficult preoperative case at a regular medical school conference. At our monthly mortality and morbidity conference, invited guests critique our approach, and we review any untoward events. We identify problems, plan solutions, and assign certain physicians to implement those solutions. Yearly, we have an outcome review, in which our current mortality and morbidity data are compared to those of all previous years for possible trends."

Gustavo Kuster sends every surgical patient a follow-up letter or questionnaire six months after the operation and every year thereafter. "I have about twenty different kinds of questionnaires, coded according to the operative procedure. These questionnaires allow me to be precise in answering questions about our operations and to improve my patient care. Through the questionnaires, for example, I found that in repair of hiatal hernia, it was postoperative bloating that made the patients most unhappy. I reviewed this technique more carefully, visited other medical institutions, and then modified my techniques slightly by making the fundal plication extremely loose around the esophagus. That practically eliminated the unpleasant side effects of the procedure."

The outcome of medical treatment may be more difficult to measure because it is usually more protracted and less well circumscribed than surgical procedures. Nevertheless, valuable data may be obtained. Alvin Mushlin conducted an outcome study in which the central measure was the patient's own report of his symptoms, activity limitation, and anxiety. He sent follow-up questionnaires to a sample of patients with upper respiratory infections, sore throats, and urinary tract infections. For 57 per cent of the patients with unsatisfactory outcomes, a review of medical records indicated definite errors in treatment, including missed or delayed diagnoses, unrecognized complications, and treatment administered without adequate indication. For patients with acceptable outcomes, on the other hand, definite errors were found in only three per cent.[17]

"To understand your practice," Mushlin explained, "you cannot review only specific diseases seen; you must look at the problems also—the complaints, signs, and symptoms, and their impact on the patient. For this purpose, an index by problem as well as by patient name is invaluable. What you are interested in is whether, for example, you incorrectly diagnose 20 per cent of your patients with coughs as having pneumonia or whether you missed, and left untreated, 15 per cent of the patients with bacterial pneumonitis who needed antibiotics. We index by problem (complaints, symptoms, and signs), and then devise fairly simple goals for treating that category of illness. We try to define how the disease affects patients and, most important, at what period we would like to see significant improvements. We have short questionnaires that are easily administered over the telephone to discover patient outcomes. To understand the disease completely, you must try to understand the reasons for the poor outcomes. Some of these can be uncovered by looking back at the medical records, but to get the most out of the study, you have to re-evaluate some of the patients with poor results. You must keep track of the data because patterns emerge only with an accumulation of cases.

"We found, for example, that many patients had prolonged respiratory tract illnesses from overuse of antihistamines. On the other hand, we saw people who came in with upper respiratory tract infections, but who, in fact, had bacterial infections with ample clues for their early detection. This highlighted the pitfalls of a relatively cursory look at patients with upper respiratory tract infections.

"The most important point is to have systematic follow-ups on patients. Questions should be asked about efficacy, adequacy of follow-up, and patient participation in follow-up. These are challenging issues in primary care, but the most challenging are in diagnosis—following up undifferentiated problems and complaints of patients and deciding which ones need further attention. The only way to do this is to look first at the problems, not the diagnosis. When you see patients with a cough, you must determine whether it is caused by a postnasal drip or by *Mycoplasma pneumoniae*. To determine if your diagnosis is correct, you need follow-up data."

*****

To profit the most from experience, physicians must know what their practice consists of and what results they obtain. The methods of study outlined in this section are, unfortunately, used by relatively few physicians. The potential dividends in improved patient care and physician satisfaction, however, are great and well worth the investment of time in practice analysis. To be most useful, the physician's experience should be compared with that of others as reported in publications, at meetings, and in discussions with colleagues.

We suggest that physicians not now involved in analysis of their practices consider establishing a simple method of indexing patient charts by problem or diagnosis and periodically review the charts with a respected colleague to discuss diagnostic approaches and therapeutic plans for specific common conditions, such as hypertension. In addition, physicians can profit from keeping simple notations on cards, like those designed by Paul Wood, on one or two conditions or procedures that interest them. The "black book of mistakes" described by John Fry is also simple, not time-consuming, and helpful in reinforcing lessons learned. With a data base defined by the physician, the office typist can conduct a procedural audit. Moreover, several physicians can cooperate in an analytic audit of one another's charts, with any disputes solved by a review of authoritative publications. The creation of a detailed profile of experience, including problems seen, drugs prescribed, and studies ordered, will be facilitated when the computer becomes a part of every medical office.

References

1. Latham, Peter Mere. General remarks on the practice of medicine. In: Martin, Robert, ed. *The Collected Works of Dr. P. M. Latham.* London: The New Sydenham Society, 1878:466.
2. Budd, William. *Typhoid Fever. Its Nature, Mode of Spreading, and Prevention.* New York: George Grady Press, 1931. Reprint of 1874 original.
3. Pickles, William Norman. *Epidemiology in Country Practice.* Baltimore: The Williams and Wilkins Company, 1939:9.
4. Mackenzie, Sir James. *Principles of Diagnosis and Treatment in Heart Affections.* London: Joint Committee of Henry Frowde and Hodder and Stoughton, Oxford University Press, 1916:1-2.
5. Wilson, R. McNair. *The Beloved Physician: Sir James Mackenzie.* New York: The Macmillan Company, 1926:51-52.
6. Fry, John. Information for patient care in office-based practice. *Med Care* Apr 1973;11(Suppl 2):35-40.
7. Fry, John. On the natural history of some common diseases. *J Fam Pract* Oct 1975;2(5):327-331.
8. Fry, John. *Common Diseases: Their Nature Incidence and Care.* Ridgewood, New Jersey: George A. Bogden & Son, Inc Publishers, 1983.
9. Reid, Robert A.; Lantz, K. Holley. Physician profiles in training the graduate internist. *J Med Educ* Apr 1977;52(4):301-307.
10. Eimerl, T. S.; Laidlaw, A. J. *A Handbook for Research in General Practice*, 2d ed. Edinburgh and London: E. & S. Livingstone Ltd., 1969.
11. Froom, Jack; Culpepper, Larry; Boisseau, Vincenza. An integrated medical record and data system for primary care. Part 3: The diagnostic index manual and computer methods and applications. *J Fam Pract* Jul 1977;5(1):113-120.
12. Baker, Collin; Schilder, Marvin. The "E-box": An inexpensive modification of diagnostic indexing. *J Fam Pract* Apr 1976;3(2):189-191.
13. Moorhead, Robert. A general practitioner's study of his own workload and patient morbidity. *Med J Aust* 26 Jul 1975;2(4):140-145.
14. Arnon, Amos. *My Practice in My Pocket.* Charleston: Medical University of Southern Carolina, 1978.
15. Osler, William. The student life. A farewell address to Canadian and American medical students. *The Medical News* 30 Sep 1905;87(14):629-630.

16. Codman, E. A. *A Study in Hospital Efficiency: As Demonstrated by the Case Report of the First Five Years of a Private Hospital.* Boston: Thomas Todd Co., 1918:8-9.
17. Mushlin, Alvin I.; Appel, Francis A.; Barr, Daniel M. Quality assurance in primary care: A strategy based on outcome assessment. *J Community Health* Summer 1978;3(4):292-305.

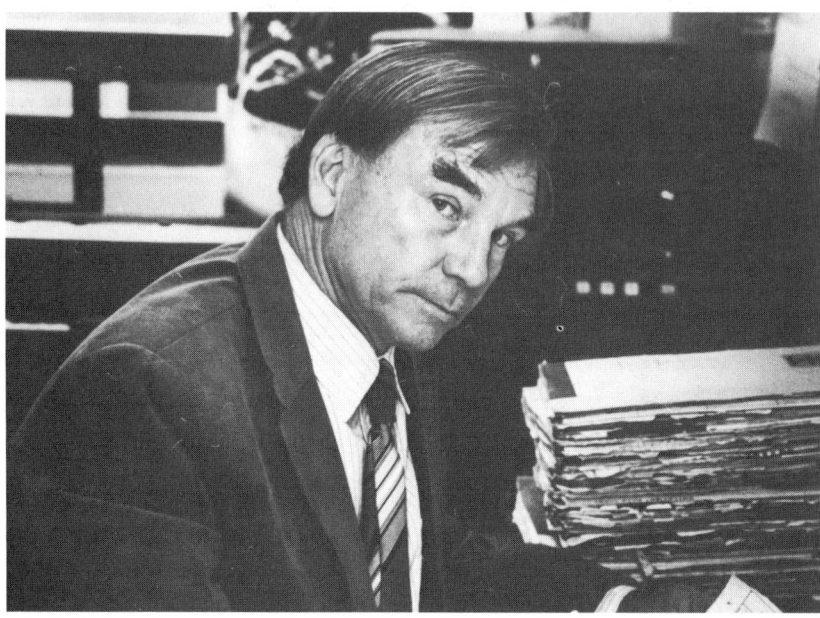

An impeccably constructed record should be educational for both the recorder and the users of the record, should encourage preservation of basic clinical skills, and should be a model for medical students.

Ian R. Mackay, M.D.

Dr. Mackay's early research in plasma protein abnormalities led to his interest in autoimmunity and autoimmune disease. He was instrumental in developing the concept of autoimmunity in liver disease and collaborated with Sir Macfarlane Burnet on a monograph, *Autoimmune Diseases*. Subsequent research interests included immunological aspects of demyelinating diseases, aging, and cancer. Current research activities include investigation of pathogenesis of different types of chronic hepatitis and their treatment, immunogenetics of autoimmune disorders, immunology of multiple sclerosis, and the immune response to cancer, particularly melanoma. His lifelong interest in competent medical-record-keeping is exemplified by the development within his research unit of a problem-oriented medical data base, useful not only for clinical care but also for medical research. A former Chairman of the Medical Staff Association of the Royal Melbourne Hospital, Dr. Mackay is the Australian representative on the Clinical Immunology Committee of the International Union of Immunological Societies. His bibliography includes more than 300 published papers and two monographs.

Dr. Ian R. Mackay, a world leader in autoimmune diseases, was the first person to recognize clearly that autoimmunity was a central component in some forms of chronic liver disease. His penetrating analytical skills have helped him identify

Personal Essay

Ian R. Mackay, M.D.
Head, Clinical Research Unit
The Walter and Eliza Hall Institute of Medical Research
and Royal Melbourne Hospital
Parkville, Victoria, Australia

The Standard Medical Record—
Perusal Is usually not an Educational Experience

The medical record, although central to medical communication within hospitals, is an unloved document that generally lacks intrinsic teaching value. Because the clinical data base is generated under pressure, legibility declines; as the data increase, their organization becomes more haphazard, and the rationale for critical management decisions, because often transmitted verbally, may be unrecorded and so not amenable to audit. Weed's comments[1] in 1969 hold true today: "There is in existence at the present time no body of literature on how to structure the medical record, particularly progress notes on long-term problems, and so there is no framework within which discipline can develop." Weed contended: "The medical record must completely and honestly convey the many variables and complexities that surround every decision. . . [and] must faithfully represent events and decisions so that errors can be detected and proper corrective measures taken when lapses in thoroughness, disciplined thought, and reasonable follow-up occur." Perhaps Weed was overoptimistic when he viewed the medical record as "the natural extension of the

---

the central core of a problem with great rapidity and depth. His capacity for lateral thinking, sharpened, no doubt, through his close collaboration with Sir Macfarlane Burnet for more than a decade, helped him to make the mental leap required for an entirely new look at aetiology of disease. Ian Mackay's mind is very organized; all his work is beautifully documented, his clinical records largely computerized, the administrative decisions recorded and filed, and this great organizing ability has rubbed off on many of Mackay's juniors, who have uniformly benefited and mainly gone on to stellar careers of their own. Ian Mackay is an intensely loyal person; his loyalty to his institution and to his director has been an enormous source of strength. Ian Mackay is also a compassionate person. This has been of signal benefit to his many patients, many of whom have chronic diseases that require interaction with physicians for years, and a holistic human understanding of the patients' problems. The compassion is also noteworthy when junior colleagues fall into personal or professional difficulties. They will have no stronger advocate than Ian Mackay.

Sir Gustav Nossal, M.D.

basic science training of the physician; in short, it must be a scientific manuscript."

Understandably, the educational value of a medical record, provided it is legible and organized, will depend on the medical knowledge of the writer; even for mature clinicians, this still represents only a small proportion of what might become known. Aware of this discrepancy, the physician tends to be guarded in drawing conclusions or interpretations from the clinical data available or tends to leave implicit what should be explicit. He may not, or perhaps cannot, specify the rationale for various decisions and actions. If the reader of the record cannot decide whether decisions were made on the basis of authentic data, sound experience, or hunches, his learning from the record becomes prejudiced.

How Medical Records Can Contribute to Education

The medical record can contribute to education in the hospital in several ways by encouraging a commitment to quality, organized structure, informative consultations, problem-solving, and decision analysis.

Commitment to Quality

A commitment to quality implies a systematic thoroughness in the construction of the clinical data base. According to Wilbush,[2] this should include data presented by the patient, data elicited by direct interrogation of the patient, and data derived from physical examination. An impeccably constructed record should be educational for both the recorder and the users of the record, should encourage preservation of basic clinical skills, and should be a model for medical students.

Organized Structure

Complex medical cases should be educational, but as the amount of recorded data increases, the less attractive the clinical record becomes as a learning document. Computers may overcome the bulk, but so far electronic records have made little impact on their organization.

Appropriate application of the three orientations used in the construction of medical records makes them more effective and educational. First is the traditional *time orientation*, that is, chronologic order of accession from the first contact with the patient. Second, and now increasingly used, is *data orientation*, that is, accumulation of similar data in one place in the record, exemplified by flow-sheets from biochemistry and hematology laboratories. Such organization permits the physician to review changes with time in laboratory data from radiology, nucleide scanning, electrocardiography, and histopathology and to relate them to clinical changes. Third is *problem orientation*, for which there is still no consensus on optimal implementation,[3] nor objective evidence of patient improvement.[4] Problem orientation requires not merely a "signposting" of data in the record, but a synthesis of all available data into possible decisions based on rigorous clinical logic. The problem-oriented record should generate incentives to consult authoritative texts or mentors to produce optimal clinical decisions.

Problem Orientation

The problem-oriented medical synopsis (POMS) was developed in Melbourne in 1970[5] as an extension of Weed's principle of a problem-oriented record, with aims of improving patient care, providing better educational uses of the medical record, facilitating communication among health-care professionals, allowing for ready audit of medical activity, and setting the stage for computerized records.

The major features of the POMS are that a problem list is constructed on a specially designed form on the patient's admission to hospital; this problem list is validated by appropriately summarized data from symptoms, signs, or laboratory reports, and these data are aligned on the POMS form alongside each specified problem. No problem can be specified without substantiation by clinical evidence, and no symptom, abnormal sign, or laboratory test can stand without a problem attached. Thereafter, all investigations, consultations, and treatments are entered into a POMS form, aligned to the relevant problem. The POMS is continually updated and amended, as necessary; existing problems become substantiated diagnoses and new problems are coded and elucidated as they develop. On discharge of the patient, the POMS form goes to a typist-clerk as the basis of a problem-oriented discharge summary.

Because POMS is a document added to the conventional "archival" medical record, its construction is viewed negatively as labor-intensive—more "paperwork." Since the POMS requires totally explicit medical documentation, however, it has decided advantages. It has great potential for teaching students the background of medical decision-making, particularly in providing insight into the balance of "documented knowledge" and "experienced intuition", in creating diagnoses, in selecting investigations, in prescribing treatment, and in conducting audit. The POMS form is handled with widely varying degrees of expertise by interns and residents, satisfactorily by informed medical staff and perfunctorily by those who dislike "paperwork," those who dislike exposing their opinions to scrutiny, or those who cannot adapt to the demanding and quality-controlled climate of contemporary medicine.

Informative Consultations

However records are organized, the opinion of the expert consultant will always represent an important educational component, even though the consultant's oral opinion may have more value than what he writes in the record. The old-fashioned consultation, based on a personally performed and recorded full history and examination, is now seldom seen in medical records. Nevertheless, specialty consultations (neurology, cardiology) should include details of history and examination relevant to the specialty and should show how conclusions can be derived from these data. Such information encourages users of the record to assimilate the skills of the expert consultant.

Unfortunately, time constraints may preclude the general availability in hospitals of opinions from chief consultants, responsibility being passed down the line to subordinates or fellows. Consultant activity is thus seen to have as much educational value for those giving as those receiving the consultation. Recommendations for effective consultations have been described by Goldman, Lee, and Rudd.[6] Automated consultations, through computerized medical data banks such as the PROMIS system, will undoubtedly become common before long.

Problem-solving and Decision-analyses

The extent to which clinical records should reflect medical problem-solving is uncertain. The record specifies the decision, but seldom indicates how the decision was reached. I do not suggest that the average medical record should include examples of Bayseian diagnostic analysis, decision-trees, or probability estimates of "profit and loss" outcomes from therapeutic options, notwithstanding their educational value. Medical problem-solving and decision-analysis, however, are legitimate subjects of academic inquiry,[7] and the medical record should make such studies feasible, when needed. It remains to be seen whether technology will hinder this process by information overload or facilitate it by use of microcomputers.

References

1. Weed, Lawrence L. *Medical Records, Medical Education, and Patient Care: The Problem-oriented Record as a Basic Tool.* Chicago: Year Book Medical Publishers, 1971:vi-vii.
2. Wilbush, Joel. Clinical information—signs, semeions and symptoms: discussion paper. *J Roy Soc Med* Sep 1984;77(9):766-773.
3. Goldfinger, Stephen E. The problem-oriented record: a critique from a believer. *N Engl J Med* Mar 22 1973;288(12):606-608.
4. Fletcher, Robert H. Auditing problem-oriented records and traditional records: A controlled comparison of speed, accuracy and identification of errors in medical care. *N Engl J Med* Apr 11 1974;290(15):829-833.

5. Gledhill, V. X.; Mackay, I. R.; Mathews, J. D.; Strickland, R. G.; Stevens, D. P.; Thompson, C. D. The problem-oriented medical synopsis: applications to patient care, education, and research. *Ann Intern Med* May 1973;78(5):685-691.
6. Goldman, Lee; Lee, Thomas; Rudd, Peter. Ten Commandments for effective consultations. *Arch Intern Med* Sep 1983;143(9):1753-1755.
7. Elstein, Arthur S.; Shulman, Lee S.; Sprafka, Sarah A. *Medical Problem Solving: An Analysis of Clinical Reasoning.* Cambridge, Massachusetts: Harvard University Press, 1978.

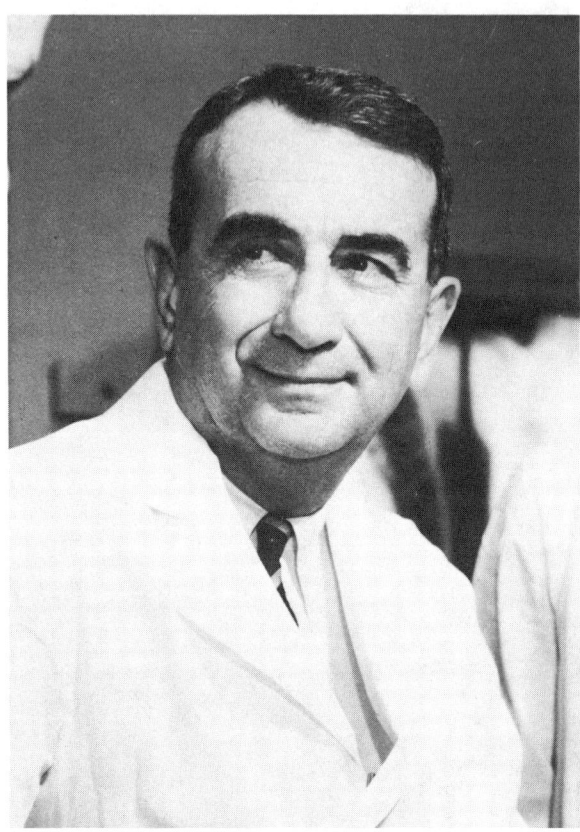

You can learn a great deal from your own cases if you share your experiences with others.

A. McGehee Harvey, M.D.

Dr. A. McGehee Harvey, Distinguished Service Professor of Medicine at The Johns Hopkins University School of Medicine, has long been a leader in medical circles, having served as President of the Association of American Physicians and the American Clinical and Climatological Association. Recipient of the Kober Medal from the Association of American Physicians, the Distinguished Teacher Award from the American College of Physicians, and the Robert H. Williams Award from the Association of Professors of Medicine, Dr. Harvey recently relinquished the editorship of *Medicine* after twenty-five years of distinguished editorial service. He is editor of *The Principles and Practice of Medicine* and author of *Differential Diagnosis* and various other books relating to the history of medicine. His major research contributions have concerned systemic lupus erythematosus and myasthenia gravis.

Personal Essay

A. McGehee Harvey, M.D.
Distinguished Service Professor of Medicine
The Johns Hopkins University School of Medicine
Baltimore, Maryland

To be a good physician, you have to make medicine your number one priority. You cannot enter medicine with the soul of a moneychanger. You must love it and must develop your own expertise through creative scholarship. That ideal alone will make you an outstanding physician. It is a matter of developing the habit of learning so that it becomes second nature and not something you turn on and off at certain times. If you can keep your curiosity about medicine alive, it will sustain you when you are in the middle of a difficult problem.

Personal Responsibility for Learning

Education must be pursued actively, not through the passive receipt of information distilled by someone else. I require all students, during their medical quarter, to choose a clinical problem that has no ready answer but for which an answer is possible by examination of patient records or by review of the literature. At the end of the quarter, they present the results of their studies to their classmates. This exercise establishes education as primarily the student's responsibility. One can motivate the student to make the most of his experience by adding to it the experience of others, as recorded in the literature or in other medical records. That principle was enunciated by William Henry Welch and later became a precept of the Western Reserve experiment in the mid-1950s.

When a physician goes into practice, he becomes a member of the medical community. If each physician presented his experiences on a particular subject to his colleagues at a local medical meeting, physicians would

---

A. M. Harvey brings to bedside teaching a profound understanding of human form and function in health in an astonishingly diverse array of pathological conditions. To understand such vast, up-to-date learning in an unpretentious, soft-spoken scholar steeped in history, literature, and the lore of baseball is to find a central aspect of Dr. Harvey's character: a lifelong, unquenchable thirst for knowledge. Dr. Harvey also brings to differential diagnosis a blend of sagacious empiricism and the scientific method, a combination that reflects a second great feature of his motivation: an abiding devotion to the dispassionate exercise of logic and reason.

Sherman M. Mellinkoff, M.D.

have a continuing flow of information, which would not only improve their medical care but would constantly emphasize the need to keep abreast of new knowledge. Special courses are important, but what you get out of them is governed largely by your motivation and the time and effort you invest in them.

Making self-education a habit—a part of your routine activities—is important. The foremost principle is that no one else is going to provide your continuing education; you must do it yourself. One way to do this is to select certain key journals for regular review. Another is discussions with colleagues, whether at lunch or at other times. You can learn a great deal from your own cases if you share your experiences with others.

Puzzling Cases

We used to keep a puzzling-case book and a mistake book at our weekly resident rounds. It was surprising how often another case would later come along about which you could learn something by referring to the previous one. By presenting your mistakes to your colleagues for discussion, you can often find out why you made the mistake and you can avoid a repetition of it.

Medicine is an exercise in problem-solving, and the same basic techniques used in the scientific laboratory to approach an unknown are applicable to the solving of clinical problems. In differential diagnosis, you have to gather information systematically from the moment the patient enters the room. You can get ideas each step of the way, and those, in turn, will create new questions to be answered.

Most important for students to understand is that they must remain curious, alert, and eager for new information. Learning to organize, assess, and transmit information clearly to consultants is a distinct advantage. A teacher can provide motivation and an environment for learning, but it is still up to the student to be an *active* learner.

11

Enlisting Help in the Analysis of Practice

> Nothing is so difficult to deal with as a man's own Experience, how to value it according to its amount, what to conclude from it, and how to use it and do good with it.
>
> *Peter Mere Latham*[1]

Most people find it threatening to have their work reviewed. For professionals, the threat may be real, since society often judges their shortcomings harshly and may devise regulatory, even punitive, solutions. A few physicians may, indeed, require regulatory sanctions, and all can benefit from reminders of their errors of omission and commission. Careful, constructive analysis of events in practice can motivate physicians to continue their education, whereas draconian penalties may drive some underground. The data on their practices then become unreliable, and their opportunity to profit from experience is lost. We distinguish clearly between formal external quality-assurance mechanisms and the improvement in medical practice that ensues from a well-motivated physician's voluntary analysis of his practice.

We explore here some of the methods by which medical organizations, consultants, or peers may "coach" physicians. Although some of the techniques were designed for external quality assurance, they may also uncover educational deficits through the self-study of practice. Most of the methods are still developmental; some are cumbersome; and all need to be refined before they are put in general use. We present these descriptions to give physicians a background for judging methods that may evolve. Physicians who do not wish to spend time designing methods to analyze their practice may wish to employ a consultant for this purpose. Although qualified consultants are difficult to find today, ultimately medical societies and medical schools will probably provide such consultations for physicians.

William Felch lists the following information to be expected from a consultation on practice analysis: (1) a practice-profile, which outlines the kinds of patients seen (by demography and diagnosis); (2) a summary of the quality of care provided to patients and, when possible, its comparison with that of others insofar as drugs prescribed, tests ordered, and diagnoses made; (3) a list of deficiencies or performance gaps; and (4) suggestions for their correction, presented as educational objectives. A second assessment some time later will determine whether performance has improved.

Specific Programs

Individual Physician Profile

Several experimental continuing education projects have been tailored to practice profiles. Sivertson and Meyer's Individual Physician Profile[2] was derived from information that physicians dictated into a tape recorder after each patient evaluation, including initial symptoms, notable findings, major diagnoses, diagnostic tests ordered, and disposition. Thereafter, the participating physicians were given a knowledge-test of 125 questions derived from the profile and had an interview with an educational consultant from the medical school. Together, the physician and consultant reviewed the practice profile and test results, after which they developed a study program to meet the physician's specific needs identified.

Practice-related Educational Program

Under the auspices of the College of Physicians of Philadelphia, Bowler and associates devised a Practice-Related Educational Program (PREP) similar to the Individual Physician Profile except that the profile was derived from data that the physician recorded on an abstract form rather than into a tape recorder.[3] On the basis of the resultant practice profile, the physician took a self-assessment test in the clinical subjects most often encountered in his practice. If his score indicated weaknesses, the physician selected self-instructional materials from those compiled by the program staff on the subjects of his weaknesses, or he was offered help in finding appropriate courses. After having studied these materials, the physician took another test to determine his progress in that subject.

In a feasibility study of primary care physicians from an urban area and a rural area, post-test scores for both groups increased significantly over pre-test scores. In the post-program subjective evaluation, only one physician gave a negative rating on the overall evaluation of the program.

Although Bowler considered the concept of PREP to be sound, it was not financially feasible. "The attempt to cover the entire field of primary care was too ambitious, requiring a great amount of self-instructional material. With the new copyright law of 1978, it became too expensive to stock the learning materials needed. Furthermore, too much effort and money went into (1) the development of the pre- and post-tests for each of the thirteen problem subjects in primary care (2,600 test items having been finally approved) and (2) the equivalency and validation studies of these tests."

External Analyses

In an unpublished report of a Connecticut ambulatory care study in 1973, Daniel Hamaty demonstrated the feasibility of external analysis of office practice, in which medical-record technicians developed practice profiles from 100 to 200 charts randomly selected from patient files. With the help of a project physician, the participating physician drew up diagnostic, therapeutic, preventive, or rehabilitative criteria that could be determined from the medical records. The participating physician then agreed to acceptable standards for each criterion. The development of the criteria and standards was itself considered educationally beneficial, but the physician's performance was judged by his conformity to criteria established by external chart audit.

Some years ago, with the concurrence of the Hawaii Medical Association and the Hawaii Hospital Association, Beverly Payne introduced an experimental design for objective measurement of the quality of medical care and its ultimate improvement. Explicit standards of performance were developed. Twenty-two clinical conditions were chosen from medical, surgical, and gynecological-obstetrical practice. Data from the medical records were collected from 22 Hawaiian hospitals, as well as from the office records of the participating physicians. Performance was judged by standards established in advance, and scores reflecting the degree of conformity to those standards were recorded.

Thereafter, representative physicians, administrators, trustees, and nurses from four of the participating hospitals were invited to a series of seminars, in which they were asked to study the data collected from their hospitals and physician-staffs. The experience was startling. Identification of specific deficiencies led to plans for improvement, and scores five months later disclosed minor, but positive, changes in performance. The investigators were later to find that notable behavioral change requires more time. In a similar study in Michigan about five years later, improved performance over a ten-month period approached a full standard deviation in the scores. In Michigan, as in Hawaii, physicians readily accepted this effort to improve medical care.

Private Initiative in Quality Assurance

William Felch and Paul Sanazaro tested the feasibility of measuring internists' performance in the Private Initiative in Quality Assurance (PIQuA). Assessment included: (1) objective substantiation of diagnosis, (2) identification of severity and risk factors, (3) validated medical treatment, (4) monitoring of treatment, and (5) patient response to treatment. Trained observers abstracted patient records in hospitals and physicians' offices and telephoned patients to ascertain their status and satisfaction with care. Peer reviewers examined the data and rated the physician on conformity to the current national standards of internal medicine. Deficiencies in performance identified by this method can be considered educational needs. Research by the American Society of Internal Medicine Assessment of Performance (ASPERF) has also explored audit techniques similar to those of PIQuA.

American Board of Family Practice Office Record Review

Part of the recertification process of the American Board of Family Practice is an office record review. Nicholas Pisacano described the program thus: "The physician selects the condition or activity to be studied from 20 chronic conditions, such as diabetes, coronary artery disease, chronic heart failure, depression, normal pregnancy, well-baby workups, or geriatric care, each of which requires long-term management. If the physician selects diabetes, for example, he must review several patient charts to answer an extensive questionnaire on diabetes management for each patient. The most important segment of the data sheet concerns the continuity of care. The questions were devised by a committee of experts who developed acceptable criteria for the history and diagnostic studies.

"The physician's answers are compared to the national norm of all other participating physicians who selected the same disease category. When we return the results to the physician, we include tutorial feedback for problems that have been identified, in the form of statements prepared by the committee with appropriate citations from a reference guide. When oral hypoglycemic agents are used, for example, the physician is cautioned about prescribing other drugs that can adversely alter the effect of the oral agent."

> Example:
>
> Tricyclic antidepressants should be prescibed with caution as they have been shown to have a variable effect on blood glucose levels and to increase the risk of hypoglycemia.[4]
>
> Example:
>
> In the past, some physicians have used the two-hour postprandial glucose determination. However, the FPG is now accepted as a more reliable test in establishing the diagnosis.
>
> The National Diabetes Data Group of the NIH recommends the use of fasting plasma glucose levels for diagnosing Diabetes Mellitus. The Data Group further recommends that the OGTT be

restricted to two groups: non-pregnant adults with hyperglycemia but in whom FPG levels were equivocal (i.e., less than 140 mg/dl) and hyperglycemic pregnant females with no previous diagnosis of Diabetes Mellitus.[4]

"The program is intended to be constructive, not punitive," said Pisacano. "Once the physician has received the reference guide and the questionnaire, we hope that he will incorporate the questionnaire items in his routine patient records and that the program will thus establish lifetime habits to improve medical records and patient care. We have emphasized the program's teaching potential and have had only favorable feedback from physicians."

Professional Competence Assurance Program

At the University of California San Francisco, Gullion, Watts, and Adamson developed a practice-based CME program known as the Professional Competence Assurance Program (PROCAP).[5] Its first trial was in hypertension education. External auditors compared the physician's performance as recorded on the patient record with specific criteria established by a panel of academicians and practicing physicians. The physician was then provided an assessment of his compliance with the criteria and of his performance as compared with the peer group. Participants received an educational packet; most took part in an hour-long instructional telephone conference call with other participants and a faculty member; and a few attended a small-group meeting.

Since faculty members had been given information about the participants' performance, they were able to base their instruction on specific needs. Reassessment at twelve months showed that the patients of physicians who scored in the highest third of the group on the initial audit showed no change in blood-pressure control, whereas the patients of the remaining two-thirds showed statistically significant improvement. The authors speculated that physicians with initially high scores had fewer changes to make and so were not as likely to increase their scores appreciably.

Since medical record data are less reliable for criteria related to patient behavior and compliance, physicians also sent surveys to their patients, who returned them to the PROCAP office. Physicians received a printout comparing their patients' responses with those of their peer groups. This feedback prompted the physicians to improve patient education. In evaluating a recent diabetes trial, participating physicians said they were unaware of their patients' knowledge in the care of their feet. On the reassessment, both physicians and patients showed statistically significant improvement in compliance with criteria related to the care of the feet.

As a result of the survey data, one group of physicians persuaded the administrators of their community hospital to hire a half-time nurse-educator for patients. Another physician who was conscientious about educating his hypertensive patients was surprised when a considerable number said they did not understand or regularly follow their low-salt diet.

The PROCAP patient survey is also being used to measure patient satisfaction, and the information obtained is being applied to improvement in physicians' communication with patients. Future applications include the use of medical data from computerized records for appropriate educational activities.

Data Collected by Insurance Companies

Some medical societies working with insurance companies have pioneered methods of assessment based on adverse events in practice. Analysis of these events should lead to discovery of their causes and to specific remedial education. The concepts were first developed in the California Medical Insurance Feasibility Study sponsored by the California Medical Association and the California Hospital Association and under the leadership of Don Harper Mills.

The 1970s brought a crisis in medical malpractice suits. Since most costly liability litigation is brought by patients with adverse outcomes, Don Harper Mills introduced a reporting system that focused on adverse outcomes such as cardiac arrest, decubitus ulcers, drug reactions, infection, neurologic impairment, and wound disruption. The outcomes are tabulated when they occur rather than retrospectively from charts. The Notification System does not lead to assessments or actions, but simply reports the aggregate data to the appropriate hospitals, thus acting as an automatic monitor of the frequency and trend of such problems. The hospital quality-assurance coordinator and committee review the printout of outcomes and formulate a plan of corrective action. This action may consist solely of education, or it may result in altered policies or procedures or removal of privileges.

"When frequent cardiopulmonary resuscitation in the hospital carries a high death rate," said Mills, "the chances are that the medical staff has never come to grips with the 'do not resuscitate' concept, that is, terminally ill patients are being improperly subjected to resuscitative attempts. The solution is staff-wide education and a staff policy approving 'do not resuscitate' orders under certain circumstances."

Physician-practice in Hospitals

William Fifer and colleagues implemented a similar program for periodic evaluation of physician-practice in hospitals. Said Fifer, "We cross-index the problems by practitioner to produce a performance profile to guide periodic recredentialing. Events that are potentially compensable, such as readmissions to the hospital, returns to surgery, or unexpected retrograde transfers to an intensive care unit, are identified. Physicians receive a score comparing their rate of adverse patient outcomes to that of their study group. For example, we will collect wound infection rates over a three-to-six-month period and send department heads a printout on those data for all practitioners in their departments. Any problems found are studied for cause and possible remedies.

"We believe that such pattern analysis provides insights not evident from peer review of individual patient records. The value of feedback in guiding the practitioner's continuing education has been impressive, but we go beyond that by using performance profiles to delineate clinical privileges. So the practice profile becomes a form of quality control in the hospital."

Medical Management Analysis

The Medical Management Analysis (MMA) System[6] was also based on the Mills study.[7] A committee of physicians and medical-audit experts devised 20 generic outcome criteria that were applied retrospectively to more than 20,000 records from 23 representative California hospitals. The purpose was to determine the types and severity of adverse events occurring in hospitalized patients. In 1976, Joyce Craddick adapted the California Medical Insurance Feasibility Study criteria as a professional liability warning system for hospitals and individual physicians. The MMA system is currently being implemented and refined by more than 100 hospitals around the country, as well as by several physician-owned professional liability companies.

The system incorporates concurrent screening of all patient records for detection of potential adverse events and record-documentation deficiencies, immediate professional review of all serious occurrences, documentation of all adverse events for identification of recurrent problems, and centralization of responsibility for reporting of findings and for establishment of criteria for corrective actions.

All patient charts are screened, regardless of diagnosis or reason for admission, according to a set of objective outcome criteria developed by a committee of physicians and medical-audit experts. Each criterion serves as a "liability sensor" for adverse events. Records failing one or more criteria are further analyzed by peer physicians. Comprehensive screening of all patient records discloses patterns of substandard care that may not be related to one diagnosis or one service and may not be detected by audit criteria pertinent only to specific diagnoses or procedures. Inadvertent injury of an organ or structure during operation, for example, would not often be detected by a diagnosis-specific audit.

Because outcome-screening can be conducted during the patient's hospitalization or immediately after discharge, adverse events are uncovered sooner than by a routine retrospective audit. The coordination of data retrieval and full chart review reduces, and may even eliminate, multiple reviews of individual patient records.

Adverse events detectable by the MMA system include surgical techniques that frequently required repeated operation because of bleeding, medication errors traced to a nurse from a temporary agency, or a defective product that remained in use after having caused the death of a patient.

The MMA system is also used for review of an individual physician for Medical Insurance Exchange of California (MIEC), a physician-owned professional liability insurance company, and by some hospitals for review of "problem physicians." With the consent of the physician involved, a specified number of recent consecutive patient records are screened retrospectively by a trained records-technician according to specified criteria. Defective records are then reviewed by the MIEC physician consultant and a peer physician from the appropriate specialty. A comprehensive written report is used in the counseling of the physician, as well as in decisions about malpractice insurance. In addition to the hospital charts, office records are evaluated whenever necessary (especially in the review of family practice).

"Problem physicians" are identified by the underwriting department of MIEC on the basis of serious or frequent claims, performance of high-risk or controversial procedures, or concerns of other insured physicians. Remedial actions have included recommendations for correction of practice problems, voluntary limitation of privileges, proctoring, recommendation that the physician obtain insurance elsewhere, or removal from the staff. These studies confirmed the impression that preceding almost every serious adverse event with evidence of negligence is an identifiable trail of lesser events that could have been interrupted by corrective intervention.

During the past three years, a series of "control physicians" from most major specialties and subspecialties has been studied by the MMA method. Composite data from these control studies are used as community standards for comparison with data obtained on problem physicians. These studies clearly show a difference in practice patterns and risk factors between the two groups. After corrective measures, the incidence among "problem physicians" of actual and potential patient injuries, as well as the number of deficiencies in documentation, has fallen. Properly applied on a broad scale, the system has a chance to make a difference. Examples of results:

1. A general surgeon took a CME course in intestinal surgery, after which reassessment showed significant improvement in his performance.
2. An obstetrician who took a course in fetal monitoring showed improvement in handling the distressed fetus as well as in documentation.
3. A family practitioner whose "fear" of using digitalis in therapeutic dosages resulted in frequent readmission of his patients for congestive heart failure called cardiology consultants until he learned how to use digitalis properly.

4. A family physician who practiced obstetrics but showed almost no knowledge of modern prenatal care and delivery was persuaded to delete obstetrics from his practice.

Analyzing the Products of Practice

In an experimental program developed at the University of Southern California, products of practice, such as copies of prescriptions, almost automatically identified certain educational needs.[8] Physicians wrote prescriptions on forms with pressure-sensitive paper attached, noting also the reasons for the prescriptions and the other drugs being taken by the patient. The identity of both patients and physicians was concealed from a committee that reviewed the information for possible problems in prescribing. Seven major categories of problems in drug-prescribing that have educational remedies were identified: inappropriate indications; overly frequent prescriptions for certain drugs; prescription of drugs with abuse potential; inadequate patient instructions; excessive dosage, especially in elderly patients; prescription of ineffective drugs; and potential drug interactions. The physicians responded favorably to the individualized instructional packets designed to remedy the identified problems. With further refinement, this method may obviate costly, time-consuming, and less automatic methods.

*****

Although continuing education is part of a quality assurance program, it should remain a separate endeavor from more punitive approaches that may sometimes be needed to ensure quality. Nevertheless, some methods described here may be used to identify educational deficits during evaluation of quality assurance. For maximum and sustained educational value, the identification of educational needs from events in practice should avoid intimidating programs that may lead to defensiveness and inhibit the physician's willingness to participate in assessment of performance. Preserving a buoyant spirit in physicians is important, so that they will continually strive to offer their patients better care. External auditors must therefore be careful not to stifle enthusiasm for practice.

References

1. Latham, Peter Mere. General remarks on the practice of medicine. In: Martin, Robert, ed. *The Collected Works of Dr. P. M. Latham.* London: The New Sydenham Society, 1878:465.
2. Sivertson, Sigurd E.; Meyer, Thomas C.; Hansen, Richard; Schoenenberger, Adeline. Individual physician profile: Continuing education related to medical practice. *J Med Educ* Nov 1973;48(11):1006-1012.

3. Bowler, Francis L.; Brading, Paul L.; Burg, Frederic D.; Finestone, Albert J.; Hubbard, John P. A practice-related educational program. *JAMA* Mar 28 1977;237(13):1346-1349.
4. American Board of Family Practice. *Diabetes Mellitus*. Reference Guide 9 of the Office Record Review Project, 1981.
5. Gullion, David S.; Adamson, T. Elaine; Watts, Malcolm S. M. The effect of an individualized practice-based CME program on physician performance and patient outcomes. *West J Med* Apr 1983;138(4):582-588.
6. Craddick, Joyce W. The medical management analysis system: A professional liability warning mechanism. *QRB* Apr 1979;5(4):2-8.
7. Mills, Don Harper. Medical insurance feasibility study: A technical summary. *West J Med* Apr 1978;128(4):360-365.
8. Manning, Phil R.; Lee, Peter V.; Denson, Teri A.; Gilman, Nelson J. Determining educational needs in the physician's office. *JAMA* Sep 5 1980;244(10):1112-1115.

11. Enlisting Help in the Analysis of Practice

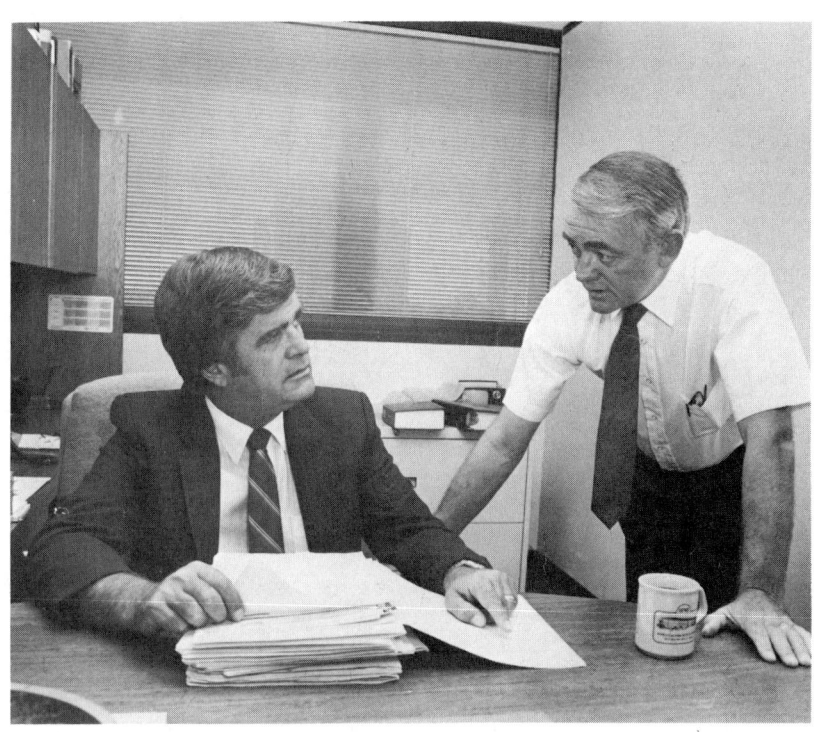

Once a month we close the office and call in a consultant for our own grand rounds. Using the diagnosis index, we assemble the records of patients with a specific problem and go through them with the consultant.

Warren L. Williams, M.D. (right)
Englewood, Colorado

12

Social, Ethical, and Economic Problems in Medicine

> The exceptional advances of modern medicine have restored to productive life many patients with previously fatal or disabling diseases, but these very successes have raised a host of troubling ethical and economic questions. Reconciling society's increasing demands on medicine with the realities of inflation, governmental regulations, changing social values, and an aging population poses knotty problems.
>
> *Michael E. DeBakey and Lois DeBakey*[1]

Opportunities for Involvement

The methods and approaches physicians use to learn from their clinical experiences not only perfect their skills, but heighten their personal satisfaction and passion for practice. Such activities can no longer be limited to the study of clinical findings, diagnosis, and therapy, for extraordinary medical innovations have raised a rash of problems— economic, social, legal, moral, and ethical. Can we afford the advances? How do we control the escalating costs? How do we provide the new services for the economically deprived? How do we reconcile society's ever-increasing demands and expectations of medicine with its increasing criticism of rising costs? What role should medical and professional judgment play in ethical quandaries? How do we define the difference between prolonging living and prolonging dying? All segments of society have become interested in these questions and problems.

"These issues have raised physicians' interest in the problems and have stimulated the desire to learn," said Philip Lee. "The changing responsibilities have begun to affect physician attitudes. I believe that the time has come to address these questions actively. Physicians must learn what the problems are and seek objective information, not base their judgments on the often biased discussions provided through give-away journals or special-interest journals. Physicians must seek out other sources of information, review and evaluate them, and then make their own decisions."

"Medical ethics is fascinating and important," in Albert Jonsen's view, "but the way it is now taught to physicians poses some problems. Because ethics is based on academic philosophy, it can be, and often is, presented purely theoretically. Moreover, when the ethicist has little clinical experience, his approach may be abstract and simplistic. Competent teaching of medical ethics requires concreteness and practicality. It should result in broadening of vision as well as have clinical relevance." Physicians can use some of the methods discussed in this book to address economic, social, and ethical issues. How can they proceed?

Individual Involvement

Bruce E. Zawacki, who took a year's sabbatical from his busy burn service to study ethical and social problems in medicine, found three resources particularly helpful in staying abreast of the problems confronting medicine: (1) regular participation in hospital ethics conferences (ethics committees in some institutions); (2) reading *The Hastings Center Report*, *The Journal of Medical Ethics*, and *The New England Journal of Medicine*; and (3) teaching medical ethics.

"Consult with other physicians or professionals regarding particular ethical problems you face in caring for individual patients," advised Philip Lee. "Some physicians in university medical centers may consult with chaplains or philosophers, or others with particular expertise in ethics. For example, this method may be used to address questions about a decision not to resuscitate a patient who may have cardiac arrest. When should the decision not to resuscitate be discussed with the patient? When should the family be involved? In the case of a hospitalized patient, when should the nurses or other members of the staff become involved? In short, the very process of deciding who should be involved in the decision, what rights the patient, family, hospital staff, and attending physician have will help to educate the physician about the issue."

Thomas Hunter pointed out the need for physicians to educate other groups, both lay and law, to the realities of medicine and biological science and for physicians to listen to the concerns of these groups. "The trust in physicians and scientists has been badly eroded for many reasons beyond our control, partly because of the general mistrust of authority since the sixties. But our resistance to participation by the laity in policy decisions has also played a part. We need to accept the fact that ultimately we are responsible to the public and that we must work actively with them in formulating ethical and social policy."

Zawacki suggested that "the most influential 'significant others' for young physicians, the attending staff, should be encouraged to include such considerations in their daily bedside teaching."

Organized Medicine

Robert Glaser has urged organized and academic medicine to help physicians follow ethical, social, and economic problems by sponsoring seminars, symposia, and conferences on these topics. "The professional media also have a role in publishing thoughtful, informative articles on these subjects."

County and state medical societies offer the physician the opportunity for grass-roots participation on committees studying and formulating policies in social and economic problems that affect the practice of medicine. Philip Lee thinks that physicians often deal with the broader issues through professional organizations such as county and state medical associations, the American Medical Association, and specialty societies. "These bodies often conduct policy studies and communicate the information to the member physicians for more consideration of the organization's policy position and for consideration with respect to the impact on an individual physician's practice. The mechanisms for representing the views of physicians, although imperfect, exist and fit very much with our pluralistic approach to public policy and the kind of influence accorded special interests, including the medical profession."

Most medical societies have capable staffs to research pertinent issues and distribute bulletins and newsletters to their constituencies. The AMA, for example, publishes the *American Medical News*, and the American College of Physicians publishes *The Observer*. These publications help the busy physician who cannot spend time reading all published material on these subjects.

*****

Advances in medical science and practice, while improving patient care, have also raised countless social, ethical, and economic problems. Their significance demands that physicians devote some time to studying the issues and contributing to their solutions. When ethical problems arise in the care of individual patients, the physician should discuss the issues with colleagues, the clergy, the patient's family, and in certain circumstances, an ethicist. Formal consultations may be in order. The leading medical journals now have regular features that discuss the issues authoritatively, and the public media also devote considerable space to these topics, so the physician can be aware of current thinking on important issues. Medical societies are becoming increasingly involved; some have formulated formal positions on specific issues, and most publish news-

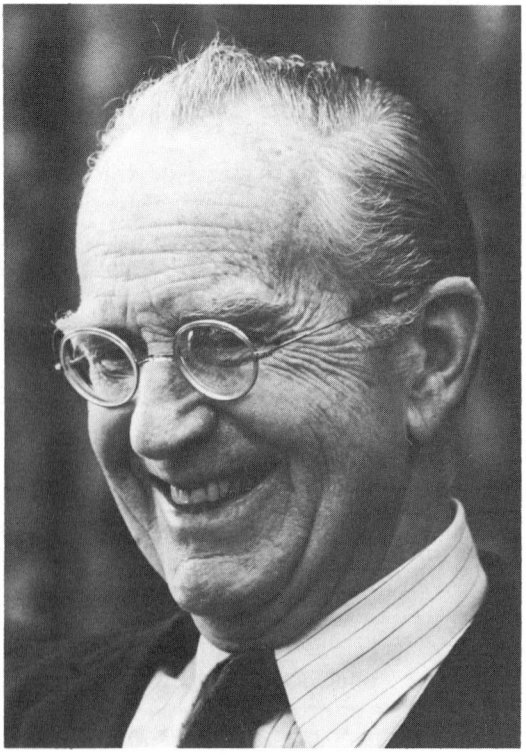

Medicine is a grand and rapidly possessive discipline that requires a lifelong interest in things human. If you give that up at any time in your practice, you are lost.

Irvine H. Page, M.D.
Director of Research Emeritus
Cleveland Clinic Foundation

12. Social, Ethical, and Economic Problems

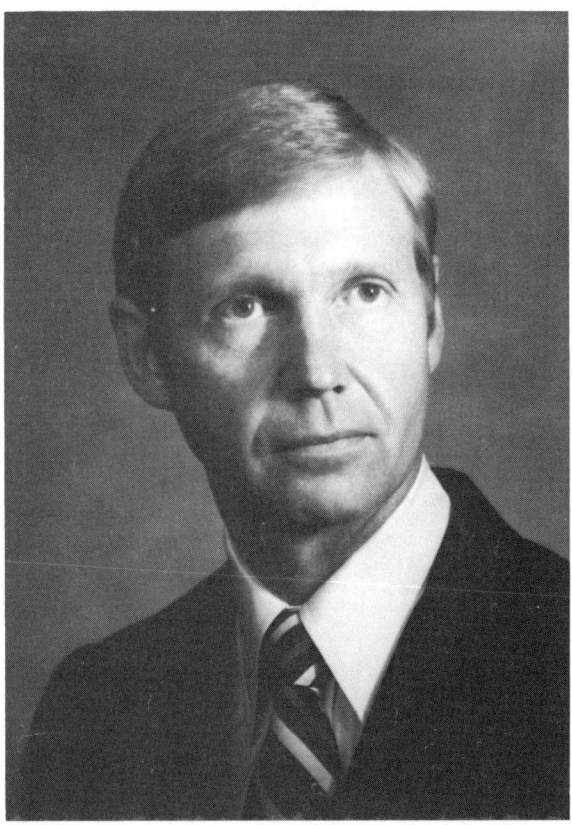

Inquisitiveness is the hallmark of a good physician and provides its own rewards throughout one's professional career.

Robert E. Rakel, M.D.
Chairman, Department of Family Medicine
Baylor College of Medicine

letters and bulletins to keep members informed. Despite time limitations, physicians must actively participate in the solutions of social, ethical, and economic problems in medicine if they are to remain effective advocates for excellent patient care. In Saul Farber's words: "We are part of a great profession; we must work to preserve it."

Reference

1. DeBakey, Michael E.; DeBakey, Lois. The ethics and economics of high-technology medicine. *Compr Ther* Dec 1983;9(12):15-16.

13

The Doctor-Patient Relationship, Physical Examination, and New Procedures

> The relationship between doctor and patient partakes of a peculiar intimacy. It presupposes on the part of the physician not only knowledge of his fellow men but sympathy. . . . This aspect of the practice of medicine has been designated as the art; yet I wonder whether it should not, most properly, be called the essence.
> *Warfield T. Longcope*[1]

Gene Stollerman, editor of *Clinical Experience*, would like to see continuing medical education designed to emphasize clinical skills.[2] He deplores the growing gap between medical technology and clinical skills, in which advice based on the interview and examination is replaced by the results of technical procedures. The development of clinical skills, he pointed out, enables physicians to obtain a better understanding of the patient's problems and to gain confidence in their own ability to determine what technologic tool is required to substantiate the clinical findings and what consultations would be to the patient's advantage. Learning about new tests and procedures, unfortunately, is much easier than discovering how better to examine a patient.

Doctor-Patient Relationship

Many patients feel intimidated by the very presence of a physician and are reluctant to ask questions or even discuss fully the nature and extent of their complaints. They may hesitate to impose on the physician's time; they may be embarrassed to expose their inner selves; or they may be fearful of the consequences of their illness. Eliminating these patient inhibitions requires special skills in interviewing and communication.

Doctor-Patient Relationship as a Therapeutic Tool

The doctor-patient relationship is, of course, a powerful therapeutic tool that the physician should learn to use adroitly. Richard Reitemeier gave this example of the importance of the doctor-patient relationship: "Dr. J. Arnold Bargen was one of America's pioneers in the study and management of inflammatory bowel disease. When he began this interest in the mid-1930s, he recognized the terrible plight of such patients and did all he could to help them. Because of that interest, many patients were referred to his care. I suspect they were referred with some gratitude on the part of their own physicians, since the management of the disease was a terrible challenge and usually very frustrating. Dr. Bargen welcomed the opportunity to care for such patients, and, as one of his assistants in the hospital in the early 1950s, I recall so well seeing a remarkable demonstration of the effect of that kind of welcome on an ill person.

"A young woman with severe ulcerative colitis of several years' duration was admitted to St. Mary's Hospital several days before Dr. Bargen was to begin his term as the consultant in charge of such cases. She arrived emaciated, with a high fever, considerable abdominal pain and the usual raging diarrhea. We did all that we could to make her comfortable, but her symptoms continued without change until the morning Dr. Bargen met her. He walked across the room and stood at the bedside of this patient, reaching out to grasp her right hand with his and placing his left hand on her forearm. Looking her straight in the eye, he said, 'I am so glad you have come! We are going to make you better!' He then went on with the usual interrogation of her history and a physical examination. However, we all noted that the very moment that he greeted her with that welcome assertion, she seemed to relax. As the day wore on, I was gratified and intrigued to watch all of her clinical signs improve. The fever abated, her diarrhea and abdominal pain quieted down, and indeed she did get better. I have always thought that the magic of his greeting was transferred to that woman through the warmth of his handshake and his evident honesty. He really did care about her."

Understanding the Patient's Point of View

The patient's perception of the hospital may be quite different from the physician's, as Francis Moore learned. "As a senior resident in a Boston hospital in a largely Italian-speaking neighborhood, I encountered a woman admitted for headache. Because all the simple tests were negative, she was scheduled for the more rigorous tests that we had in those days, including an encephalogram and a ventriculogram. One morning, as I was coming around with my white-suited junior resident troupe behind me, she said, 'Doctor, you know, I think I am just too sick to be in the hospital.' There was no response from the dumbfounded residents. She continued: 'I would like to go home for a few days until I feel a little better. Then I will be happy to come back to the hospital for the tests. But right now, I am just not feeling well enough.' How many patients she unwittingly spoke for."

"One incident served to teach me," recalled Kunio Okuda of Japan, "that things that seem trivial to the physician may have great significance for the patient. As a young resident at the Chiba National Hospital, I was in charge of a ward room with five middle-aged women with chronic diseases. I made it a rule to see them in the morning, starting from the right side of the door. One day, for no reason and without thinking, I started seeing them from the left. I later learned from the nurses that the woman on the right whom I used to see first and the one on the left whom I saw first that particular day had a big fight in the afternoon. I realized that I had been concentrating on the patients' diseases, and had been negligent of their feelings and personalities. I learned an important lesson."

Most physicians are relatively content with their clinical skills, not realizing that even basic skills need to be analyzed to avoid bad habits and omissions. There is even need to improve continually one's ability to listen intently and actively to patients. A common mistake made by medical students is to refer to the patient as "a poor historian." "Walter Cherny, former Professor of Obstetrics and Gynecology at the Duke University School of Medicine and now Chief of the Department of Obstetrics and Gynecology at the Good Samaritan Hospital in Phoenix, Arizona, has always been a stickler for precise language," said Arthur C. Christakos, M.D. "Whenever students or residents make the mistake of referring to the patient as a historian, Walt is always quick to remind them that the one who records the history is the historian, and most of the time, he agreed, the historian was poor."

The doctor-patient relationship, moreover, is constantly changing in response to societal changes as patients become more aware of medical matters. To adapt to these changes, the physician must be ever alert to the human side of medicine. Thus, daily learning must include opportunities to become more skillful in the doctor-patient relationship as well as in the physical examination and new procedures.

Methods that Promote Growth of Clinical Skills

SEMINARS. Michael Balint pioneered research seminars to study the psychological implications in general medicine. His discussion groups, first organized at the Tavistock Clinic in England, consisted of eight to ten general practitioners and two psychiatrists. Balint noted that at first the general practitioners tried hard to entice the psychiatrists into a teacher-pupil relationship, but for many reasons it was thought advisable to resist this. Instead, Balint strove for a free give-and-take atmosphere, in which everyone could discuss clinical problems and receive assistance based on the experience of the others. The chief purpose was an examination of the ever-changing doctor-patient relationship. Physicians' recent experi-

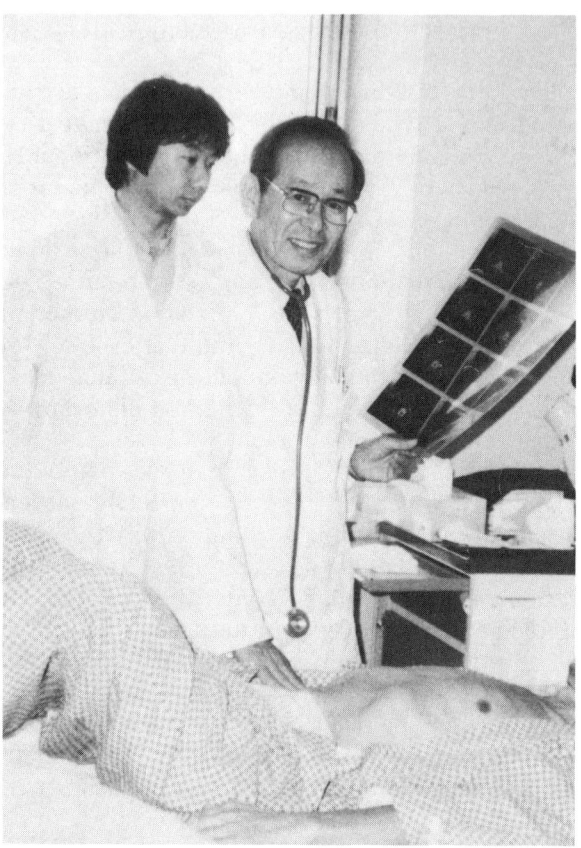

Things that seem trivial to the physician may have great significance for the patient.

Kunio Okuda, M.D., Ph.D.
Director, Department of Medicine
Chiba University
Chiba City, Japan

ences with patients, reported by the doctor in charge, provided the material for Balint's discussion groups. The doctors reported freely on their experiences, using clinical notes and including an account of their emotional responses to patients.[3] Many physicians now participate in seminars based on the principles devised by Balint.

FILE OF CLINICAL BIOGRAPHIES AND WRITING. In addition to participating in seminars that focus on doctor-patient conversations and interactions, G. Gayle Stephens also maintains a file of "clinical biographies" of patients in his practice—narrative descriptions of patients' longitudinal experiences with illness. He also teaches and writes about interviewing and the doctor-patient interaction.

KEEPING ABREAST OF CHANGING ATTITUDES. Physicians need ways of ensuring that they are reacting constructively to the changing attitudes of their patients toward medicine. G. Gayle Stephens recommends that physicians develop a circle of friends who are *not* physicians and listen to their stories about doctors and hospitals. Reading articles on health for the consumer in newspapers, magazines, and books and watching television programs and advertisements about health and related issues can be helpful. Stephens advocates a nonjudgmental listening style so that patients will be uninhibited in their conversations with physicians. Never should a physician deride or humiliate a patient for doing something unorthodox.

"Listening is the most important way to learn what the changing attitudes are," said Jonathan Rodnick. "I serve on the Board of Directors of a community-based health organization that has predominately 'consumers' on its Board, and listening to their views makes me aware of the public's attitudes. If I were unaware of my patients' changing attitudes, however, I would hope that they or my staff would constructively point out my inappropriate assumptions and actions."

John Geyman advocates self-study to improve knowledge about patients' attitudes. "Increase your knowledge of the community, the occupational settings, and the home environments. If, for example, you practice in a logging town, visit the local lumber mill and make occasional home visits. Encourage your patients to take an active role in the decision-making concerning their health care."

VIDEOTAPING OR AUDIOTAPING DOCTOR-PATIENT ENCOUNTERS. Each physician should have the benefit of being videotaped periodically, or at least audiotaped, while interviewing a patient and having the tape reviewed later with an expert. Both profit from the exercise. The human interaction that takes place in medicine is too important to be neglected in lifelong learning. Some medical schools offer courses in this subject, but hospitals and specialty societies could do more in this regard.

I. R. McWhinney considers videotapes of the doctor-patient encounter to be the most powerful learning tools we have. "The ideal is for a learner, whether student, resident, or practicing physician, to review his tape with a colleague skilled in the art of the interview."

SELF-OBSERVATION. For those physicians without access to videotaping facilities, self-observation can be useful. John Geyman periodically audits himself during a patient encounter. "I remind myself of the need for a relaxed, approachable manner; open-ended questions and active listening; and avoidance of distractions. I try to learn something new about the patient as a person in each encounter, that is, beyond information related to his medical problems. I also ask myself whether the patient has had sufficient opportunity to participate in decisions about further diagnostic steps, management, and follow-up. In addition to self-audit techniques, it is useful to observe the patient's reactions to me as a physician as well as the reactions of residents and students to me as a teacher."

TEACHING. Observing and teaching medical students at the bedside increases the physician's understanding of the basic techniques of the doctor-patient relationship. As part of the family practice residency program in which Jonathan Rodnick teaches, the residents are observed and videotaped while interacting with patients. "By observing young physicians with patients, analyzing their styles, and trying to give constructive feedback, I subsequently analyze my own office behavior. This self-analysis gives me ideas to improve communication in my practice and helps me understand both verbal and nonverbal doctor-patient communication. The adage that the teacher learns as much as the students is certainly apt in this situation."

The Physical Examination

A master clinician can gain astonishing information from a physical examination. "I often think of the best teaching that I ever had in medical school," said Marvyn L. Elgart. "It was the introductory demonstration by David Barr, Professor of Medicine at Cornell University. An eminent clinician, Dr. Barr told us that he was going to show us all the things that we could learn from a patient without his taking his clothes off. He then had a patient come into his office, stood up to greet him, and then stopped and turned to us. For the next 40 minutes, as he and the patient remained standing, he pointed out from an unending fountain of knowledge all the things he had discerned about the patient's eyes, skin, touch, and gait, as well as all the disease possibilities that had entered his mind during those few minutes. It was remarkable. In novels, only Sherlock Holmes came close."

Bill Bennett recalled the considerable influence that Howard P. Lewis, an outstanding physical diagnostician, had on the medical careers of every student he touched. "Twice weekly at a two-hour conference with interns and residents, Dr. Lewis would elicit a history and do a physical exam-

13. The Doctor-Patient Relationship

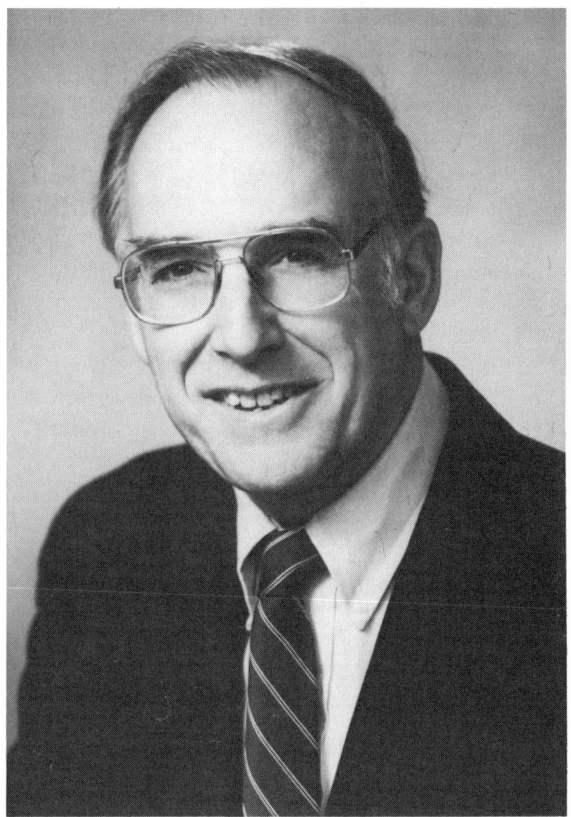

I remind myself of the need for a relaxed, approachable manner; open-ended questions and active listening; and avoidance of distractions.

John P. Geyman, M.D.
Chairman, Department of Family Medicine
University of Washington

ination on a patient. He would construct a differential diagnosis brilliantly and would predict findings that would be found at operation or on chest x-ray. One need only recall the dullness over Kernig's isthmus, signifying scarring from tuberculosis, or percussion of dullness over Traube's space, signifying enlarging of the spleen, to realize his lasting impact on a young intern. It would be interesting to pit this consummate clinician's physical diagnostic skills, painstakingly developed over a career, against modern imaging devices. In cost-effectiveness, I suspect that Dr. Lewis would win hands down. After retirement about fifteen years ago, he remained very active in the teaching of physical diagnosis to medical students and house officers. It is clinicians like Dr. Lewis who signify excellence in the art of medicine.''

Once a physician has completed formal training, he has few opportunities to improve his techniques of physical examination. Proctor Harvey offers excellent courses on cardiovascular diagnosis, but most formal courses do not address this problem. Physicians who teach learn from the shortcomings of students and residents, but many physicians slip into faulty habits that can easily be corrected. Being observed by a colleague while performing a physical examination helps the physician avoid careless and sloppy approaches to physical diagnosis.

Experts' Need for Advice on Fundamentals

One might wonder if being videotaped during a patient interview and being observed in performing a physical examination is not too basic for experienced physicians. Everyone, however, can profit from expert advice and exhortation. In athletics, coaches help team members perform their best. In sports such as tennis, even the champions continue to receive instruction from coaches. In 1964, Charles MacKinley and Dennis Ralston were preparing for a Davis Cup match at the Los Angeles Tennis Club with the help of Pancho Gonzalez. MacKinley, Wimbledon winner the previous year, was considered the number one tennis player of the day. Watching the great Pancho Gonzalez, one of the masters of the game, give a lesson to two champions offered spectators the promise of learning some of the fine points of the game. But Gonzalez's first remark to MacKinley during a rally was the basic ''Watch the ball,'' followed a little later by the admonition, ''You're not bending your knees!'' So even champions need reminders about the fundamentals.[4]

Louis J. Kettel received a valuable reminder from a patient. ''Recently, I volunteered for an evaluation of my history, physical examination, and diagnostic skills using the patient-instructor program put in place for competency evaluation of our medical students and house officers. This program uses patients with well-established illnesses, physical findings, and considerable knowledge of their diseases along with a validated, structured, gradable analysis form. In the process, I fully expected to find that I lacked some skills, since I have been an administrator for a number of years. I was taken aback, however, by the major critique. In analyzing my overall

13. The Doctor-Patient Relationship

skills, the patient informed me that I had neglected throughout the examination to recognize that he was, in fact, a human being and on no occasion had I called him by name. What a depersonalizing experience for the patient! Were I to function in the role of Dean in the absence of so simple a social grace, I would surely deem myself a failure. I assure you I corrected that behavior."

Dr. Peter Lee cited an example of the value of being observed. "For his discussion of the doctor-patient relationship with medical students, Dr. Seymour Pollack, then a young faculty member in the Department of Psychiatry, asked if he could accompany me while I made ward rounds on my Medicine service. I agreed, assuming that he would compliment me on my sensitivity and skill. Feeling that I was in need of some positive reinforcement, I took his invitation seriously. One morning after I had recently returned to clinical medicine from several years of almost full-time administration, Dr. Pollack accompanied me on rounds. I was naturally somewhat anxious in the presence of my resident, who was somewhat intimidating in his skillful use of roundsmanship. He and I and two interns went from bed to bed, followed by Dr. Pollack, reviewing the problems of the patients, discussing the appropriate literature, and recommending plans for diagnosis or management. At the end of the rounds, Dr. Pollack and I stepped into a conference room, and I asked him for his observations. His first sentence I remember vividly to this day: 'Pete, I'm shocked.' He then described the several ways in which my behavior on rounds had not only been rather oblivious of the feelings of patients but, in some cases, actually offensive. Some specific instances included my examining a woman patient in a ward with four or five other patients without pulling the curtains around the bed. In another instance, I made what I felt was an appropriate witticism across the bed of another patient, not at the expense of the patient, but the patient had no way of knowing that the joke did not relate to him. In another case, a resident and I discussed the problems of a certain patient who acquired tapeworms from working in unsanitary mines directly across the supine body of an anemic patient in whom the question of some esoteric tapeworm disease had arisen.

"The impact of this honest description of my behavior at the bedside of patients was profound. Over the succeeding 20 years, I have been followed by the ghost of Seymour Pollack as I have made rounds. There is no question that the sensitivity I gained from having my own ward rounds observed by a friendly critic changed my way of making rounds and my bedside behavior for the better."

New Procedures

Physicians have too few opportunities to learn procedures that were developed or perfected after their formal training. A surgeon usually "scrubs in" with a colleague trained in the procedure. A few specialty

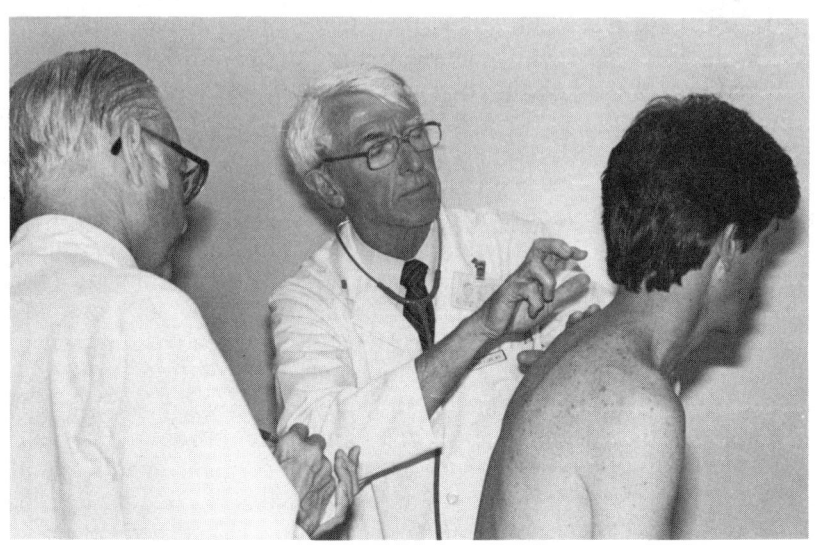

Having a colleague observe me helps me improve my performance and prevents my falling into faulty habits.

Peter V. Lee, M.D. (center)
Chairman, Department of Family Medicine
University of Southern California

13. The Doctor-Patient Relationship

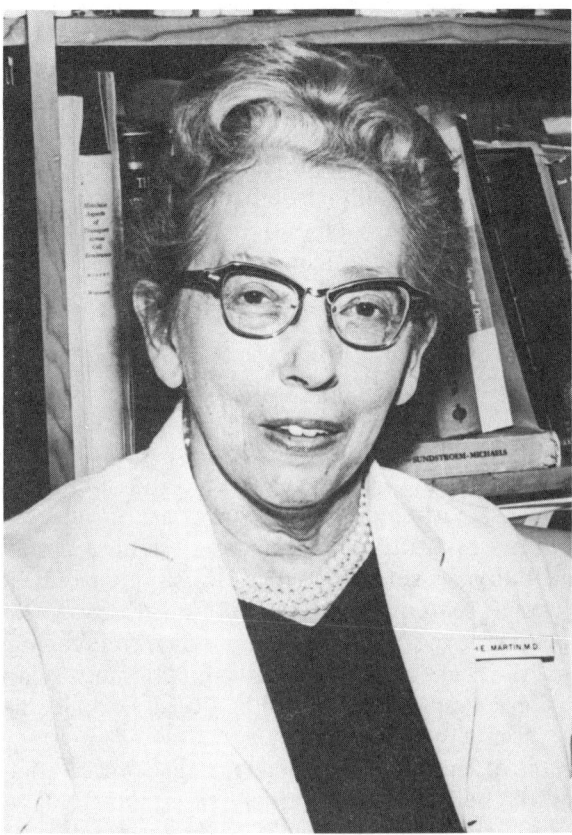

In the past, a fine classical education may have made it easier for physicians to be more broadly informed, but even today physicians can advance their intellectual and cultural development by a lifelong personal learning program.

Helen E. Martin, M.D.
Emeritus Professor of Medicine
University of Southern California

societies offer programs for this purpose. Since 1977, for example, the American Academy of Orthopaedic Surgeons has included laboratory components in courses on surgical skills, with hands-on experience. Programs include Rotary Instability of the Knee, Intramedullary Nailing, Shoulder Disorders with Arthroscopy, and Arthroscopy of the Knee. In 1983, 33 courses in the use of chymopapain in the treatment of herniated lumbar disc disease drew 6,300 participants. In addition to lectures and film presentations, "hands-on" laboratory sessions with special manikins and image intensifiers helped participants learn the essential skill of needle placement.

When considering attendance in a course on a procedure, keep in mind the experience of Irwin Schatz. "It was 1958 and I had just returned from a year in London, after internship and before starting a residency in internal medicine. The British cardiologists' expertise at auscultation had been astonishing; Paul Wood, John McMichael and Aubrey Leatham demonstrated that important data could be detected by careful auscultation of the heart. During the early months of my residency, I discovered that the cardiologists at my institution—all of them talented clinicians—either scoffed at this ability or were apathetic. I was convinced, however, that auscultation was an extremely useful skill, and I desperately wanted to learn how to become expert at it. One day, while rummaging in the storeroom of one of the wards, I found a still functioning, relatively mobile Sanborn phonocardiograph machine, which I boldly decided to use to teach myself auscultation.

"After a week of fumbling with leads, I discovered that recording a clean tracing at the bedside was relatively easy, and so immediately after my physical examination of every patient I saw, I would record the heart sounds, look at what should have been heard, and then reexamine the patient. The other physicians, nurses, and aides on the wards thought I was doing a special research project and would often help me in hooking the patient up to the machine. I taught myself to distinguish splitting of the second heart sound, increased intensity of pulmonic closure, mitral opening snaps, differences in intervals, systolic murmurs in various positions, and more. These auscultatory skills are, of course, commonplace now, but in 1958 detection of these phenomena, particularly in the United States, was unusual and often derided. This experience taught me a lesson: don't depend on someone else to *teach* you something—you can *learn* it yourself." An inherent weakness in any course is that physicians learn best when they are confronted with a real problem in their own practice.

*****

In all professions, basic skills need to be refined. But pressures of practice and embarrassment prevent most physicians from actively seeking to hone their skills in interviewing or doing a physical examination. Few formal courses address these issues. Physicians can, however, ask a skilled colleague to observe them during these activities and then solicit suggestions for improvement. Observing a videotape of oneself in action and noting the problems recorded can also be instructive. New procedures may be particularly difficult for the average physician to learn, but colleagues are usually willing to help, and medical societies are becoming more active in providing such instruction.

References

1. Longcope, Warfield T. Methods and medicine. *Bull Johns Hopkins Hosp* Jan 1932;50(1):20.
2. Stollerman, Gene H. Care of your clinical skills. [Editorial] *Clinical Experience* Mar 1984;1(1):11-12.
3. Balint, Michael. *The Doctor, His Patient and the Illness,* 2nd ed. New York: Pitman Publishing Corporation, 1964.
4. Manning, Phil R. Continuing medical education, physician competence, physician performance. *Federation Bulletin* Aug 1978; 65(8):227-235.

14

Problems in Practice Unrelated to Medical Knowledge

> If anything can go wrong, it will.
>
> *Murphy's Law*[1]
>
> Murphy was an optimist.
>
> *O'Toole's commentary on Murphy's Law*[1]

The physician who reviews his practice continually will serve his patients well, but good health care requires more than medical knowledge. At every step, extrinsic phenomena, errors, and omissions may adversely affect medical practice despite the physician's superb knowledge. "The best performance is built upon sound information," said George Miller, "but sound information is no assurance that it will occur." John Williamson found, for example, that highly informed physicians often did not respond to an unmistakably abnormal laboratory report.[2] About two-thirds of the abnormal results of three routine screening tests (urinalysis, fasting blood glucose, and hemoglobin) elicited no response from the physicians in his study, even after they attended a specially designed continuing education workshop and received reminders about the problem. The simple device of obscuring the abnormal findings on the laboratory report with a piece of removable fluorescent tape, however, significantly improved the response.

Starfield and Scheff illustrated that many of the problems interfering with patient care are unrelated to the physician's knowledge.[3] In only 14 of 53 children with low hemoglobin identified by a review of medical records and home interviews was the abnormality recognized, diagnosed, and treated, and the test subsequently repeated. The reasons for the oversights in the remaining 39 children varied. The low hemoglobin was unrecognized in 24 patients, was recognized but undiagnosed in six, was diagnosed but untreated in one, and was treated but not re-examined in four. Four patients were diagnosed correctly, but did not keep their subsequent appointments. Patient care can thus go wrong at any stage.

Morehead and Donaldson, after studying the care of patients with serious diseases in 40 neighborhood health centers, concluded that major problems resulted from failure to follow-up on abnormal laboratory or roentgenographic reports, failure to implement the suggestions of consultants and others, and poor patient compliance.[4] In a study of emergency room care in an inner-city hospital, Brook and Stevenson reviewed the medical records of patients referred to the radiology department for upper gastrointestinal series, oral cholecystography, or barium-enema study.[5] Of 136 patients for whom adequate data were available, 30 (22%) did not receive appointments for treatment after completion of diagnostic procedures. Of the 106 patients who did receive appointments, only 54 (51%) kept them. Furthermore, only 37 (38%) of 98 patients interviewed who had had radiologic examinations could recall being told the results. The authors concluded that effective care had been provided to only one-fourth of the patients.

Gonnella and co-authors studied the detection of urinary tract infections at a university outpatient clinic.[6] An interview designed to elicit historical information about symptoms and signs of urinary tract infection was used on 133 patients, and urine samples were obtained from all of them. Thereafter, all patients were seen in the medical clinic by the regularly assigned student-attending team, which was unaware of the preliminary study. Eighteen patients with significant bacilluria (10^5 colonies/ml urine) were discovered by the preliminary history and screening, whereas only eight had correct diagnoses on the regular clinic routine. Yet when the knowledge of staff members was tested, their average score of 83% on the diagnosis and treatment of this condition showed that the problem was not primarily a lack of knowledge but failure to perform.

These and other studies show that medical practice is subject to oversights, lack of follow-up, and poor communication between physician and patient. Such quality-degrading incidents occur in any complex organized system, whether involving medical practice or a large engineering project. According to Chris Kraft, former Director of the National Aeronautic and Space Administration (NASA), a constant vigil is maintained in the space program to prevent errors of omission, misinterpretation, and lack of inspection: "After our initial years of experience, we recognized that redundancy checks were required to prevent termination of an otherwise perfect mission. Hundreds of examples of human error can be cited, including the problems of the Space Shuttle.

"We used color coding on liquid gas transport lines to warn of their contents and to ensure proper attachment. In the Space Shuttle, we even used different threads at junctions to prevent technicians from assembling the support equipment improperly. Unfortunately, they misassembled them anyway, forcing the lines together and causing damage to the system.

"In many instances parts were omitted from an assembly, despite required inspection points and a recording as each step was completed. When such an omission occurred in a pressure regulator of a space suit, we had to cancel a planned event on a 1982 Space Shuttle flight. We have had parts assembled backwards, an error that eventually caused a profuse leak in a system and, in one case, required the complete redesign of a hydraulic actuator at great cost because of a psychological effect of 'no confidence' that it left on the space team."

A powerful analogy to this diminished effectiveness in complex organized systems, whether medical practice or space missions, comes from the relation of chemical thermodynamics to molecular behavior. According to the second law of thermodynamics, energy spontaneously becomes less concentrated, that is, more diffused, in closed systems, and inanimate matter tends to become random rather than remaining neatly ordered and organized. As Frank L. Lambert, Professor of Chemistry Emeritus at Occidental College noted: "Complex human activities are inherently subject to becoming disorderly—just as orderly groups of molecules in a high energy system are unstable."

Aspects of patient care have a similar tendency to become less orderly and more random if left alone. Constant monitoring and constant feedback are essential to maximal efficiency. Considering the analogy to systems governed by chemical thermodynamics, we should not be surprised by this tendency. Physicians act as critical catalysts in superior medical care. The need for rigorous control is recognized by physicians who must continually check on themselves and others to ensure proper handling of even routine matters. We cite the analogies of the space program and the second law of thermodynamics to emphasize that the tendency for a system to become more disorderly is universal and constant. The physician must therefore be ever alert not only to medical but to nonmedical problems in practice.

The Physician as Manager

How can physicians intervene to correct the tendency for the system to become disorderly and thus less efficient? Joseph Gonnella sees the physician as a manager, constantly monitoring the patient's care to ensure that everything is proceeding as it should and attending to each problem as it occurs. Almost all physicians interviewed acknowledged that numerous difficulties arise in medical practice that are unrelated to medical knowledge, and almost all made conscious efforts to combat them.

History and Physical Examination

Most physicians guard against the incomplete review of systems and physical examination by following an outline, preprinted form, or checklist, even though they may know it by memory. Others have a nurse or secretary scrutinize the chart after the examination and return it to the physician for any omissions.

Warren Williams has his office staff go over his charts for important oversights in the history or physical examination. Several years ago, as an experiment, he discontinued these procedural audits only to find that in two to three months his workups again had some omissions. The second law of thermodynamics is always operating. Physicians who use checklists may also write occasional notes on the progress sheet, such as, "Next time do pelvic examination."

Overbooking patients' appointments increases the risk of omissions and inadequate recordings. Rushing through an examination because appointments are overbooked or because the patient or doctor is late can be a major cause of incomplete physical examinations and of failure to record findings accurately and legibly.

Laboratory Data

Laboratory Studies Unordered, Unperformed, or Unreported

Some physicians use a checklist of possible laboratory studies as a reminder of relevant studies to order. The temptation to over-order, which such a list may carry, must be resisted. Other physicians set aside charts on difficult patients for review at the end of the day, call patients back for further tests, or write notes on progress sheets to order certain tests. Still others ask new patients to return to review their laboratory reports with them, and at that time note any needed tests that were not done.

To discover any unperformed or unreported laboratory studies, physicians can advise patients of the tests ordered and, at the next visit, ask them what was actually done: was blood drawn or a roentgenogram taken? Having the office staff check tests ordered and completed can also minimize laboratory omissions. Writing laboratory orders in a specific place in the patient chart, such as the left margin, facilitates checking. Some physicians review each day's laboratory reports and ask patients either to call or to schedule another visit to receive the reports.

Lost Laboratory or Radiology Reports

Since loose data are liable to become lost, all laboratory reports should be filed in the patient's chart promptly or kept in a special box for the physician to review and initial before being filed. A master file of all laboratory reports is useful in case of a misfiled or lost report. Some laboratories and departments of radiology send a second report on all significantly abnormal studies, or telephone to ensure that a seriously abnormal study has not been lost or gone unnoticed. A backup report on "critical findings," such as suspected cancer, can prevent medical disasters.

Ideally, all serious findings should be called in to the physician's office as well as reported in writing.

Failure to Note or Act on Abnormal Laboratory Results

A report that contains a single abnormal result seems most likely to be overlooked. Physicians use various techniques to avoid oversights, such as a red "Alert" stamp on all abnormal laboratory findings, highlighting abnormal studies in red and leaving the laboratory sheets on the physician's desk until he dictates a letter with the results to the patient, or Sequential Multiple Analysis Computer (SMAC) reports that list results in a low, normal, or high column.

Many physicians require their initials on all laboratory data before the office assistant places reports in patients' charts. Other physicians look over the chart for recent laboratory and roentgenographic reports while they are seeing the patient on a re-visit, to make sure that abnormal studies are followed properly. Partners sometimes review one another's hospital charts before a patient's discharge to ensure that all abnormal results have been noted.

Flow Sheets

The advantage of a flow sheet, which can now be generated by a computer, is that you can see the data at a glance. "When it occupies four or five pages," said Telfer Reynolds, "you have lost the benefit of the flow sheet. A flow sheet for a liver patient contains results of the major studies needed to treat liver diseases, just as that for a fluid and electrolyte patient has the fluid and electrolyte data. The flow sheet also has a couple of columns for important clinical information. For a general internal medicine patient, the flow sheet should be adaptable, with blank spaces for the physician to write in whatever he wants to follow."

Medical Records

Incomplete or Illegible Records

Physicians avoid forgetting pertinent facts by making notes during the patient visit, but illegibility can cause problems, particularly if the physician's writing deteriorates as he becomes busier, more rushed, or older. Many physicians dictate their records for later transcription. Physicians generally agree that charting can be improved in most practices. Discipline and determination may provide the only solution, although the monitoring of records, particularly in the hospital, has lessened the deficiencies.

Consulting the Wrong Chart

Consulting the wrong chart does not happen often, but physicians should check the patient's name on the chart at each visit. A safeguard used in some offices is to have the patients record their names, dates of birth, and telephone numbers at each visit and then to match that information against that in the chart. Writing the name of the patient on every progress sheet is also helpful, and when more than one patient has the same name, the charts can be labeled in a way to alert the physician, nurse, and file clerk.

Lost or Misfiled Records

Patient records are more likely to be lost or misplaced in group practice than in solo practice. Computerized appointment systems are said to be an aid in this regard. In most clinics, charts are not supposed to leave the building or to be out of file overnight. Outcards can be inserted into the file to indicate where the record is at all times. Misfiling is more likely to occur in hospital practice, but medical record administrators can help immensely.

Lack of Follow-up of Patients

At the end of each day, Murray Salkin's nurse gives him the charts of patients who missed their appointments. He evaluates the records and gets in touch with patients with serious problems. To facilitate rescheduling, Cathleen Caton uses an FTKA (fail to keep appointment) stamp for patients who do not show up or who cancel appointments. Some physicians use a card file to make sure that patients with certain diseases are followed, and others have a secretary keep a separate list of seriously ill patients and their diagnoses to minimize loss to follow-up. Still others send cards to remind patients of a follow-up visit and, if the condition is particularly serious, they may telephone or wire the patient. In addition to contributing to poor care, lack of follow-up on patients can cause physicians to have an inaccurate perception of their results. (See Chapter 10 about sending follow-up questionnaires or letters to patients.)

Patient Noncompliance— Failure to Fill a Prescription or Follow Directions

A physician should never assume that patients are following instructions. Instead, he should ask his patients on each visit how they are tolerating their medications, if they have finished their supply, and other questions to determine if treatment is being followed. Seeing chronically ill patients every few weeks allows the physician to note symptoms and tolerance to drugs, to adjust dosage, and to encourage compliance. A special form for medications can be kept in the chart, to be updated at each visit when therapy is discussed with the patient. William Hart has his patients make a list of their medications and dosage, to be reviewed on each visit. He re-emphasizes the need for medication, explains the reason for the schedule, and relates the possibilities of drug interactions and adverse effects.

A good doctor-patient relationship facilitates compliance. When Page McGirr finds that a patient is not complying with his prescribed treatment, he restates the medical need, warns of the consequences of omission, and enlists the patient's cooperation, but avoids intimidation. Talking to other members of the family can also be useful.

Noncompliance can be a serious problem in patients with chronic diseases, such as diabetes and hypertension. As long as patients are feeling well, they may not exercise the self-discipline necessary for long-range health preservation. Follow-up visits may be needed to reinforce the importance of treatment and to provide encouragement.

Misunderstanding instructions is a common cause of patient noncompliance. Making the instructions simple, having patients repeat them, and writing them out reduce such misunderstandings. Some physicians keep a copy of written instructions as a reminder of what was communicated, and others ask the patient to bring all medications to the office. Elderly patients, in particular, need additional attention, written instructions, and more frequent office visits.

Inattention of the Patient

Patients, of course, need to give their full attention during conferences with the physician. You may need to ask distracting children or other relatives to remain in the waiting room when the patient is called in to see you. On the other hand, enlisting the aid of a spouse or relative can often help the patient understand. It is your responsibility to individualize your explanations and instructions to the patient's needs, to be extremely careful in delivering them, and to use language the patient understands. Roger Stickney likens a good physician to a good teacher who can hold the attention of a class.

Patient Denial

Patients who are frightened and distracted by anxiety often fail to recognize or accept a serious diagnosis. The patient may use a psychological defense to reject what he does not want to hear. The physician may give a clear description of the patient's problem and its possible solutions or prognosis, only to find that the patient has not absorbed or has totally misconstrued what was said. The physician may therefore have to rephrase the information and even schedule another appointment to ensure that instructions are being followed. Pressing for complete patient understanding immediately is not always wise, since denial can offer the patient psychological protection initially. Where education is essential to the patient's well-being and longevity, however, a thoughtful, compassionate, articulate, and attentive physician can usually deliver the proper message.

Factors Limiting Physician Effectiveness

Inattention of Physician

Perhaps the most significant barrier in the doctor-patient relationship is the physician's failure to give full attention to the patient. He may need to reduce his patient load to provide unrushed time for patients. Patients are receiving the physician's full attention, according to Steven Hamman, when he allows them to tell their tale while he actively listens and before he begins asking specific questions. The ability to listen and filter carefully is a great asset in medicine. Fred Turrill warned that, "Some physicians look at their patients and make a snap diagnosis without giving the patient time to say everything he has to say. Listening may teach you something new about a disease, and the patient will always feel better for having been heard out." Paul Bohannan, Dean of the Social Sciences and Communication Division of the University of Southern California, recommends paying attention to what is being said instead of planning your next statement while the patient is still talking. Try to discipline yourself to give full attention to your patients, including their "silent messages" and body language.

Sometimes the messages will not be so silent if the physician gives the patient a chance to speak and express his views. "The late Conrad Wesselhoeft of Harvard Medical School told a classic story," said Francis Moore, "and the moral of the story was simply that the physician has to think of a diagnosis before he can make one, and listening carefully to the patient is often the most important part of the examination. He illustrated the point with the account of a man who lived on an island in Boston Harbor and was stricken with a disease which made it difficult for him to open his mouth. The physician ministered to him, giving all the pukes, purges, and perspiring agents fashionable at the time, and confiding to the patient all the various diagnoses that came into his mind, ranging from diphtheria to glandular fever, quinsy sore throat, and epileptic seizures. Finally the patient, dying and hardly able to open his mouth, muttered, 'Doctor, don't you think I might have lockjaw?' To which the physician replied, 'Doggonnit, my good man, why didn't you think of that before?' "

Many of us are so busy asking the patient questions that the patient can never tell a complete story. M. Kenton King recalled that "The housestaff at Washington University customarily saved the most puzzling and perplexing case on the ward for presentation to the Chief about once a month. Accordingly, Dr. Carl Moore was brought to the bedside of an elderly lady with neurological findings plus abnormalities in many other systems. About 20 house officers were gathered around the bed. A young, eager, well-meaning house officer presented the case in a rather dull and rambling manner. Finally, the house officer finished and everybody looked at Dr. Moore, who turned to the patient and asked: 'Ma'am, what do you think your diagnosis is?' She replied, 'Well, when I visited Dr. Wintrobe about 20 years ago in Salt Lake City, he said that I had pernicious anemia before he started treatment.' Dr. Moore, realizing that it all fit together, said, 'My dear lady, why didn't you tell these doctors?' To which she replied, 'I tried to, but they told me to be quiet and answer their questions.' "

William Bardsley is convinced that the physician's interest in and attention to his patients are sharpened by his own good health, proper diet, adequate exercise, and adequate sleep. Interest is also enhanced by a certain amount of teaching and medical student discussions, since constantly listening to complaints is abnormal and can become tedious and stressful. Occasionally, something about a patient may arouse resistance in the physician. If the physician cannot resolve the matter, he should refer the patient to a more compatible colleague.

Distractions Diverting Attention from the Patient

Telephone calls should not be allowed to interrupt the doctor-patient conference unless they are extremely important. Many physicians try to take calls between patient visits, whereas others leave an opening in their morning and afternoon schedules to accommodate calls. When the physician must interrupt a patient interview to take an urgent call, it is best for him to leave the consultation room and to return afterwards, ready to be fully attentive to the patient.

"I have come to realize that the level of expertise a physician develops may be altered significantly by various factors, including fatigue, poor equipment, frequent interruptions, and emotional disturbances," said Francis S. Buck. "I now try to examine my most difficult diagnostic problems in the morning hours when I am mentally alert and most efficient."

Rushing through an Examination

Cotton Feray allows a certain number of appointments for acute problems, a certain number for physicals, and a certain number for follow-up appointments. The receptionist asks the patients what problems they are having, and Dr. Feray provides her with a list of patients who need longer appointments because of multiple problems. By allowing certain slots for physicals and other examinations, he never has to do a complete physical and Pap smear in a 10-minute slot. He schedules acute problems in the morning and all office surgery in the afternoon.

Some physicians schedule patients to arrive fifteen minutes before their appointments. The physician, however, also has an obligation to be prompt. If the physician finds himself rushing through examinations, he obviously needs to plan his schedule better and establish priorities. Because unexpected events may sometimes force physicians to "play catch-up," some schedule "catch-up" periods.

Physician Denial of Significant Data

Occasionally, physicians may psychologically deny significant data or fail to absorb what a patient is saying because they do not wish to accept the evidence that the patient has a life-threatening or socially unacceptable disorder. A long physician-patient relationship may intensify the resistance. The physician must, however, recognize that venereal disease, cancer, child abuse, AIDS, and other serious disorders exist and, regardless of his own discomfort, should look for them during his evaluation.

Acting on Insufficient Data

Some believe that pressure to reduce the cost of patient care has encouraged physicians to act on insufficient data. It puzzles Roger Stickney that some patients seem to prefer his treating them on instinct rather than factual data. There is no substitute for an excellent physical examination and penetrating analysis of the medical history and symptoms. To avoid acting on inadequate data, Page McGirr asks two questions: (1) "Do I have enough data on this patient to make everything clear to another physician should I become ill or go on vacation?" (2) "If the case ends in death or legal action, will my data support my actions?"

Colleagues

Strained Relationships within the Health Team

Unfortunately, strained and even destructive relationships can develop between physicians, or other health professionals attending a patient, just as they can between any two human beings. Resolving the problem at the earliest possible moment serves the patient's interest best. Avoidance or delay usually worsen the situation. In Osler's words, "[W]hen any dispute or trouble does arise, go frankly, ere sunset, and talk the matter over, in which way you may gain a brother and a friend."[7] The willingness of the physician to listen carefully to all concerned is crucial, and frequent team meetings can maintain rapport.

Reporting of Errors and Omissions

"It is a major responsibility of physicians," Richard Reitemeier believes, "to report to the proper authorities all significant errors of commission and omission by the professional staff." Because physicians do not always do this, either for want of time or fear of criticism, simple, remediable problems may accumulate and become chronic. Reitemeier relates three incidents involving personal or institutional responsiveness in identifying and reporting problems. The first occurred when, during the middle of a hot summer, reports of prothrombin time at a hospital were unexpectedly high. The residents on the service had stopped believing the reports or using those data. Neither the residents nor the attending physicians supervising them, however, had initiated an inquiry into the cause of the abnormal prothrombin values. "When I came on the service," said Reitemeier, "I validated that the prothrombins were clinically inconsistent and then advised Walter Bowey, head of our coagulation laboratory. Walter sent one of his technicians to draw blood from a patient whose prothrombin time we knew should be normal. He gave part of the blood to the laboratory at the hospital and took the rest to the laboratory at the clinic, where a normal prothrombin value was reported. The sample processed at the hospital, transported in the regular fashion to the laboratory, was reported as abnormal.

"Upon investigation, it was discovered that the technicians assigned to draw blood from patients throughout the hospital often did not return to the laboratory for two to three hours. During that time the tubes with the blood samples were kept in racks on their carts, and the prothrombin became degraded as a result of the summer heat. Walter Bowey simply provided each cart with a styrofoam container filled with dry ice to hold the blood samples, and the problem was immediately corrected. In addition, the incident led to a review by the laboratory of all studies that might be influenced by the ambient temperature.

"The next incident occurred when I saw a sturdy, tough Wyoming rancher weeping at his bedside on the morning he was to have colon surgery. He had had some 22 enemas in the preceding two and one-half days and told me that he was simply demoralized and could not endure having another one. Several months earlier the gastrointestinal surgeons had complained that the patients' colons were not completely free of feces at operation. This spurred the nurses who performed routine preoperative preparations to subject patients to increasing numbers of enemas. A serious lack of communication among nursing supervisors resulted in an occasional comment about the inadequacy of the preparation, which led, in turn, to

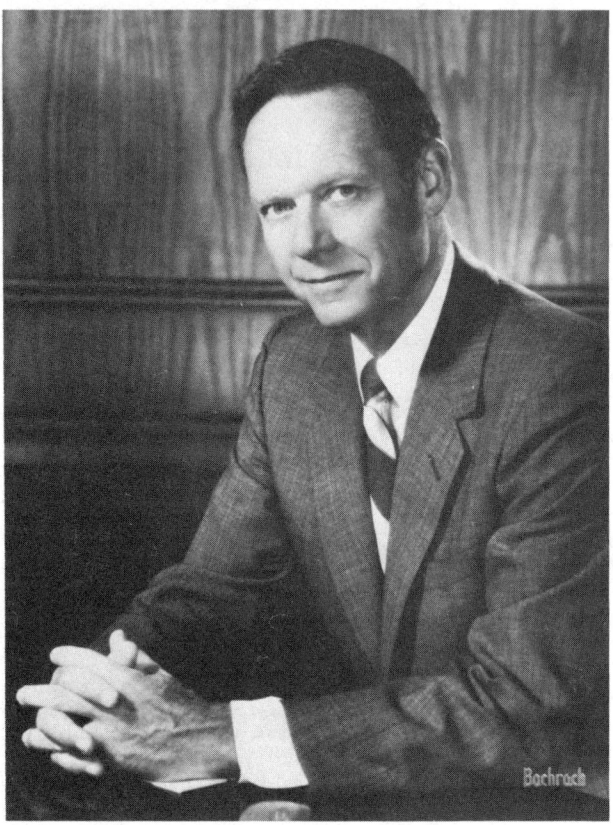

It is a major responsibility of physicians to report to the proper authorities all significant errors of commission and omission by the professional staff.

Richard J. Reitemeier, M.D.
Consultant in Gastroenterology
Mayo Clinic

an effort to cleanse the colons completely. Large amounts of total body sodium and potassium were probably washed from these patients in unnecessary procedures. A meeting with each group involved in such decisions led to the conclusion that each patient needed only a few enemas for cleansing, and a much more humane and comfortable preparation was put into effect.

"The third example occurred while I was Chairman of Medicine. I continued to hear complaints that, although we might be able to put a man on the moon, we could never successfully collect three-day stool samples from a patient. I asked the administrative assistant in the Department of Medicine to solve the problem. He assigned two young men with Master's degrees in business administration to find out what was wrong and what could be done. They discovered that no one felt personally responsible for the collection of the stools or the handling of the samples. The administrative assistant implemented a program that included methods to identify clearly the samples and give specific directions to all involved about how to move the material, where it was to go, and who was responsible. For the first time in the history of the institution, we had successful three-day collections of stools."

Solutions

Clement McDonald, who recognizes man's limited ability to process information, designed a computer program with protocol-based reminders for physicians.[8] Once a week for two months, physicians received computer suggestions. As a result, they detected, and responded effectively to, twice as many clinical events and data as previously.

Monthly meetings for clinic and hospital staffs to discuss problems in practice due to systems difficulties and not lack of scientific knowledge should allow physicians and other members of the health care team to identify, confront, and solve many of the problems outlined in this section.

*****

The tendency for a complex system to go from a state of order to a state of disorder is a serious and frustrating reality in medical practice. A lost laboratory report can sometimes be more devastating to good patient care than a lack of medical knowledge. Computer reminder-and-monitoring systems can help prevent omissions, oversights, and inattention to abnormal findings and can thus lessen disorder in practice. Without such assistance, physicians must themselves constantly monitor and guide the care given their patients.

As Peter Mere Latham wrote: "[I]n medicine. . . it requires as much labour and time fairly to lay hold of an error, and uproot it, and have done with it, as to learn and settle a truth, and abide by it."[9]

References

1. Bloch, Arthur. *Murphy's Law and Other Reasons Why Things Go Wrong.* Los Angeles: Price Stern Sloan Publishers Inc, 1982:11, 12.
2. Williamson, John W.; Alexander, Marshall; Miller, George E. Continuing education and patient care research: Physician response to screening test results. *JAMA* 18 Sep 1967;201(12):938-942.
3. Starfield, Barbara; Scheff, David. Effectiveness of pediatric care: The relationship between processes and outcome. *Pediatrics* Apr 1972;49(4):547-552.
4. Morehead, Mildred A.; Donaldson, Rose. Quality of clinical management of disease in comprehensive neighborhood health centers. *Med Care* Apr 1974;12(4):301-315.
5. Brook, Robert H.; Stevenson, Robert L., Jr. Effectiveness of patient care in an emergency room. *N Engl J Med* Oct 22, 1970;283(17):904-907.
6. Gonnella, Joseph S.; Goran, Michael J.; Williamson, John W.; Cotsonas, Nicholas J., Jr. Evaluation of patient care: An approach. *JAMA* Dec 14, 1970;214(11):2040-2043.
7. Osler, William. The master-word in medicine. *Bull Johns Hopkins Hosp* Jan 1904;15(154):7.
8. McDonald, Clement J. Protocol-based computer reminders, the quality of care and the non-perfectability of man. *N Engl J Med* Dec 9, 1976;295(24):1351-1355.
9. Latham, Peter Mere. General remarks on the practice of medicine. In: Martin, Robert, ed. *The Collected Works of Dr. P. M. Latham.* London: The New Sydenham Society, 1878:382.

15

Women Physicians and Continuing Education

> Man may work from sun to sun,
> But woman's work is never done.

Time Pressures on Women Physicians from Multiple Roles

Because of multiple roles as physician, wife, mother, and homemaker, some women physicians face different and more difficult problems than men in finding time for continuing education. Women have to set priorities, especially in assigning time for education, sometimes at the expense of recreational activities.

Jacqueline D. Miller believed that she faced a larger problem than younger women, since mores have changed somewhat. But when she questioned younger associates and friends who work in other occupations, she concluded that women with homes and families generally have more responsibilities than their husbands. "Even when the husbands help," she explained, "the daily responsibilities for the home and the family continue to rest largely with the wives. A woman physician's attention is divided between practice and home, whereas a man's primary concern is his practice and only secondarily duties in the home. This situation may lead women to feel torn, and the stress becomes more acute when they have children who are having problems."

Time is the major problem women physicians face, acccording to Marjorie Price Wilson. "They do more than full-time housewives in the same socioeconomic circles. When they enter medicine, women do not abandon any of the traditional roles of mother and household manager. As I look back on my life, I realize that although my husband shared the time with the children, I actually spent more time than he did with them while never compromising my professional duties. His life would have been the same if I had been a full-time housewife. I have maintained a fairly traditional lifestyle at home; even with a great deal of good help I still managed the 'helpers' and the household. Most women who assume multiple roles, regardless of their profession, perform them all with great intensity. Professional men, on the other hand, often feel a greater intensity about their profession than their families."

Surgeon Laurel Weibel traces the major difference between men and women physicians to the fact that few women can go home from their medical offices and relax—read journals, listen to the radio, or watch television. "There are always meals to prepare, children to counsel, and after-dinner chores to do. Even when there is an evening meeting to attend, the family must first be fed. And in the morning, babies have to be bathed and fed, or lunches have to be made."

This "time-vise" has troubled Eileen Duggan. "Being locked into a schedule makes me feel as if I am compressing my professional and private spheres too much. Medicine can be extremely seductive, especially to someone who likes to think of herself as indispensable. Because of the wear-and-tear on my physical and mental health, I have had to set priorities in my work. Mornings with my children are special times, and so I do not attend early rounds, even though my associate does. I make my commitments at work very specific and manageable. I also schedule three to five meetings each year for education. Most are two- or three-day meetings and are inspiring and invigorating. Getting away for a fresh perspective is necessary, I believe. Women physicians should not begrudge paying part of their earnings to another person to do housework. My friends who insist on doing their own housework seem dissatisfied with themselves unless it is done perfectly."

Women physicians are vulnerable to interruptions by husbands, children, and household responsibilities, and this vulnerability makes it difficult to establish a "do not interrupt" period. Whereas men physicians face interruptions from medical emergencies, women face interruptions from multiple sources.

There is still great reliance on women for housecleaning, cooking, laundering, and shopping, as Lailee Bakhtiar observed. "Few husbands want their day interrupted with household chores. A live-in housekeeper can help with some of these tasks, but this is only a partial solution. Housekeepers quit, children get sick, and the final responsibility for organizing usually falls on the woman. Organization, strength, and a spouse willing to share can all help."

Karin Jamison also sees multiple roles as a major problem. "Add to the list any personal interest the woman has outside of medicine and her family, and the demands on her time and energy create a real conflict. Only the housekeeper role can be delegated, not that of the 'homemaker.' A responsible male physician will also have conflicts if he takes his roles as father, husband, son, sibling, friend, and neighbor seriously, but his role of physician coincides with his role as husband/father, since a traditional aspect of both has been to be a good provider. So he does not experience the same 'shortage' of time or the same degree of inner conflict. For a woman physician, fatigue is a constant companion."

Motherhood accentuates the problem. Lailee Bakhtiar sees flexibility and physical well-being as two desirable qualities of a woman physician. "A pregnant woman can work until delivery, and her husband can be supportive, loving, and helpful. But the man married to a woman physician pays a toll as her professional life and the size of their family grow. The difficulty in striking a balance probably accounts for the high divorce rate among women physicians. An extended family, with a solid bond among parents and in-laws, can help with problems arising from the mother's absence at meetings or work. Women are often superior in caring for the sick, but their personal relationships with men suffer as a result. Community recognition of an outstanding woman may further alienate the husband."

During pregnancy, Linda Shortliffe had some physical incapacitation, but it did not affect her daytime work. "I worked up to the time of the delivery and was not bothered much by pregnancy, but I was not as efficient in reading and writing in the evenings. I took four weeks off after delivery and found it difficult to return to work after that. Being physically present in the hospital during the day was not a problem, but the chronic fatigue from rising every two to three hours for nursing was. It was difficult to find opportunities to freeze breast milk during the first several months after I returned to work. During that time, many of the routine home chores such as laundry, cooking, grocery-shopping, and housecleaning were taking valued time from our baby. As a result, we now have a live-in 'nanny.' We have delegated some of the household chores to her so that we can have more time to spend with our child and still fulfill our professional responsibilities."

In the opinion of Beverly June Gregorius, younger women will do much more than she has. "But it still tends to be a man's world, and a woman is required to work harder to prove herself. Sometimes this requires sheer physical stamina, for it is hard to remain in surgery for hours or stay up all night. I go into everything wholeheartedly; I participate in resident conferences three times a week, give community talks, and speak to women's groups, in addition to my regular obstetrics-gynecology lectures, all of which require reading and research."

Interruption of Practice by Childbirth and Children's Rearing

For six years, while Karin Jamison's children were in high school, she closed her private practice and worked only two days a week at an Air Force Base outpatient clinic. "Because I was free of the heavy responsibility of a solo family practice, I was able to attend many medical meet-

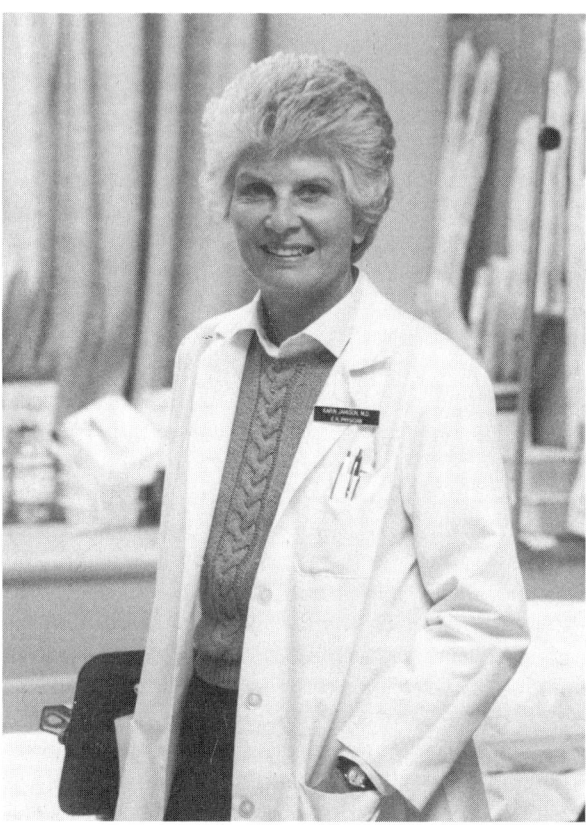

It is not too hard to be a doctor or a mother of four or a lifelong student. Indeed, each is challenging, personally rewarding, and even fun. It is the coordination of the three that is difficult and even painful at times.

Karin E. Jamison, M.D.
Lompoc, California

ings. The patient contact at the Air Force Base helped me maintain my clinical skills, although I had no acutely ill patients to care for at that time. When I returned to private practice, I wanted to do emergency medicine and so took some intensive courses in that field. I also studied a great deal on subjects for which I knew I would have responsibilities."

When Jacqueline Miller had a child just a few weeks after she completed her residency, she stayed away from work for a year. "I enjoyed my child and did not keep up with medicine, so I found it very difficult when I went back. I don't think I did any of it quite right. I would now recommend that a woman do everything possible to maintain her intellectual activities and her contact with medicine. You can get out of touch in a year. One thing that helped me catch up was that I had not yet taken my clinical pathology boards. I settled down and prepared myself for them, spending the better part of a year in intensive study. I did my studying after the baby went to bed. During that time I had household help and considered it a wise investment."

Kit Chambers stopped working as a physician and stayed home for six years when her children reached 11 and 13 years of age. "Before returning to practice, I read copiously, attended grand rounds in my specialty every week at the University of Southern California and the University of California at Los Angeles, and attended all resident lectures at UCLA from 4:00 to 6:00 p.m. daily, after having worked from 8:00 a.m. to 4:00 p.m. I also went to as many postgraduate courses in my specialty as I could in the Los Angeles area." Her advice: "Learn to budget time, and learn to live with fatigue and stay healthy."

Because Barbara Buchanan's third child had a congenital anomaly requiring surgery and a prolonged recovery period, she took off six months from medicine. "I never thought it was difficult to 'keep up' during the months I took off, or to 'catch-up' once I started practicing again. If anything, I had more time to read journals and books during that time."

Some women physicians do not take time off for childbirth. Susan Tully went back to work within a couple of weeks after her children were born. "I paid people to look after the children and was never out any longer than my scheduled vacation."

Enlisting Support

"The first thing a young woman physician with a family needs to acknowledge," in Jacqueline Miller's view, "is that she cannot do everything herself and do it as well as she would like. Physicians in general, and women physicians in particular, are perfectionists, and it is difficult to acknowledge that you are not going to be superb in all your efforts; there is simply not enough time. You must accept your need for help. My own solution has been to recognize that I will not have as much spendable income as I might expect, because I must employ help. Skimping on household and babysitting help is a mistake. Concentrate your energy on what you consider to be important. The woman physician may want to spend a few more hours a week at the office or hospital than a man, since she can do some of her studying there. I can get a lot done from 5:00 to 6:00 p.m., or from 5:30 to 7:00 p.m., whereas when I go home, I get little or no work done. Sharing the responsibilities at home with others as much as possible is very helpful."

Of paramount importance to Alice Bessman, when one's children are young, is strong family support (grandparent type) or reliable full-time help—someone to be home during the illnesses of children, at the end of the school day, and for errands. "I never worked full-time after my training period until the youngest child was at the junior high-school level. Until then, I worked half-time or less."

Career women need to have realistic expectations for the home, according to Bernice Z. Brown. "To me, being a career woman means settling for standards at home that are not the highest, but are acceptable. I try not to look in corners or under beds." Genevieve Burk agreed: "To attempt to satisfy one's mother-in-law regarding household duties is folly. Mine once expressed dismay that I did not save my grease to make soap! Set priorities and stick to them."

Gail Clark identified three major parts of her solution: "(1) a true partnership with your husband at home concerning *all* duties (house and children), (2) working in an academic setting where lectures and day-to-day conversations with interns, residents, and colleagues keep you in touch with prevailing ideas in your specialty, and (3) setting your priorities and realizing that you cannot be an A-1 wife, mother, *and* physician everyday, but that your best should be satisfactory for you, your family, and your patients' well-being. You are not an island, and there is backup all around you if you will accept it."

"Those who combine marriage and medicine have a very difficult time meeting the needs of both," said Ruth Bain. "Some do it, but it isn't easy. They must have an understanding husband who is willing to share what is usually seen as women's duties." "An understanding husband," in Dame Sheila Sherlock's opinion, "is a most important aid for the woman physician."

For Maureen Sims, "Choosing a housekeeper is very important and deserves top priority. I would advise my colleagues to interview several candidates and be prepared to pay top dollar for the type of services you expect. Above all, be able to communicate with the housekeeper. Many unpleasant situations with long-term ramifications can develop if inappropriate choices are made, especially in the early developmental phases of child-rearing. If an inappropriate choice is made and difficulties cannot be worked through successfully, it may be necessary to dismiss the housekeeper and start over. If your own employer is not understanding, it can lead to frustration and a difficult situation. Fortunately, my boss and my colleagues have been in similar situations and understood. Working

15. Women Physicians and Continuing Education

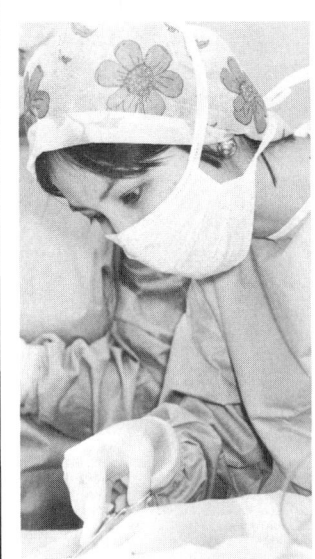
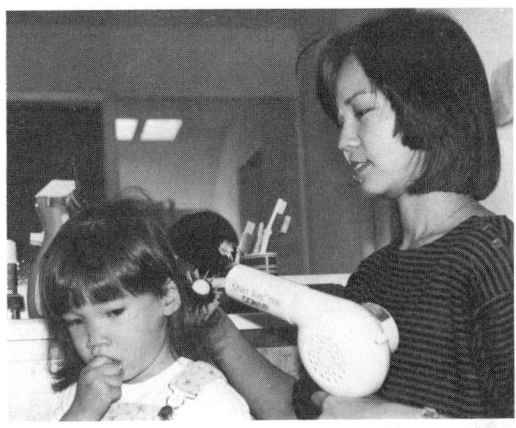

We now have a live-in "nanny." We have delegated some of the household chores to her so that we can have more time to spend with our child and still fulfill our professional responsibilities.

Linda D. Shortliffe, M.D.
Chief, Urology Section
Veterans Administration Medical Center, Palo Alto

with people who have had or are currently having children-work conflicts is helpful."

Collegial Relationships

Collegial relationships within the medical community are as useful to women physicians as to men. In Marjorie Price Wilson's words: "Most of my colleagues are men, and I have always been accepted by them. Women in the health professions, however, do not always have the same status as men. The 'old boy' network has left me out politically more than once, even when it involved close friends. Nevertheless, I have good learning experiences from collegial relationships. The 'old girl' network, on the other hand, is not yet very effective. Women can be unduly competitive with one another. In recent years, I have formed some close associations with three or four other professional women, and I know that we can go to one another for support, but it is not really a network, only close friendships that have developed over the years."

Rodanthi Kitridou agreed that the relatively small number of women in universities has prevented the establishment of effective networks within specialties. "As a rule, male colleagues have been helpful in providing information and suggestions. Of course, an occasional physician will flaunt his knowledge and try to make a female colleague look ignorant, but he will do the same with male colleagues, because his insecurity and self-aggrandizement supersede a productive exchange of information."

"I enjoy the exchange of ideas and discussion of interesting cases with colleagues in the surgery lounge," said Laurel Weibel, "and have never felt excluded because of my sex. Unfortunately, I am frequently assigned to committees to investigate female problem-physicians because 'You're not so prone to be vindictive or biased' or 'You can be the devil's advocate.'"

Lailee Bakhtiar would like to see women physicians and men physicians share in one fraternity, without prejudice. "My experience (limited to Los Angeles) has been that common specialties and common membership in professional societies support collegial groups. For some unknown reason, however, many women do not enter collegial groups. The 'old boy' network has not excluded me from appointment or election in medical societies. For problems unique to women, the 'old girl' network could be helpful, but I have had no personal experience with it."

Jacqueline Miller has obtained support from belonging to a group. "If you are in a group, you never feel alone, and you learn how to have a productive relationship with your peers. I have practiced only with an occasional woman physician, so I have had little experience with the 'old girl' network. I have not felt any direct prejudice from men, although on occasion I have observed some reservations about women in medicine. If you sit back and relax, however, it goes away."

Linda Shortliffe, practicing in the male-dominated specialty of urology, has not had any specific collegial difficulties. "My best professional relationships have been with residents with whom I have worked. Probably the most important professional advantage has resulted from interactions with a male faculty mentor, who, fortunately, appears to have overcome the traditional ideas about women in surgery."

Marjorie S. Sirridge's experience differed: "The 'old boy' network admits only a few women sponsored by 'old boys.' I have struggled hard to become part of collegial groups but have usually felt excluded. There have not been enough women to organize and perpetuate 'old girl' networks, and few women have yet acquired the necessary skills to make them work. Most women do not feel secure enough to help other women; they seem to isolate themselves. They may form support groups as a defense mechanism to sustain themselves. I have been most comfortable with women's support groups, but they have contributed little to my lifetime learning, which has been active, continuous, and isolated. My husband is a physician, and I have been included in some groups through that relationhip. Most collegial associations have resulted from my status as a presenter on professional panels and programs, where I am usually the only woman."

In Ruth Bain's experience, you become a full participating member of the 'old boy' network by doing your best at every committee or other assignment. "Many young women seem convinced that they will not be accepted or allowed to participate in organized medicine; that simply is not true. We tend to find what we look for; in expecting problems, many young women really create them."

The Single Woman–physician

The main advantage for a woman physician who is single, in Marjorie Price Wilson's view, is that her time is more her own. "She can plan more deliberately. When you have a family, you must set priorities; that is the dilemma. On the other hand, the single woman may miss the joys of children and a family." Although unmarried men and women should be able to organize their continuing education more efficiently, motivation is a highly individual matter, and they may not always do so. Kit Chambers observed that "Single women can devote more time to their work and have more leisure time to develop hobbies. They can travel more freely to postgraduate courses, whereas husbands of women physicians are not always willing to take trips for the benefit of their wives' medical interests."

Satisfaction from Multiple Roles

The time demands described by the women physicians interviewed justify the question: "Is it worth it?" The following represent typical responses from our interviewees.

"Professional activities such as clinical teaching and participation in professional organizations expose one to new experiences, people, ideas, and aspects of life outside medicine," said Bernice Brown. "If one believes that we have only one 'go-round' in life, it makes sense to pack in as much as possible and make it as meaningful as possible in the time we have. Being a professional woman leads to a hectic, busy, often overextended life, and a woman physician must strive to save moments for herself so she does not become a machine. A medical career is fulfilling and stimulating, but being a homemaker and having children are also fulfilling, although when the children grow up and lead their own lives, it creates a void for the woman who has dedicated herself solely to her children. This is where the rewards of a rapidly changing, ever stimulating profession are greatest. A profession can then give one a feeling of self-worth, of making a contribution to society, and of keeping the brain cells working.

"A real source of pleasure in being a physician, wife, and mother is that your children and husband are proud of your accomplishments and let you know it now and then, in sometimes amusing or offhand ways. They do not treat you like a 'has been' or someone not to be reckoned with, as many children seem to treat parents. Once after I repaired a deep laceration on my younger daughter's ankle (she was 13 years old) in a backwoods place where we were vacationing but where there were not good medical facilities, she turned to me and said, 'Say Mom, you're not a half-bad doc.' "

The human element is the most rewarding factor in the medical career of Kit Chambers. "I enjoy helping and caring for people. Allaying their anxiety is a large part of my contact with patients, as well as explaining what they can expect from me."

For Beverly Gregorius the practice of medicine is the best thing that ever happened to her—with the exception of marrying her husband and having her daughter. "One cannot have a better mood–elevator, energizer, or ego-builder than seeing patients. They are always glad to see me and are fond of me as their physician. I can't imagine anything more interesting, exciting, and fulfilling than the practice of medicine."

Karin Jamison, with her four children grown and almost out of college, is practicing from 24 to 48 hours a week in an Emergency Room. "This is far and away the happiest time in my professional life because the sometimes agonizing conflict between the legitimate demands of my family and my medical career is over.

"The benefit of the busy life a woman physician leads is that she is able to fulfill Robert Louis Stevenson's idea that: 'The purpose of life is to become what one is capable of becoming.' The woman physician with a family is able to realize her intellectual, physical, emotional, creative and spiritual potential in a way few others are privileged to do. I would here acknowledge that our dear husbands play a vital part in facilitating this. However, if one has an intrinsic interest in medicine and people, all the effort is richly rewarded."

Linda Shortliffe has enjoyed several benefits from the lifelong associations made through her medical career: "It is gratifying to attend meetings and recognize old friends and acquaintances with whom I can discuss research ideas or academic problems. In addition, there is a fulfilling relationship with residents and young people. Perhaps the most important satisfaction is a constant association with new ideas, and later seeing those ideas turned into action. It is exciting to see hypotheses become study protocols, then experimental research, and then accepted as fact or routine treatment. Watching and participating in the evolution of ideas are most gratifying."

As Jacqueline Miller looked back over the past 35 years, which included years of postgraduate training and practice, she found that she had been extremely happy in her choice of medicine as a profession. "Each day has been stimulating and interesting, full of intellectual challenges and interesting cases. My professional associates and companions have been intelligent, motivated by concern for their fellow man and compulsive in their desire to excel. This kind of association is well worth the sacrifices. The most difficult problem is the inability to do as much as you would like for and with your family. This leads to a pervasive sense of guilt, with which one must learn to live. The variety of experiences from combining a marriage and family with a career is nonetheless a satisfying life."

In Alice Bessman's view, academic advancement should not be the physician's only goal. "An oft-heard dissatisfaction is that women do not advance as rapidly as their male colleagues. In many cases, however, outside distractions may limit productivity. The contributions to the social structure in general and to the family in particular should more than outweigh this lack of academic advancement. My satisfaction from having contributed to increased medical knowledge and to the replenishment of the younger generation of physicians is satisfaction enough."

*****

Since most women physicians have more diverse responsibilities than men physicians, they feel time-pressures more acutely. Organization of time and development of efficient study methods are therefore even more critical for women in medicine than for men. All the women physicians we interviewed agreed that it is mandatory to rely heavily on outside or extended family help for household tasks and child care. A woman physician who marries would do well to discuss with her prospective husband the time difficulties that are certain to occur and to come to some conclusions and agreement in advance. If the woman physician plans carefully, sets realistic goals for each of her roles, and accepts skilled household help to permit the best use of her time, a medical career can offer her great opportunities for service and fulfillment, and this rich professional life can go hand-in-hand with an equally rewarding personal life—one enhancing the other.

16

Can Families Help?

> [Osler's] *Aequanimitas* is a medical classic and was a bedside book of mine. In it he preaches the virtue of the quiet mind, "do the day's work and let tomorrow take care of itself." But like most preachers he did not always practise what he preached. His wife, in a memoir she wrote of him, says something to this effect. "It was all very well of William to preach Aequanimitas but I noticed that when there was trouble at home, . . .he invariably had important engagements elsewhere and left me to cultivate the quiet mind—if I could.
>
> *Alfred Cox*[1]

The time pressures in medical practice can stifle the drive for daily study, especially if responsibilities at home are equally demanding. On the other hand, families can help the physician sustain the flame of interest and still share a full and satisfying family relationship.

Attitude

Of her physician-husband's continuing education, Babs Gordon said: "Alan's studying and journal reading is so much a part of his life, and ours, that I never give it special thought. It is something that he must do to remain the fine physician he is. From his medical school days through all the years the children were growing up, and even today, Alan has studied. A great deal of it he does in the early morning and in the evening after dinner. He has never deprived us of his 'prime' time, but his study hours are his 'private' time. During those hours I manage to do chores that don't involve him; the children have also always respected this time. I, too, enjoy time to myself, as do the children. The only way I have consciously facilitated Alan's 'lifelong learning' is by allowing it to be a natural part of our lives."

Dorothy Brooks became reconciled many years ago that there was a certain part of her husband's time she could not share. "I try as best I can to fill that time with activities of my own that are enriching and interesting. In that way I don't feel cheated. In other words, his education time allows me time to participate in activities he might not be interested in. I have not, however, always felt so generous. When our four sons were growing up, my attitude was quite different—then the burden was on me, and I certainly wasn't free to think about myself. But we got through those years beautifully; the time my husband spent with the family was quality time. There are no secrets to time management. It is a matter of attitude and the right spirit on the part of the spouse. Individual management of time and shared family time can be made a learning experience for young children, too."

"Include your husbands and children in your planning of household chores," advises Kit Chambers, "so they can better understand the problems."

Making Time for Study

Elizabeth Ramirez-Rodriguez asked: "How can I say this without sounding like a martyr? It has simply been a matter of taking over responsibilities, as much as possible, whenever my husband decided he wanted to take a course. I must admit, I haven't always accepted it with grace, but, as a nurse, I understood his need to keep abreast of the newest knowledge in his field." The nonphysician spouse can take charge of arranging the social and personal calendars, thus allowing more time for continuing medical education.

Joan Burns was able to relieve her husband of any household duties such as paying bills, income tax, insurance, car maintenance, and garden work. She could schedule airline travel and usually did the driving between home and St. Louis or Kansas City, allowing him time to work. Because she did not work outside the home, she felt it was easy for her to adjust her own schedule to help him.

Gee Pei, a mechanical and materials engineer, is supportive of his wife's medical career. "I have learned one thing about being married to a physician—you can't expect your spouse to be on time. I do not get frustrated about that, even if my wife does not call. It is important for a husband to understand the extent of a physician's time commitment, and to have some interests of his own. My wife has had some tough times with on-call schedules, but this has not bothered me, for I can occupy myself in the evenings she is on-call. We make it an unwritten rule that we don't talk about work at home. Granted, my wife does have interesting things to tell me, and I enjoy listening to her stories, but we simply try not to dwell on our work. I do quite a bit of the shopping because my wife does not have the time. I also enjoy cooking and feel that it is important to have dinner together. Even if my wife is going to be late, I will wait for her."

From our interviews, women physicians may not always find their husbands so helpful. Said one woman surgeon, "Like so many other men of his vintage, my husband feels that a woman should be allowed to do anything she wants—as long as she takes care of the home and family and does not try to get him to do any housework. He will make his own breakfast and lunch if I'm not home, but carrying his dishes into the kitchen and leaving them in the sink is his contribution to helping me with the housework. I hire my own housekeeper, but because of the children I have little at-home study time."

Daniel and Cecelia Essin, both pediatricians, share the household responsibilities. "In order for my wife to pursue her activities, I manage the house and take care of our child on the weekends she is on call. Usually, when a man is a physician, his wife is expected to manage the household but may never understand the time demands of her husband's career. It must seem like an imposition to the wife—and I admit, it sometimes seems like an imposition to me. But my spouse and I have a common background so I understand and accept the career pressures."

During the week, "homework" can be the first priority, and quiet evenings are arranged to facilitate study. Spouses must, first of all, accept the fact that physicians require at-home study time. A spouse who takes on tasks inside and outside the home will give the physician more time to read and study.

Aiding Study

> [I]n May 1844, I married, and began to enjoy that happiness of domestic life which has already lasted without a break, without a cloud, for 39 years. From this time, the "being alone" was the being alone with one who never failed in love, in wise counsel, in prudence and in gentle care of me. With her it was easy to work and be undisturbed by anything going-on around me; a habit which I can advise every one to learn. . . . she wrote for me, copying for the press my roughly written manuscripts, sitting with me till midnight or far into the morning.
>
> *Sir James Paget*[2]

"After 31 years of marriage, my problem is less one of facilitating Ralph's continuing education and more one of planning time for him to play and relax," said Betty Wallerstein. "When he gets up early to work, I cooperate by sleeping late. When he says he must be alone to work, I

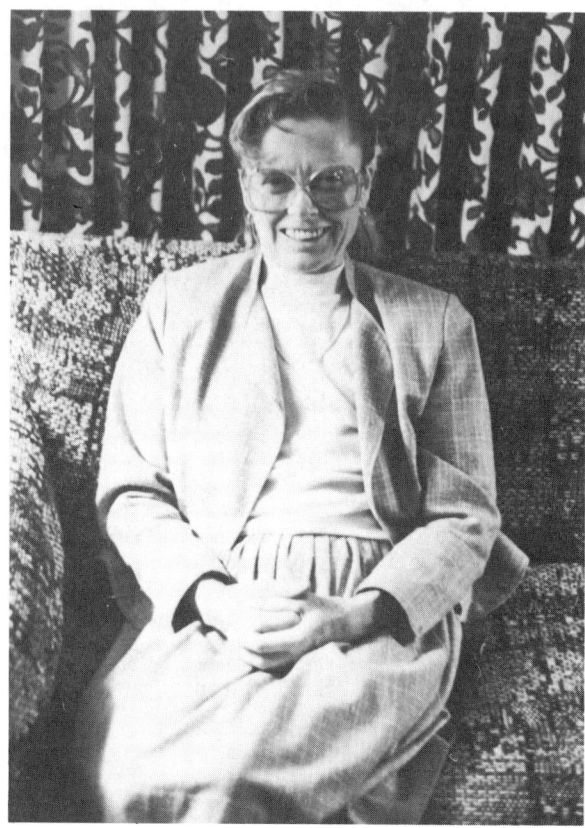

Include your husbands and children in your planning of household chores so they can better understand the problems.

Kit Chambers, M.D.
North Hollywood, California

16. Can Families Help?

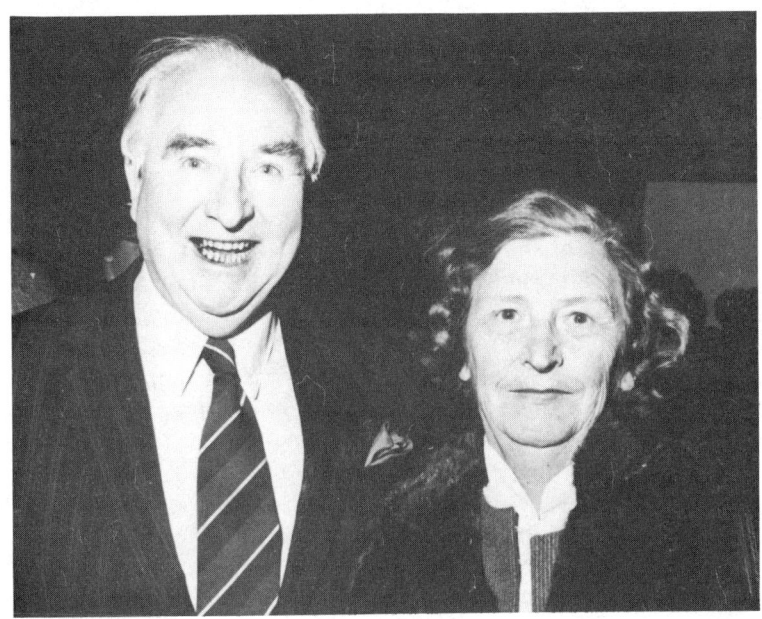

An understanding husband is a most important aid for the woman physician.

Dame Sheila Sherlock, M.D.
Emeritus Professor, The Royal Free Hospital
London, England
(with husband D. Geraint James
Dean, Royal Northern Hospital)

leave him alone and make no demands on his time or energy. On cross-country flights, I do not talk to him, so that he can read reprints." Marjorie Bird recognizes that her husband's career and "the ultimate survival of our family demands his consistent and purposeful continuing education. Everything that we can reasonably do in that pursuit is important, and if a course or conference can be combined with vacation pleasure, so much the better."

Louise Hart considers patience to be essential in a physician's spouse. "Time alone for my husband to read all he has set out for himself (often too much) was my aim, and it did take time from family activities when the babies were growing. Now that they are off at college or married, I am 'alone' (after all my volunteer work). I long for some adult conversation with the man I married, but he still has to read medical material! This reality makes me try to help him by keeping him informed on timely topics, family events (and trivia), and friends' news and events. I enjoy worthwhile continuing education meetings, where we can enjoy each other's company while he is learning. I also think it is important to entertain his medical colleagues at home, so that they can discuss medicine."

Some spouses actively assist in continuing education by filing notes or articles, either by computer or manually. Janet Grignon, a nurse, often studies with her husband, since they attend many of the same sessions. "I also quiz him on subjects I have just studied or want to know about. Both of us are always reading and studying medicine, history, or anthropology."

Lynn Pittier has noticed depression in the nonworking wives of housestaff members. "Because I was employed during his residency, our busy schedules seemed to provide a common platform for communication—fatigue, challenges, goals, mutual outlets. After his residency, he continued to put in many hours a week keeping current on the literature. Because I teach nursing, we study together and have converted one of our larger bedrooms into a medical library. We decorated it to lure us into its quiet ambiance as the most restful room of our house. We often have lunch together so we can talk uninterruptedly for about an hour. This reduces the need to interrupt his nightly reading sessions. I believe that my 50-hour work weeks have been very useful for Mike's busy schedule. We see a lot of each other and continue to have empathy for the fatigue, stress, and occasional drained states we experience. When he is on-call, I love to dive into writing or household activities. These arrangements have encouraged his keeping abreast of medical literature, medical politics at our local hospital, and involvement in continuing medical education."

Pediatricians Daniel and Cecelia Essin pursue their lifelong learning together. "Whenever one of us has a difficult case we discuss it in the evening and decide what books or consultants may be helpful. We try to attend the same conferences, and have combined our at-home reference library." J. Douglas and his wife, also both doctors, often attend seminars or meetings together while family members care for their children. "When one of us goes alone," he said, "the other partner stays home to look after the family." Physician couples in partnership practice can cover both medical and household responsibilities in one member's absence.

*****

Physicians whose practice is organized to provide optimal educational benefit from experience can have a full family life and still allocate time each day for study. The professional demands on the time and energy of physicians, however, are real and should be discussed fully before marriage. Most spouses of physicians assume greater responsibilities in the home and offer encouragement and support for continuing study. When the spouse is a physician or nurse, studying together can be fun. Nonphysician spouses, on the other hand, are sometimes grateful for the free personal time the physician's studying allows them, and they arrange their activities accordingly. Postgraduate programs given in vacation areas and scheduled to permit free time are rewarding for physicians and their families. Physicians who enjoy studying regularly are excellent models for their children. Families that understand and accept the heavy demands of medicine can contribute greatly to the physician's sense of well-being and sustain the spirit of lifelong learning. The physician's enthusiasm and zest can be infectious, and the entire family can benefit.

References

1. Cox, Alfred. *Among the Doctors*. London: Christopher Johnson, 1950:134.
2. Paget, Sir James. In: Paget, Stephen, ed. *Memoirs and Letters of Sir James Paget*. New York: Longmans, Green, and Co., 1901:128.

17

The Computer: Aid to Learning and Satisfaction from Practice

> Technology is preparing a world in
> which we may be learners all life long.
>
> *George B. Leonard*[1]

By analyzing their clinical activities and linking their education to real events in practice, physicians can enhance not only their skills but their satisfaction from practice as well. Many of the effective methods we have described can be facilitated by the computer. Some physicians, and all hospitals, have access to computer services for financial and administrative activities, and many are now also using personal computers to analyze their practice, access medical information, and expedite communication with colleagues. They are now seeking guidance in diagnosis and therapy to improve their patient care.

Because the computer can provide information at the time and place the physician needs it, it reduces unrealistic reliance on memory. In Lawrence Weed's words, "The computer links thought to action." Even though the complete information system necessary to do this is not yet available, the computer's assistance in organization and retrieval of information can save the physician's time, and will ultimately mitigate the suppression of intellectual curiosity ensuing from disorganization. Used properly, the computer can facilitate communication among colleagues, encourage deeper understanding of practice, allow more time for listening to patients, and promote a more zestful professional life.

The application of computers in the physician's office, hospital, and medical library to promote practice-linked education will probably occur in three stages: First, some conventional functions that are now being recorded on paper will be performed electronically. Second, new methods of information management will be devised that can be performed best, and sometimes solely, with the computer. Third, entirely new and unpredictable methods and approaches to clinical problems will be developed in the future.[2]

Enhancing the Personal Information Center

Computers will make the personal information center more productive and efficient for physicians. Moreover, the personal computer, equipped with modem, telephone line, and communication software, will permit physicians to do the bibliographic searching and screening traditionally done by librarians.

Keeping Notes on Reading and Indexing Articles

The advent of the microcomputer has revolutionized journal note-taking. Donald M. Switz now reads journals while sitting at his Apple computer. Using a computer filing program, he enters citations and data while he reads, easily cross-referencing and storing the information. A 5-1/4-inch floppy disk will hold about 300 references. "When you want to look up that forgotten bit of clinical information," said Switz, "the computer will find it in a flash if the information was coded correctly. For example, a notation of a recent article might read:

> *GUT* 1982;23:A910. ERCP* in primary biliary cirrhosis. E Hamilton et al. 22 Pt with PBC; 17 Panc duct seen and abnl in 1. DV sclerosing cholangitis -3 have chr panc. 7 or 19 PBC pts CBD show caliber variation & irreg.[3]
> *Endoscopic Retrograde Cholangiopancreatography

"Our minds are wonderfully effective at association and synthesis, but some of us are not very good at recall. I am forever wondering 'Where was that marvelous article on. . .?' Now, after I have referenced it on a disk, I no longer have to wonder." The user creates the abbreviations in such an abstract, but it would be useful if multiple users agreed upon common abbreviations.

Computer cross-indexing facilitates Eric Sohr's use of his personal reprint file. "Many articles have more than one topic of interest. Suppose I read an article on dog bites that discloses a good method for injecting xylocaine painlessly, discusses the advisability of suturing various animal wounds, reviews the flora of the mouth of a dog, and presents current information on tetanus and rabies prophylaxis. If I have multiple file folders keyed to various topics, such as the chapters in a medical textbook, the question is 'Where should I file that article?' Multiple categories are difficult to manipulate manually. All manual systems require a lot of time and effort. If, for example, you want to use eight key words to describe an article, you must pull all eight cards and enter the information on each.

"A computer program may contain all key words in the computer memory. You must enter them before use, but you can enter a new key word during the indexing of a particular article. The only writing needed is the recording of an accession number on the actual reprint. You can describe the article briefly by use of the text-editor and can index it rapidly by entry of the first few letters of the key words.

"The computer dictionary is user-defined. The dictionary used by a cardiologist will differ from that of a family practitioner. Once a key word is defined, it remains on the program disk, and may allow for synonyms as well. Several searching routines can be provided so that the user can examine his dictionary instantaneously. The real power is the relative ease of entry combined with the ability to do Boolean searching faster than with other data bases."

A Boolean search, which uses the key words in combination with three connectors, *and*, *or*, and *not*, rapidly and economically achieves a level of access that could never be reached in manual systems, even with extensive cross-referencing. In a search for articles on cats and dogs, for example, one may ask for a list of articles about 'cat *and* dog,' and the system will produce only those articles with both key words. Asking for articles with 'cat *or* dog' will produce citations with either word. Using *not* excludes a certain component of the search subject; asking for 'dog *not* cat' will produce a listing of all articles on dogs except those about both dogs and cats.

Sohr emphasized the searching speed of computer indexing. "To search a diskette for all articles that apply to cardiology takes less than two seconds. To search it for articles that apply to cardiology and pediatrics and fever and differential diagnosis takes less than four seconds. Compare that with using a manual system and pulling out cards for cardiology, pediatrics, fever, and differential diagnosis and then examining them for articles that appear on all four lists. Cross-indexing makes it possible to obtain information immediately, at the time of a patient visit, if desired, and reduces the risk of missing material within the file that cannot be located when needed." Storing notes on articles read, cross-indexing, and recalling articles filed in the personal reprint file are thus simplified, and the easy access permits the physician to apply the information immediately to the problem at hand.

Accessing National Data Bases

The computer expands the opportunities for accessing medical references from national data bases. If the query is properly designed, a physician can sit in his office and in a few minutes gain useful information from MEDLINE or other data bases. Abstracts can also be displayed on the screen.

Thus, the physician can now perform functions traditionally carried out by librarians. Rand Corporation's Barbara Quint noted that user-friendly data bases in medicine are now operable by one "flat language" and do not require a lot of time and effort. "You indicate that 'I wish to search such-and-such,' and the machine translates your request into the protocol of the system. The more complicated search systems require fairly constant use, so you will not forget certain basic procedures. Searching will, however, continue to become easier, and subfiles will be developed." Martha Williams, Professor of Information Science, College of Engineering, University of Illinois, agreed. "More systems in medicine will be tied together. Ultimately, the person who knows nothing about command languages and structural files will be able to extract information. Much has happened in the past ten years, and more will happen, to make information retrieval easier at the doctor's desk. Expert systems already exist that answer specific questions on problem patients, but only in limited domains. It takes five to ten man-years to develop one expert system for one narrow field. Ultimately, the physician's computer will be connected to an 'expert' system that will provide guidance in diagnosis and treatment. The physician will then be less reliant on memory, but he will still have to make the ultimate judgment. Computers that accept voice commands, now available experimentally, will also eventually become available commercially, not only for general question-and-answer programs but for access to systems."

Nancy M. Lorenzi, Past President of the Medical Library Association, noted that microcomputer links will allow physicians at their homes or offices to notify hospitals about patients arriving for emergency care, scan medical records, and transmit pertinent data and orders to emergency rooms, and, by use of a "paper-chase"system, will also permit them to search publications in relevant knowledge bases. "Library collections may become available on video or optical disks, and linking of a medical center's computer with cable television networks may eventually give library users access to the collection 24 hours a day."

The Institutional Medical Library of the Future

If these predictions are accurate, what will happen to the institutional library? Nina Matheson predicted that "Specialized electronic browsing will replace the reading of paper journals. Every morning when physicians turn on their computer terminals, they will find a series of headings and brief stories on their fields of interest, in a specialized newsletter. Thus, documents such as the *Medical Letter* will be available on computer by subscription. Telefacsimile transmission of text from remote sites to the physician will be common.

"An electronic journal will be linked automatically to the physician's automated patient record system or the hospital record system. When the patient history and diagnosis are recorded, the subscription will automatically drop in any pertinent new key concepts, discoveries, tests, or treatments for the physician's review. The physician can leave the information at that, track back to the fuller report in the newsletter, or back further to the research report, which will be cited in the subscription. The electronic journal will take longer than the newsletter to be developed and widely accepted. In the meantime, linkages to tumor registries, genetics data banks, and the like will be available for the two-way transfer of information."

Matheson pointed to the positive effects on medicine of easy access of information: "The computer can shift the burden of 'fact banking' from individual memory to electronic data bases, and human skills can be concentrated on pattern recognition, problem analysis, intuitive comprehension of problems, and human relationships—functions that machines do not do well. The forces for change will include improved technology but also heightened expectations of the patients."

Wilfrid Lancaster sees computers and telecommunications as changing not only the economics of access to information, but also all previous notions of collections, libraries, and librarians. "A medical research 'library' of the future need not contain any printed materials; it may be a room containing only a terminal. Apart from archival repositories of the printed records of the past and institutions designed primarily to lend inspirational/recreational reading materials, libraries as we know them are likely to disappear.

"The librarian of the electronic age does not need to function within a library. Librarians will be able to apply their professional skills in searching information sources and in answering questions wherever they can plug in a terminal. They can freelance from their homes or can form group practices, as physicians and attorneys do. These trends are already evident in the profession. During the past several years, some de-institutionalization has occurred, as illustrated by freelance librarians, information brokers, and librarians serving on health care teams. These information specialists, identifiable through on-line directories, will provide complete literature searching and will deliver text and other data to the physician's terminal after evaluation and synthesis. A physician who needs to consult an expert outside his field will also be able to use on-line directories to identify such a person on the network.

"Rapid growth of information resources in electronic form may greatly reduce the value of the library structure, but it will greatly increase the efficiency of information services. The magnitude and diversity of the electronic resources available will mean that skilled information specialists will be in great demand."

Robert Cheshier, director of a busy inter-library lending service among academic health science libraries, finds that each new technologic advance increases acquisition and archival functions. He believes that traditional library roles, made more efficient by computer technology, will continue in the forseeable future, in addition to the newer electronic services.

Facilitating the Collegial Network

Discussions with colleagues about puzzling patients and various diagnostic and therapeutic approaches are an important part of continuing medical education. Many of these discussions are dependent on chance encounters in hallways, in the doctors' lounge, or over lunch, but some physicians are now using the computer for information exchange.

Donald Lindberg finds two features of electronic mail (see page 259) to be useful in this respect. "First, unlike telephone calls, computer messages can stack up without interrupting the addressee. Physicians can read their electronic mail when it is convenient. Knowing this, they will feel free to send colleagues queries that would not warrant a telephone call because it would interrupt the person called. Second, computer mail systems are usually coupled with electronic bulletin boards. For example, members of a formal special-interest group of physicians on hypertension can use an electronic bulletin board to exchange information on a new drug, its effectiveness, and toxicity.

"In COMPUSERVE and SOURCE electronic exchanges, physicians can discuss a particular patient problem and request assistance or references. Subsequently, comments and responses by other participants will provide the literature references. This is not, of course, proper patient consultation; it is learning by an electronic collegial network. One facilitating feature is called 'threading,' by which one can pick up the trail of the conversation at any point and follow it either forward or backward because the system preserves the links between comments."

Medical Consultation

One of the difficulties in medical consultations is reaching a colleague by phone. Through computer–messaging, requests for consultations can be made, and perhaps even answered, through the computer, and time spent playing "telephone tag" can be reduced.

"Difficulty in responding to a colleague's request for assistance about a patient," noted Donald Lindberg, "usually occurs because the proper information (tests, patient history, roentgenograms) has not been gathered. If an electronic form had to be completed before the consultation is requested, the whole process would be greatly simplified."

Thus the computer can transmit the notes requesting consultation or the consultant's summarizing letter, as described on pages 102 and 107. The physician would save time in reaching the consultant, indicating the need for consultation, and presenting pertinent data. Computer messaging does not, however, obviate the personal discussions between the consultant, the referring physician, and the patient, as discussed on page 108.

Courses and Conferences

Computer analysis of the physician's practice will help identify educational needs and thus provide guidance in the selection of needed reading, consultations, courses, and conferences. If societies and medical schools announced courses on computer bulletin boards, it would be more convenient for physicians and would reduce the "junk mail" currently being delivered. Better use of patient care data collected by hospitals can help identify educational needs of the medical staff and thus improve the design and quality of hospital conferences.

The Study and Analysis of Practice

The computer will undoubtedly simplify the indexing of cases by disease and the development of a practice profile of patients' age and sex, laboratory studies ordered, diagnoses made, and drugs prescribed. Notes on salient features learned through the study of puzzling patients, as well as notes on experience and description of mistakes, can be classified, stored, and accessed more readily by computer. The computer will help provide the physician with precise recall of his clinical experience, a significant asset, since the physician's recall of his experience is not the same as his actual experience.

Charles W. Given and associates[4,5] have used information from a computer-based billing system to review the performance of family practice residents—an analysis of patient visits, their purposes, diagnoses, laboratory procedures, and treatment. The reviews permitted faculty to provide feedback and instruction to the residents.

To aid in evaluation of the work of family practice residents, Mark Braunstein and associates[6] developed a computerized system that listed patient problems; social and demographic data, including age, sex, race, and family status; medication profiles; and laboratory profiles. From such an analysis, the faculty could recognize resident prejudice in treatment of patients with obesity, evidence of diagnostic error, and difficulties in therapy.

In 1975 and 1976 the Mountain Plains Outreach Program in Denver, Colorado, designed a Family Medicine Information System with an accounts package and a practice analysis package that indexed patients by name and diagnosis to permit a review of accumulated experience. "We found, for example," Lawrence Green remarked, "that one of our physicians was spending 4 per cent of his patients' dollars on thyroid function tests. Once this overuse was identified, he changed this practice."

Frank Reed's computer system provides data on diagnostic frequency and age/sex distribution. "When you look at the top 250 diagnoses encountered, they are probably the same everywhere. Their frequencies differ, however, and that makes a lot of difference in facility planning and training. Lacerations are in the top 250 in every family physician's practice, but in mine they are third. Our data show what kinds of diagnoses place the biggest burden on the practice. It may take 1.3 visits to solve a case of otitis media, for example, but the average diabetic visits our offices nine times a year. So we are able to determine the maximum, average, and minimum number of visits necessary for a problem, and this information has been more helpful in planning educational programs than a simple rank order of diseases seen."

Fred V. Light has no written records in the office, having entered all his patients' records in the computer. "Among the eight physicians in our group, three use this system. I am also in the medical directory for the prepaid health plan, and we use the computer system for that as well. The plan includes about 27,000 patients and 180 physicians in seven counties, so I use the computer to identify problems in this total practice. We have the names, addresses, phone numbers, ages, and employment levels of the patients in the computer, and we enter the diagnosis and its code on each patient visit. In the first column of the computer form is the diagnosis, in the second column the prescriptions or injections given on that visit, and the third column the laboratory tests or roentgenograms ordered on that visit. We can look at any arrangement of data for the medical groups scattered over seven counties. We can print out data on all the patients who have had a certain complaint or diagnosis over a period of time. It is educational because it makes us look at what we do every day."

The computer aids Light and his associates in conducting procedural audits, as described on page 165. "In the prepaid group, we have four meetings a year, at which we develop new criteria for what we should have on the records. In our own ambulatory practice, we use the computer to audit charts once a month. We then review the charts to see if we are following the criteria."

Byron Oberst, a pediatrician in group practice, has a system that supplies a problem list; laboratory tests; and information on demographics, functional assessment, emotional maturity, educational capacity, social and cultural maturity, family attitude, reason for visit, patient history, immunizations, and potential problems (risk factors). He uses this material not only for analysis of the medical aspects of practice but for financial analysis. "Analysis of the statistics has led us to develop needed services. We also use it to do cost-accounting of all services in our office from vision or hearing tests to patient encounters. We know, for example, that two years ago it cost us $10.33 for a patient to walk through the door. We know now, two years later, that it costs us $11.22, so we have been able to contain costs reasonably well." Data of this type, assembled to promote cost-containment, can direct study and enhance personal involvement in practice.

Gaining Information at the Time and Place Needed

The computer can deliver needed information to physicians when they are developing diagnostic and therapeutic plans. The prototype for such a system was a computerized monograph on hepatitis with efficient indexing system devised by Lionel Bernstein of the National Library of Medicine.[7]

AMA-GTE Network

In 1983, the American Medical Association and the General Telephone and Electronics Corporation made computer-based medical information available to the practicing physician through a telecommunication network. According to Marvin Johnson, who helped conceive and design the basic structure of that system, the objective is to provide the physician with medical information at the time and place it is needed to solve a clinical problem. Johnson described the following initial information bases in the network.

The Drug Information Base contains up-to-date, commercially unbiased information on the properties and clinical uses of about 1,500 individual drug preparations marketed under some 5,000 tradenames in the United States, Canada, and Mexico. Full information about a given drug can be called up on the terminal by category, nomenclature, and use, and can be read much as one would read a book. Such specificity allows the precise information needed to be readily retrieved. An inquiry can be made, for example, for a list of drugs for asthma or rheumatoid arthritis. Information about possible drug interactions permits the physician to avoid adverse effects. Since one-twelfth of the Drug Information Base is updated each month, the profession is assured of having the most current information on drugs.

The Disease Information Base (from the AMA publication, *Current Medical Information and Terminology*) contains information on several thousand identifiable diseases, disorders, and conditions. Each entity listed is divided into eight sections: alternate terms, etiology, symptoms, signs, laboratory data, radiologic findings, course and prognosis, and pathologic findings. The telegraphic style provides the most important basic information in the briefest form. The comprehensive nomenclature index allows the user to call up all diseases that include a specific term, such as pneumonia or tuberculosis. An additional index assists in identifying specific diseases manifested by a particular sign or symptom. This synopsis of basic medical information represents a compendium of vital facts, rather than an exhaustive dissertation.

The Medical Procedure Coding and Nomenclature Information Base is a uniform coding and nomenclature system for identification of medical services and procedures. This listing of more than 6,000 procedures with the exact identifying code in medicine, surgery, or diagnostic service is based on the AMA publication, *Physicians' Current Procedural Terminology*, which is now the most extensively used reporting system for communicating with third-party payers. Eighteen modifiers can be coupled with the procedural term, and the physician can thus indicate that a service

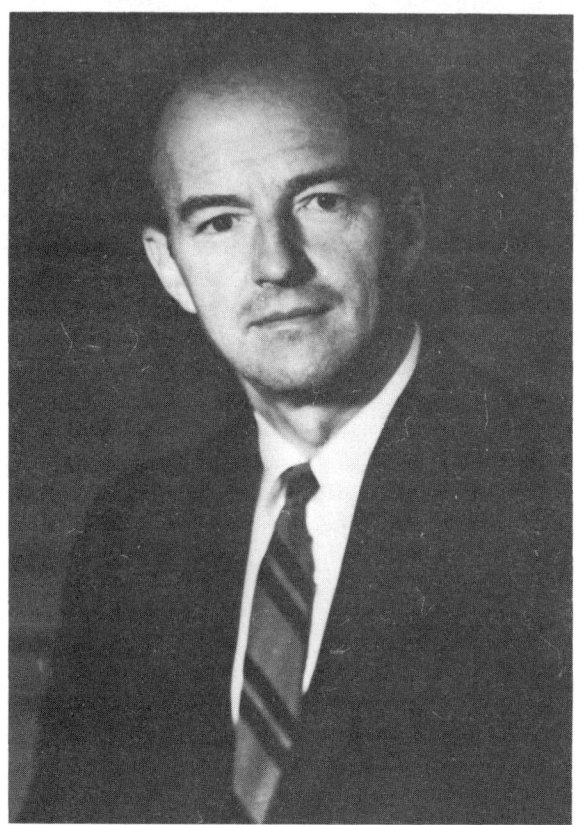

The computer links thought to action.

Lawrence L. Weed, M.D.
Professor of Medicine Emeritus
University of Vermont

17. The Computer: Aid to Learning

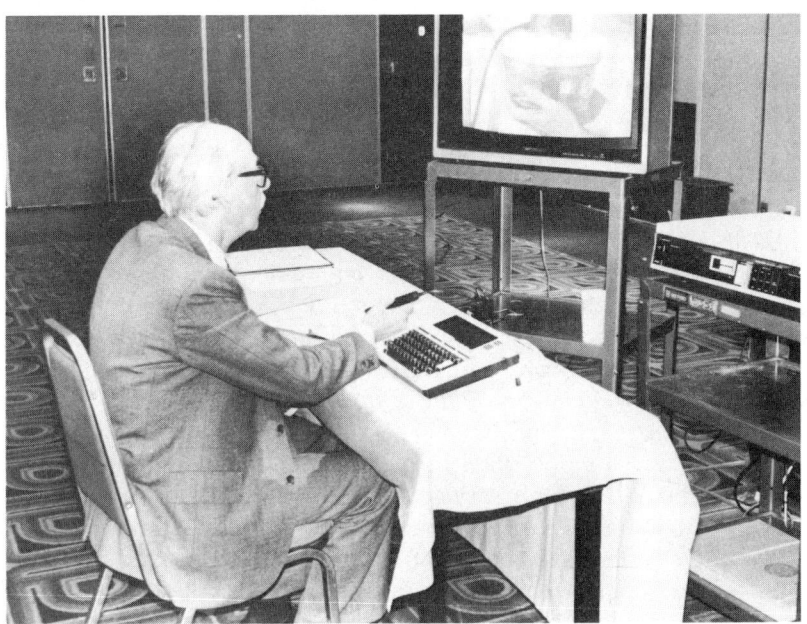

Microprocessors with the videodisc player allow interaction between the learner and the teacher.

Leo L. Leveridge, M.D.
Consultant, Interactive Audiovisual Education
Bandon, Oregon

or procedure performed has been changed by a specific circumstance. Reporting flexibility is therefore heightened without loss of standardization.

Searches are possible by procedure name, code number, or classification heading. In coding a herniorrhaphy, for example, one can call up all types of this operation and then select the pertinent code number. This feature assumes greater importance under the new fixed-fee reimbursement-by-diagnosis systems.

The Socioeconomic Bibliographic Information Base was created by the AMA Library staff from more than 700 journals on nonclinical subjects, including economics, education, ethics, international relations, legislation, medical practice, political science, psychology, public health, sociology, and statistics. More than half of these journals are not covered in the MEDLARS System of the National Library of Medicine.

The Excerpta Medica Physician Information Retrieval and Education Service (EMPIRES), a bibliographic service containing abstracts from 298 key medical journals published throughout the world, is both a current awareness and a reference service. The abstracts appear in the system within eight to twelve weeks after publication. Fifty thousand new citations and abstracts are added to the information base yearly. The current-awareness service provides, on demand and by medical specialty, articles from the past three months. Citations are cross-referenced, so that an article on pediatric neurology appears under both pediatrics and neurology. Searching is possible by subject, title, author, or key word.

The Massachusetts General Hospital (MGH) Continuing Medical Education Information Base, a collection of interactive patient-problem simulations, covers clinical management for abdominal pain, coma, and gastrointestinal bleeding. The user is presented with a clinical problem and with answers from which to choose. The correct answer brings up the next question. An incorrect answer brings a response containing the correct answer with supporting information.

American Society of Contemporary Medicine, Surgery and Ophthalmology

John Bellows described the efforts of the American Society of Contemporary Medicine, Surgery and Ophthalmology to develop a computer-based network to provide health-care information to physicians as the need arises in daily practice: "Up-to-date knowledge and information appear on-line immediately upon availability, long before it would appear in printed journals or other sources. Physicians who subscribe to the system gain access using individual passwords. The systems are designed to answer specific clinical questions as well as to provide general information. EYENET is a system designed to serve ophthalmologists. HEARTNET, soon to be available, contains information on cardiovascular disease, diagnosis, therapeutic guidance, and drug therapy. LUNGNET addresses pulmonary medicine; GUTNET, gastrointestinal medicine; and GERI-NET, geriatric medicine."

Electronic Mail

In addition to the multiple-information bases available on the AMA-GTE network, an electronic mail system provides several unique services. Any network subscriber can send a message instantaneously to any other subscriber(s) simply by entering the message with the appropriate address(es). The message remains on file until the recipient either erases it or transfers it to a personal electronic file. Information transferred to an individual electronic mailbox can be retained indefinitely. A single message may also be distributed simultaneously to preselected recipients.

Messages of general interest from a variety of sources are posted on electronic bulletin boards. A bulletin board maintained by the AMA, for example, gives detailed information on AMA conferences and seminars, whereas another lists continuing medical education courses throughout the country. The list can be searched by medical specialty, subject, date, or site of presentation. Plans are being made for the inclusion in electronic bulletin boards of special communiques from the Centers for Disease Control and the Food and Drug Administration (FDA).

The electronic mail function also provides a ready mechanism for physicians to report adverse drug reactions to the FDA. In the tragedy in which cyanide-contaminated Tylenol caused several deaths in the Chicago area, a warning, with the serial numbers of the known contaminated lots, was on the electronic network within 30 minutes of the discovery of the cause of these deaths. A network such as this is an intricate, high-speed system in which the messages are routed by computer. If any line is busy or out of service, the message is instantly rerouted by another open circuit, and it is thus virtually impossible for communication lines to be disrupted.

The AMA/GTE telenet is an ambitious program. Physicians will need to learn to use it properly, and with more experience the producers will undoubtedly simplify accessing and displaying of the information. Although developmental problems are to be expected, this service is a major advance in the improvement of information services for physicians.

References

1. Leonard, George B. *Education and Ecstasy*. New York: Delacorte Press, 1968:237.
2. Matheson, Nina W.; Cooper, John A. D. Academic information in the academic health sciences center: Roles for the library in information management. *J Med Educ* Oct 1982;57(10, pt 2):1-93.
3. Hamilton, I.; Lintott, D. J.; Ruddell, W. S. J.; Axon, A. T. R. Endoscopic retrograde cholangiopancreatography (ERCP) in primary biliary cirrhosis, abstracted. *Gut* Oct 1982;23(10):A910.

4. Given, Charles W.; Browne, Malachy; Sprafka, Robert J.; Breck, Elaine C. Evaluating primary ambulatory care with a health information system. *J Fam Pract* Feb 1981;12(2):293-302.
5. Given, Charles W.; Simoni, Lewis; Gallin, Rita S.; Sprafka, Robert J. The use of computer generated patient profiles to evaluate resident performance in patient care. *J Fam Pract* Nov 1977;5(5):831-840.
6. Braunstein, Mark. The computer-based medical record in family practice. In: Medalie, Jack H., ed. *Family Medicine: Principles and Applications.* Baltimore: The Williams and Wilkins Company, 1978:281-292.
7. Schoolman, Harold M.; Bernstein, Lionel M. Computer use in diagnosis, prognosis, and therapy. *Science* May 26, 1978;200(4344):926-931.

18

The Computer: Guidance in Diagnosis and Therapy

> The future can be extraordinarily bright for the practicing physician if we use computer technology creatively and not simply to perpetuate outmoded passive learning or learning from simulation.
>
> *Phil R. Manning*

The simplistic idea of a computer "making a diagnosis" has been replaced by the recognition that modern decision-support systems entail several related tasks: gathering data, identifying disease categories, assessing individual patient prognosis, suggesting further evaluations, and perhaps educating the physician.[1-3] Decision support is no longer an unexplored topic; innumerable articles have been published on the subject, and national and international groups on decision-support systems have been established.[4]

The source of the data in a decision-support system is of utmost importance. For the present, systems may need to rely on expert-generated "rules of thumb," despite disagreements among authorities on many aspects of medicine. Carefully designed and recorded data banks based on hard data from controlled studies are the most valid sources of information available, and these are being constructed. Study groups by the Research Committee of the World Organization of Gastroenterology, for example, are evaluating data bases from a number of nations on such conditions as acute abdominal disorders and inflammatory intestinal disease. As de Dombal pointed out, it is "Better to wait for hard data than to rush half-ready systems into service." He further warns against "unsubstantiated expert opinion and (worse) systems based on 'a survey of the literature.' "[1]

Lusted,[2] who devised guidelines for several fundamental principles of evaluation, warned that the role of the computer should be clearly defined and argued that computer systems will serve adjunctively until they become demonstrably superior to unaided clinicians. He also stressed the importance of real-life testing; some evaluations include so few cases as to nullify any practical value.

Experimental Programs

Several experimental programs suggest what we can look forward to in clinical computer programs.

MYCIN and ONCOCIN

Edward H. Shortliffe developed two of these, MYCIN and ONCOCIN.[5] MYCIN was an early experiment in the application of artificial intelligence techniques to medical decision-making. The domain of application was the selection of antimicrobial therapy for patients severely ill with septicemia or meningitis. The program was validated in formal experiments and provided recommendations that compared favorably with those of acknowledged experts in infectious disease.[6] "We worked on that system between 1972 and 1978," said Edward Shortliffe, "during which time the program expanded to include about 500 rules that summarize expertise in the subdisciplines of infectious disease. The program's ability to explain the basis for the reasoning allowed the user to decide independently whether to accept its advice. Because the decision in antimicrobial selection is inherently ill-structured, conventional statistical approaches were not appropriate.

"Nevertheless, we did not implement the program for routine use in the clinical setting because we viewed it as fundamental research in medical artificial intelligence, from which we learned many lessons that have had an impact on subsequent system development. MYCIN itself, however, contained information about only a few types of infectious disease, and we did not have the resources to expand its knowledge base into additional fields such as pneumonia, urinary tract infections, and endocarditis. A system like MYCIN, had it become generally available, might have had a favorable impact on continuing education. The explanations provided an educational spinoff, especially since the learning occurred in the setting of the specific patient's case under study.

"The newer system, known as ONCOCIN, was built on our knowledge of MYCIN but does not have a diagnostic component. Instead, the program is designed to help physicians select therapy and adjust dosages for patients in formal cancer chemotherapy programs, in which the oncologic diagnosis is generally made well in advance of chemotherapy decisions. The complexity of this problem requires all the rules in a given protocol to be memorized and those rules to be adapted appropriately as a patient responds to the early cycles of therapy.

"ONCOCIN has been in experimental use in our oncology clinic at Stanford since May, 1981. Physicians have gradually come to accept the program and now routinely use it when caring for a patient whose records are in the system. As we expand ONCOCIN's data into other aspects of cancer chemotherapy, we expect all treatment of clinic patients at Stanford to be guided by computer. The program, like MYCIN, offers advice about drug selection and dosage, but allows the physician to decide whether to follow the computer's advice or make minor or major changes. Experimental data indicate that the physicians accept the computer's recommendations about 75 per cent of the time, with minor modifications in most of the remaining cases.

"A system such as ONCOCIN is beneficial for individual patients as well as for optimal long-term cancer chemotherapy trials. The computer provides immediate feedback for the physician when questions arise about therapy. Data in the patient record are immediately available for statistical analysis.

"Another lesson provided by ONCOCIN is that physicians will use computers routinely if the computers are smoothly integrated into the normal activities of a clinical setting and if they provide sufficient assistance at little cost in time or money. We already have evidence that the fellows in our program learn about cancer chemotherapy through use of the system. As such systems become more readily available, their educational components will become increasingly important."

ARAMIS

James F. Fries described ARAMIS, a national chronic disease data bank in arthritis, thus: "Thousands of patients from throughout the United States are being followed on as many as one hundred observation points. Each time these patients are seen, perhaps five hundred items are stored in the computer, and each is thus described by several thousand numbers representing the course of his disease. Rheumatoid arthritis, for example, is typically diagnosed at about age fifty and is progressive in most patients, although at an extremely variable rate. It is modifiable by treatment, but the treatment may involve disadvantages, short-term toxicity, and adverse long-term effects, including the possibility of neoplasia. To make intelligent decisions about the long-term welfare of a patient with rheumatoid arthritis, you need to visualize an outcome you desire in that patient in perhaps ten years, and then develop a strategy to optimize that outcome. With such an approach, you may make quite different decisions than if you use short-term biomedical models such as lowering the sedimentation rate over the next six weeks or reducing synovitis by use of corticosteroids over the next week because the patient is complaining a lot."

CONSIDER and RECONSIDER

Computers may be useful as prompters during diagnosis. A physician cannot diagnose a disease unless he has thought of it, and the rarity of a

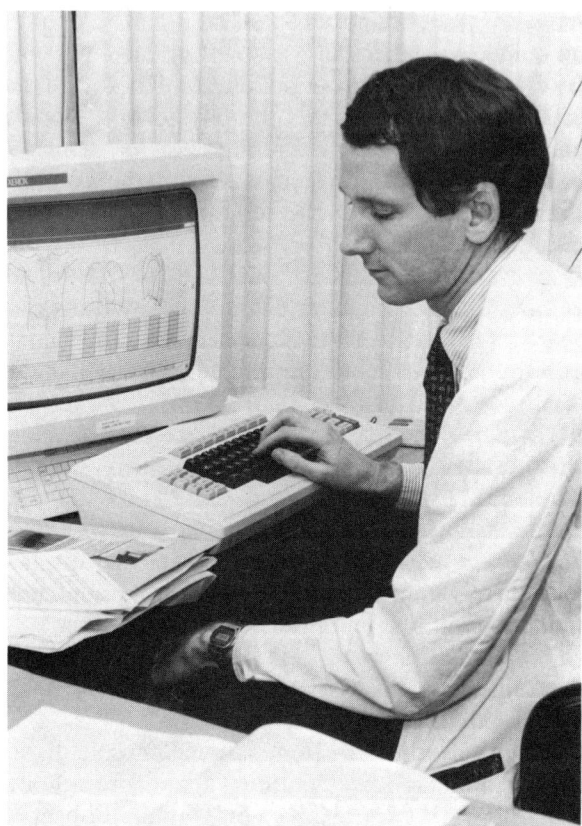

The computer provides immediate feedback for the physician when questions arise about therapy.

Edward H. Shortliffe, M.D., Ph.D.
Associate Professor of Medicine and Computer Science
Stanford University Medical Center

disease or the physician's human limitations can cause him to overlook the correct diagnosis. In 1968 Lindberg and associates designed the CONSIDER program, which matched patient attributes (signs and symptoms) with the descriptions of more than 3,000 diseases. Blois and colleagues have devised a program called RECONSIDER which, in addition to matching patient attributes to disease descriptions, ranks the diagnostic possibilities according to similarity with the patient's manifestations (signs, symptoms, and laboratory data). It also contains a synonym capability that describes attributes by more than one word, for example, "itch" and "pruritis."[7]

RECONSIDER is thus an interactive diagnostic program that uses simple retrieval techniques to alert a physician to possible diagnoses, given a list of positive patient findings. Blois and colleagues used the information in the computer-readable version of the *Current Medical Information and Terminology (CMIT)*. The physician enters into the computer the terms that describe the patient's clinical and laboratory findings. RECONSIDER then compares the terms (and their synonyms) with 3,262 different disease descriptions, and each is given a "score" based on the number and selectivity of the matching terms. The possible diagnoses are ordered by these scores to form a list from which the physician can choose a differential diagnosis.

Blois considers one of the advantages of RECONSIDER to be the large number of diseases about which it has information. When the findings of the published cases diagnosed by INTERNIST, which considers a few hundred diseases from internal medicine (see next paragraph), were entered into RECONSIDER, the correct diagnosis was listed at or near the top of the disease list. Evaluation of RECONSIDER continues, and the knowledge base is known to be out-of-date. In Blois's opinion, the timeliness and completeness of both CMIT and the synonym dictionary are serious limitations. The usefulness of computer-based diagnostic aids will be decided, he cautioned, by their performance, as well as by cost and convenience.

INTERNIST-I

Pople and Myers[8] developed INTERNIST-I, an experimental computer program that can make multiple, complex diagnoses in internal medicine. After fifteen years, INTERNIST-I comprises more than 500 individual diseases and 3,550 manifestations. When compared to the performance of physicians on examples from the Case Records of the Massachusetts General Hospital in *The New England Journal of Medicine*, use of INTERNIST-I yielded results qualitatively similar to those of individual hospital clinicians, but not as good as those of case discussion groups.

Said Myers, "If you want the profile of an internal medicine disease, whether common or unusual, I can get the information out of INTERNIST-I within 15 seconds. If you ask INTERNIST-I for all the diseases associated with an S-3 left ventricular gallop, you will have the list in ten seconds. The computer will also tell you whether causes are common or rare and will give you the frequency of an S-3 gallop in a particular entity once you know the patient has that disease."

As for the future of data bases, Myers hopes that they will be generated according to certain standards, since more than one person generates a data base: "Gene Stead's colleagues at Duke put into their data base all the data on every case of myocardial infarction and now, after many years, they have a rich store of information. That is fine for a common disease like myocardial infarction, but a data base on paroxysmal nocturnal hemoglobinuria cannot be prepared at Duke Hospital because the staff does not see many cases. So collaboration around the country will be necessary, and uniformity of behavior and interpretation thus becomes critical. We are doing our study retrospectively. We get all the data we can find on scleroderma and derive the likelihood of certain things occurring from those data. But it would be far better to do this prospectively. Someone would have to take responsibility, of course, for keeping the knowledge base up-to-date because medicine is not static."

Duke Cardiovascular DATABASE

At Duke, data on both surgically and medically treated patients are entered into the computer.[9] Coronary disease has a large number of specific descriptors that are recorded for each patient. David Sabiston described the procedure thus: "Suppose Mrs. Jones comes in today with three-vessel coronary disease, ejection fraction 58 per cent, known cholesterol level, and diabetes. In twenty seconds the computer will tell us that we have had 122 patients like that. When you ask how they have fared with medical versus surgical treatment, the computer will tell you the number alive and the number pain-free in each category. That has been a tremendous help to us because the computer does not forget. Not that we will necessarily treat the patient the way those in the past have been treated, but we can get a statistically objective idea of what happened to past patients. And when we give a paper, it is easy to obtain our surgical results in a moment because each of these patients is followed at regular intervals."

AI/RHEUM

Donald A. B. Lindberg described AI/RHEUM as a program in the advanced research stages: "It models the reasoning of the expert rheumatologist. A user can obtain a diagnostic consultation by entering information about his patient. The system asks questions of the user, with answers in the form of 'yes,' 'no,' 'unknown,' or numerical measurements. About 900 findings are understood by AI/RHEUM. Many of these are details such as 'which joints?' that are not asked unless a more general condition, such as 'arthritis' is present. The system will answer on the basis of whatever information is provided. It is possible to make a definite

18. The Computer and Medical Decisions

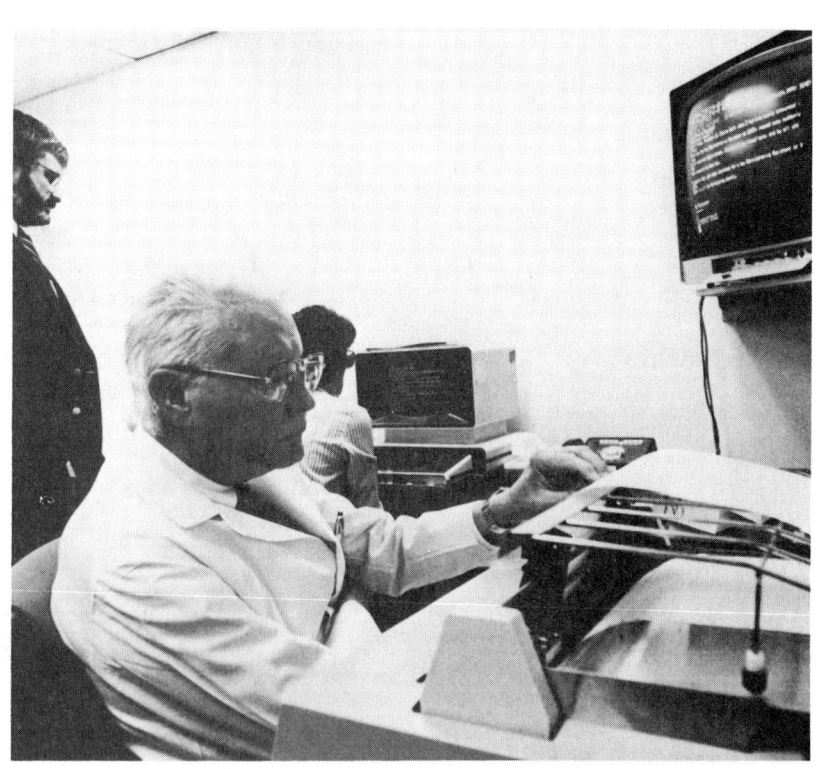

If you ask INTERNIST-I for all the diseases associated with an S-3 left ventricular gallop, you will have the list in ten seconds.

Jack D. Myers, M.D.
Emeritus University Professor
University of Pittsburgh

diagnosis with as few as six findings, provided these are the critical ones. Because the system can show tables of diagnostic criteria, the user can more easily see which findings are critical and which are irrelevant to the diagnostic decision.

"An additional feature of AI/RHEUM was designed specifically to assist in continuing education and in increasing the reliability of the user's patient observations, and hence the data he enters. If the user has any question about how the term is used by the specialist, why it is being asked of him, or how to make the observation, he need only request an expanded definition, which is available when he enters the data. These definitions include one or more references to scientific publications, which can provide further clarification.

"Lastly, the reasoning provided by this and other AI systems affords the user an opportunity for learning. When a diagnostic conclusion or management recommendation is offered by the computer system, it can recapitulate, on command, the steps leading to that particular conclusion. In the case of diagnosis, this includes enumerating the findings that supported the diagnostic conclusions, the next set of observations needed to increase the certainty of the diagnosis, and findings that are not explained by the diagnosis.

"None of these features, of course, is as useful as an unhurried conversation with an expert. On the other hand, the computer is valuable for continuing medical education because it is tireless and available for learning apart from the immediate patient care."

ATTENDING and HT-ATTENDING

Perry L. Miller, who has developed two programs to evaluate the physician's therapeutic plans before their implementation, describes them thus: "The objective of our research is to develop medical computer advisors or expert consultation systems that critique a physician's plan of medical management rather than try to tell him what to do. The physician is asked to enter a list of the patient's medical problems, a proposed surgical procedure, and a plan outlining the agents and techniques to be used for premedication, induction, intubation, and maintenance of general or regional anesthesia.

"We are using the ATTENDING system experimentally for teaching anesthesia residents. ATTENDING produces a critique of the pros and cons of various approaches, emphasizes the risks and benefits of the different alternatives, and thus ensures that the physician will be aware of all possible problems.

"In our hypertension system (HT-ATTENDING), the physician describes a patient's underlying problems that might affect the choice of drugs used for treatment of essential hypertension. Then he enters the dosages of the patient's current and proposed antihypertensive drugs. The assumption is that the patient is still hypertensive, and that now the physician wishes to modify the regimen by adding another drug, changing a drug, or increasing dosage. The system will produce a critique of that particular antihypertensive regimen for the particular patient described. Again, the computer may yield additional factors the physician might want to consider."

Diagnostic Guidance on Acute Abdominal Disorders

A clinical computer system devised by de Dombal and colleagues at the University of Leeds consists of a simple desk-top computer and an input/output writer.[10] The physician uses preprinted forms for history and physical examination information. Each patient attribute is assigned a three-digit code number, and the written medical information is thus entered into the computer. Within a few (rarely more than 20) minutes, a hard copy of the patient's history and the computer's calculations, including the diagnostic probabilities based on that information, is provided to the physician, printed in everyday English (not code). Further, the computer can compare its diagnosis with that of the physician; if they do not match, the program will automatically select, from filed information, the attributes needed to distinguish between the two diagnoses. The computer may also be called on to list, without mathematical probabilities, the rare diseases that might help the clinician in obscure cases. The computer makes no decisions about treatment, providing only the diagnostic probabilities for a subset of diseases and recommendations for the acquisition of additional information. During a five-month trial conducted with 113 cases of acute abdominal pain, senior clinicians and the computer showed virtually identical levels of diagnostic accuracy: 76 per cent and 78 per cent, respectively. The computer can thus support the physician in the statistical analysis of large volumes of data but does not supplant his decision-making.

Regenstrief Medical Record System

In Chapter 14 on "Problems in Practice Unrelated to Knowledge," we cited examples of what can go wrong at every step in medical care. The tendency for order to become disorder appears to be characteristic of all complex systems, as suggested by Lambert's description of this manifestation of the second law of thermodynamics (p. 215). Thus, errors of omission, such as failure to notice or respond appropriately to an abnormal urinalysis or hemoglobin, cause many difficulties in medicine.

Clement McDonald has developed a computerized medical record to provide protocol-based reminders that prompt the physician to react to relevant data.[11] On the preceding evening, the computer will search the records of all patients with appointments the next day, identifying the conditions for which instructions for care have been formulated. The printed reminders are given to the physician in advance of the patient visit. Examples:

> These suggestions are based on incomplete data; your judgment should take precedence.
>
> Patient: SS Age: 65 Sex: M Race: W
>
> Last potassium was high (= 5.8 on 22-AUG-83). Consider repeat potassium to verify and/or follow results on intervention.
>
> The CREATININE = 1.9, dated 21-AUG-83, was the first recorded high value for this patient.
>
> Assuming that gout, ankylosing spondylitis, and infection have been ruled out, aspirin is the usual first drug for nonspecific arthritis.
>
> Patient: JA Age: 21 Sex: F Race: W
> Trichomonas was recently observed on 29-JUL-83. If patient is symptomatic, i.e., abdominal pain, menstrual cramps, bothersome discharge, a single 2–gm dose of Flagyl is curative. It also will eliminate the obscuring inflammation that trichomonas vaginitis causes on routine pap smears. Flagyl should not be used unless patient has stable consort who can be treated. Ethanol should be avoided. (R:928, R:2426)
>
> There is no cervical pap on record for this patient. If test done but not recorded, please record date: _____ and cervical pap: _____ here.

On the premise that patients are more likely to receive effective care if the physician receives a reminder at the time of the visit, McDonald has developed more than 1,410 core statements as reminders for physicians. "The issues tend to be simple ones, such as to do a pap smear, to check for premature ventricular contractions in patients on digitalis, or to check potassium levels. The reminders have about the same effect on physicians at all levels of training but are, of course, followed most carefully by physicians who have accepted the medical principle upon which the computer advice is based."

Family Medicine Information System (FMIS)

Lawrence Green gives an example of reminders from the Family Medicine Information System for physicians:

> Dear Doctor: The risk of thrombotic disease appears to be especially great for the person using both birth control pills and tobacco. Although the FMIS users don't like to record tobacco abuse on en-

counter forms, I can find some smokers just by reviewing encounter data. I thought you would want to know if you had any patients on the pill who smoke. I checked encounter forms you completed from Jan 1 79 through Apr 30 80. Here they are:

Name*	Number	Age	HOH†	Last Visit
Jane Doe	Z10756-02	19	John	Nov 17 80
Doris Smith	Z11027-02	27	Doris	Oct 31 80
Mary Jones	Z10870-02	18	Mark	Mar 23 80
Lisa Johnson	Z10627-02	41	Lisa	Mar 10 81
Mary Tucker	Z11427-01	30	Mary	Jan 15 81
Kathy Stone	Z10876-02	25	George	Dec 14 79

*Fictitious names.
†HOH = Head of household.

Let me know if I can help with any of these patients.

Some predict that computer reminders will be more acceptable than those from peers or superiors and will reduce omissions in patient diagnosis and therapy. In Frederick Jelovsek's words, "They will help to fine-tune our behavior to desirable standards and decrease day-to-day fluctuations caused by emotions and fatigue."

Problem-oriented Medical Information System (PROMIS) and Knowledge Coupler

Perhaps the most complete medical computer system to date has been PROMIS, developed by Lawrence Weed and associates[12] and based on the problem-oriented record with a defined data base, problem list (problem stated at the physician's level of understanding rather than by diagnosis), diagnostic and therapeutic plans, patient education, and progress notes divided into Subjective findings, Objective findings, Analysis, and Plans (SOAP). PROMIS provides not only complete patient case records but current information or medical diagnosis, therapy, procedures, and guidance for use of the information. Reliance on memory is thus greatly relieved. Patient data can be retrieved by problem, date, information sources (laboratory and radiology reports), and flow sheets. The system preserves logic of all medical actions and offers feedback that can be used to improve the system and trace the outcome of medical actions.

In addition to PROMIS, Weed and Hertzberg have developed the "Knowledge Coupler," which will support diagnostic and therapeutic possibilities on the basis of the number of important features that the patient manifests. The Knowledge Coupler helps link thought to actions and does not place patient care at the mercy of human memory or the limitation of human information processing abilities at the time of action. The Knowledge Coupler system is available on microcomputer for use in the physician's office and hospital.

What Is Possible versus What Is Practical

"While the future may be 'rosy'," cautioned Frederick Jelovsek, "current programs often produce frustration because of the disparity between what is possible and what exists." He believes that physicians must learn more than the technical skills of signing on, signing off, and using data base management programs on the computer. Just as an understanding of physiology and biochemistry are necessary in making medical decisions, physicians must understand how computer programs function to use them intelligently and efficiently. Only by understanding the underlying functions will they be able to judge when an algorithm is outside its domain of knowledge.

E. E. Van Brunt cited several issues that are not clear at present and pose important questions: "One is the selection and maintenance of the materials that will eventually be included in the numerous data bases to become available over time. Aside from such issues as data accessibility and presentation, where will the information to be included in a given data base be obtained? What persons or agencies will be responsible for the selection? How will the information be validated? Who will maintain the data and ensure continuing accuracy? What role(s) will government regulatory agencies and professional organizations play as these services become established? When errors occur in data communication or presentation, as opposed to interpretation, who will be accountable for any untoward effects?" Despite these questions, we agree with Van Brunt that "The ready availability of a broad base of scientific and clinical knowledge will surely enhance the potential of the clinician; it will result in an emphasis in medical education and practice on those skills for which humans are uniquely suited, such as the elicitation and interpretation of historical, physical, and psychological data in the context of individual patients. In this way, it is conceivable that we will move closer to the 'traditional' image of 'physician' than ever before, certainly closer than the recent decades of progressive specialization have permitted."

*****

The computer and electronic transmission of information are revolutionizing the management of medical information. They will expedite Weed's linking of thought to action and will obviate the impossible responsibilities currently assigned to human memory. Information will be available faster, and guidance will be better. The computer will facilitate the implementation of the concepts used by the outstanding physicians quoted in this book. If used correctly, this tool should encourage deeper involvement and immersion in practice, and improve doctor-patient relationships.

Unless a physician wants to be a pioneer, he should not buy a computer for patient-care application until he has seen it operate with software that will perform the tasks he desires. He will need to learn how to make the computer an integral part of daily office activities. For some of the "stage one" applications, such as keeping notes on reading, creating his personal reprint file, and computer messaging, existing software packages are ready for general use. The national data bases and connecting services are expanding and improving. Computer methods of indexing patient records by problem and profiling practice by diagnosis, drugs prescribed, and laboratory studies ordered are now possible and may soon be practical enough for everyday use. Voice-activated systems will simplify computer use.

We agree with de Dombal that computer systems in medicine will not enjoy credibility unless they are based on absolutely impeccable medicine. Until they adopt the computer, most physicians will continue to be well served by the manual methods described in this book. A major risk in the promise of the computer, however, is that physicians will delay implementing simple manual methods of practice-linked continuing education while awaiting the "easy way." That would be a mistake. Additionally, it is efficient to develop methods on paper before jumping in with the computer. Start small, start with manual approaches, but start *now*.

References

1. de Dombal, F. T. Towards a more objective evaluation of computer-aided decision support systems. In: Van Bemmel, Jan H.; Ball, Marion J.; Wigertz, Ove, eds. *Medinfo 83: Proceedings of the Fourth World Conference on Medical Informatics.* Amsterdam: Elsevier Science Publishers, 1983:437.
2. Lusted, Lee B. Clinical decision making. In: de Dombal, F. T., Gremy, F., eds. *Decision Making and Medical Care: Can Information Science Help?* Amsterdam: North-Holland Publishing Company, 1976:77–98.
3. Blois, Marsden S. Clinical judgment and computers. *N Engl J Med* Jul 24, 1980;303(4):192-197.
4. Wagner, G.; Tautu, P.; Wolber, U. Problems of medical diagnosis: A bibliography. *Methods Inf Med* Jan 1978;17(1):55-74.
5. Shortliffe, Edward Hance. *Computer-based Medical Consultations: MYCIN.* New York: American Elsevier Publishing Company, Inc., 1976.
6. Yu, Victor L.; Fagan, Lawrence M.; Wraith, Sharon M., et al. Antimicrobial selection by a computer: A blinded evaluation by infectious diseases experts. *JAMA* Sep 21, 1979;242(12):1279-1282.
7. Blois, Marsden S. Conceptual issues in computer-aided diagnosis and the hierarchical nature of medical knowledge. *J Med Philos* Feb 1983;8(1):29-50.
8. Miller, Randolph A.; Pople, Harry E.; Myers, Jack D. INTERNIST-I, an experimental computer-based diagnostic consultant for general internal medicine. *N Engl J Med* Aug 19, 1982;307(8):468-476.
9. Rosati, Robert A.; McNeer, J. Frederick; Starmer, C. Frank; Mittler, Brant S.; Morris, James J.; Wallace, Andrew G. A new information system for medical practice. *Arch Intern Med* Aug 1975;135(8):1017-1024.
10. Wilson, P. D.; Horrocks, Jane C.; Lyndon, P. J.; Yeung, C. K.; Page, R. E.;

de Dombal, F. T. Simplified computer-aided diagnosis of acute abdominal pain. *Br Med J* Apr 12, 1975;2(5962):73-75.
11. McDonald, Clement J. Protocol-based computer reminders, the quality of care, and the non-perfectability of man. *N Engl J Med* Dec 9, 1976;295(24):1351-1355.
12. Weed, Lawrence L. *Your Health Care and How to Manage It.* Essex Junction, Vermont: Essex Publishing Company, Inc., 1978.

Afterword

On the basis of our extensive examination of the daily practices of exceptional physicians, we have several recommendations for you as clinicians. One is that you understand the need for two kinds of lifelong study: (1) general and (2) specific, patient-oriented study. By reading, listening to audiotapes, attending courses, and conversing informally with experts and colleagues, you can be alert to new developments and can obtain a nucleus of understanding upon which to build. Toward that end, editorials in leading journals are particularly useful. Although essential, all of these are not enough. You will also profit from consciously cultivating intellectual curiosity and from assuming responsibility for answers to specific questions arising in practice; such answers require framing the question precisely and often require accessing pertinent medical publications and consulting with colleagues. By these simple methods, you can best minister to individual patients.

You need to acquire the self-discipline and diligence to read and study every day and, because of time limitations and the flood of mediocre publications, to screen articles critically for pertinence and validity. Current medical textbooks offer a quick source of relevant information. A personal reprint file, indexed either manually or by computer, is extremely efficient in satisfying your information needs. Medical librarians can access almost anything you need if your request is specific and clear.

Participating in the collegial network of medicine permits you to benefit from shared experience and to enjoy the warm spirit of fraternity. Not only is this an excellent way to learn, but it provides recreation and will enhance your fulfillment. Teaching is an added stimulus, and even if you are not affiliated with a medical school or teaching hospital, you can profit from informal teaching sessions with colleagues, other members of the health-care team, and patients. You can avoid falling into ineffective and inefficient habits by inviting periodic observation by peers, even of routine tasks, such as taking a history, performing a physical examination, or doing a clinical procedure. Professional athletes get advice from coaches and peers, and so should physicians. Choosing one or two medical subjects for intense study, moreover, will heighten your intellectual satisfaction, spur your motivation, permit you to serve as a consultant, and thus enhance your self-confidence.

Our fervent hope is that all clinicians will one day adopt simple methods of practice analysis that will allow them to make corrective changes in their practices. It should be possible to use billing data to keep statistics on problems seen, drugs prescribed, and laboratory studies ordered. Indexing of charts by problem or diagnosis permits examination of cumulative experience; keeping note cards on lessons learned from instructive patients is equally beneficial. Hospitals, medical societies, and medical schools can help physicians interpret their experience by advocating standards, by encouraging discussions of the validity of published material, and by offering guidance in effective methods of practice analysis.

We are optimistic that the computer will help physicians implement concepts of lifelong learning. Current technology makes this possible now, but software needs to be improved, and physicians need to learn how to use this remarkable tool. The future can be extraordinarily bright for practicing physicians if they use computer technology creatively to link education to practice and not simply to perpetuate outmoded passive learning or learning from simulation. Medical schools, hospitals, and specialty societies need to foster and perfect this approach by engaging in experimentation. More important than the computer is the commitment to maximal immersion in practice, although the computer may ultimately be the best tool toward that end.

We also encourage you to be attentive to the changing social and ethical problems in medicine. Here again, it is wise to remember the two approaches: (1) general, for a framework upon which to build, and (2) specific, with consultation, for solution of problems of particular patients.

The things that human beings do best they do every day. You will therefore practice better medicine if you engage in daily study and daily evaluation of your performance.

Finally, although you need to be well-informed, many problems in practice do not relate to medical knowledge, but are caused by omission, administrative inefficiency, lost data, or lack of proper reaction to data obtained. These problems must constantly be combatted. With patient care becoming more complex, and with stronger emphasis on the team approach, greater entrepreneurial involvement, and more regulation to contain medical costs, system problems will probably multiply. To improve the quality of medical care, you must become more skilled managers of patient care rather than abrogate these responsibilities. In the words of Hippocrates:

> The physician must be ready, not only to do his duty himself, but also to secure the co-operation of the patient, of the attendants and externals. (Aphorisms. With an English Translation by W. H. S. Jones. New York: G. P. Putnam's Sons, 1931, Vol IV, p. 99.)

Afterword

If you will approach the clinical puzzles in medical practice as intellectual challenges, if you will develop the custom of reading and discussing the steady flow of new medical knowledge issuing from scientists and scholars, if you will evaluate your clinical results regularly, and if you will view each patient not as a clinical case, but as a fellow human being whose unstated fears, anxieties, and dependence associated with illness also require attention, you will be rewarded with professional satisfaction and personal enjoyment, and you will assuredly *preserve the passion* for medicine that led you into this noble humanitarian profession.

Phil R. Manning, M.D.
Lois DeBakey, Ph.D.

Interviewees and Correspondents

The following persons generously described the methods they have found useful in continuing their medical education after formal training. Most were interviewed by telephone or in person, whereas some returned written statements in response to specific questions, and others answered questionnaires distributed at courses conducted by the University of Southern California School of Medicine. The list includes world-renowned academicians, solo and group practitioners, and some spouses. The pages containing quotations from interviewees are shown next to their names. All those listed made significant contributions, but since some concepts were mentioned by many different physicians, it was not possible to quote everyone directly.

Nancy Abdou
Stephen Abrahamson, 120
James Aiyarrow
Bobby R. Alford, 137
Horace J. Anderson
Susan S. Anthony
Henry Aranow, Jr.
John Martin Askey, 138
J. B. Aust
Ruth Bain, 83, 232, 235
Carol A. Baker
Duke H. Baker, 65
Lailee Bakhtiar, 228, 229, 234
Oscar J. Balchum, 92
James J. Ball
Edwin V. Banta, Jr.
Barry Barber
Emil Bardana, Jr.
William Bardsley, 221
Marloe Bareis

R. Bareis
Anne L. Barlow
Octo G. Barnett
Jeremiah A. Barondess, 157
Howard S. Barrows
Jacques Barzun
Garry G. Becker
John S. Beedie
Paul B. Beeson, 88, 117
Roy Behnke, 11, 86
John G. Bellows, 258
Jack Benhayon
William M. Bennett, 204
J. Alfred Berend
Kenneth Berge, 87, 116
Stanley Berman
Betty Bernard
Clarence J. Berne, 161
Michael Bernstein
Charles A. Berry

Alice N. Bessman, 232, 237
Peter Best, 113
John E. Bethune, 75
Daniel C. Bird, 117
Marjorie Bird, 244
Gordon L. Black
Courtland Blake
David Blankenhorn, 62, 78
Andrew Bliss
Harry A. Bliss
Melvin A. Block
Marsden S. Blois, 265
Daniel K. Bloomfield
Baruch S. Blumberg, 3, 104
Morton Bogdonoff, 146
Paul Bohannan, 220
Eli L. Borkon
Louis G. Bove
Francis L. Bowler, 184
Marjorie A. Bowman
Tom Bradley
Robert M. Braude, 74
Mark Braunstein
Eugene Braunwald, 45, 48–51
Donald F. Brayton
Thomas H. Brem, 84
D. J. Brennan
Dorothy Brooks, 240
Arnold L. Brown
Bernice Z. Brown, 232, 236
Clement Brown
Janis Brown, 128
Barbara Buchanan, 231
Francis S. Buck, 221
J. H. Burgess
Genevieve Burk, 232
Joan Burns, 240
Thomas W. Burns, 134
Richard Byyny, 40, 86
C. A. Caceres
Arthur A. Calix
Thomas Callister, 37, 41
J. T. Campbell, Jr.
Richard M. Caplan, 112, 114
David B. Carmichael
Susan T. Carver

William J. Casarella
William B. Castle
Cathleen Caton, 218
M. E. Chaffin
Kit Chambers, 231, 235, 236, 240, 242
Wallace L. Chambers, 85
Robert Cheshier, 66, 251
Arthur C. Christakos, 201
Norman Christiansen
Gail Clark, 232
J. Philip Clarke
D. Kay Clawson
Clifton R. Cleaveland, 134
Mrs. C. R. Cleaveland
Linda Hawes Clever, 137
William A. Clintworth
Nancy Coates
Walter S. Coe
Bradford Cohn
Morris Collen
Russell F. Compton
Marilyn Cook
William M. Cooper, 155
W. G. Corey
Blake Courtland
Mitchel D. Covel
Susan Covel
David G. Covell, 38, 91, 92
Joyce W. Craddick, 189
Jean A. Creek, 85
Harold D. Cross, 11, 165
Martin H. Crumrine
Robert Cullin
Martin Cummings
Hiram Cury, 158
David J. Dahl
David C. Dale
W. Andrew Dale, 88
Walter J. Daly
William H. Daughaday
Nicholas Davies
Lawrence Davis
William D. Davis, Jr., 121
Pamela Day
John De Angelis

Michael E. DeBakey, 3, 6, 14–23, 137, 167
Vincent A. DeLuca, Jr.
Scott Deppe
N. A. Desbiens
Kenneth Diddie, 58
Preston V. Dilts, Jr.
Richard L. Dobson
James E. Doherty
John Donald
James Dooley, 102
Doris Doran
T. E. Doszkocs
J. Douglas, 244
Andrew Dow
Edgar Draper
F. Dubeck
N. L. DuBlurg, Jr.
Eileen Duggan, 228
Harriet P. Dustan
James M. Duvall
Donald Dworken
Eileen Eandi
Allan J. Ebbin, 37
Robert E. Ecklund
William H. Edwards
Richard H. Egdahl
Roger Egeberg
Hans E. Einstein
Robert S. Eisenberg
Marvyn L. Elgart, 204
Neil Elgee, 65, 85
George J. Ellis
Henry L. Ernstthal
Daniel Essin, 241, 244
T. N. Evans
Saul Farber, 5, 138, 139, 140, 141, 198
Gerald Farinola, 113
Richard G. Farmer
Aaron Feder, 106
James F. Feeney
Arthur W. Feinberg
Donald Feinstein, 116
Theodore Feit
William C. Felch, 183, 185

Alan W. Feld
Benjamin Felson
Cotton Feray, 221, 222
Thomas B. Ferguson
Daniel Ferrigno
Richard Field, 37, 141, 144
William R. Fifer, 188
Harry W. Fischer
Joseph Fischer
Winthrop Fish
Charles Fitch
Edmond B. Flink
Timothy Foley
Arthur Fox, 140
Raul Fraide
Boy Frame, 5
Richard Friedman
William F. Friedman, 49
James F. Fries, 263
K. O. Fritz
John Fry, 154, 155, 164, 169
Ronald K. Fujimoto
Jack J. Fulton
William B. Galbraith
Norman H. Garrett, Jr.
Paul J. Geiger
John P. Geyman, 203, 204, 205
Ray W. Gifford, Jr.
Nelson J. Gilman
Robert J. Glaser, 195
Charles Goldstein
Robert M. Goldwyn
Joseph Gonnella, 94, 215
Lillian Gonzalez-Pardo
Brian W. Goodell, 94, 144
J. F. Goodman
Alan L. Gordon, 42, 141
Babs Gordon, 239
Antonio M. Gotto, Jr., 135
Arthur E. Grant
Lawrence A. Green, 37, 253, 270
Robert Green
Norton J. Greenberger, 5, 9, 38, 150–151, 159
Beverly June Gregorius, 229, 236
Ward O. Griffen, Jr.

Janet Grignon, 244
James A. Grimes
Paul Griner
David S. Gullion
Rolf M. Gunnar
Warren G. Guntheroth
Jeffrey A. Hahn
Daniel Hamaty, 185
David A. Hamburg, 69
Jean Hamburger, 3
James T. Hamlin, III
Steven Hamman, 220
Richard J. Hannigan
Louise Hart, 244
William Hart, 219
A. McGehee Harvey, 178–180
Paul Harvey, 106
W. Proctor Harvey
James N. Haug
Robert M. Hayes
Ralph Haymond, 91, 141
L. Julian Haywood
Robert Hecht
Eugene M. Helveston
Bruce L. Henderson
Eva H. Henriksen
John Bernard Henry
Lester T. Hibbard
Lawrence Highman, 114
Allen Hinman
Joan E. Hodgman
Daniel Hoffman, 113
Wu Hokwang
John H. Holbrook
G. Holmes
Grace Holmes
Rita B. Hopper
Louis Horlick
Sylvan H. Horwood
Cyril Houle
James D. Houy, 129
Sidney Howard, 141
James T. Howell
Willard J. Howland
J. P. Hubbard
Thomas Harrison Hunter, 194

J. Willis Hurst, 6, 24–30
F. Ikezaki
James M. Ingram
Thomas S. Inui, 158
Julien H. Isaacs
Donald M. Jacobs, 114
D. Geraint James
Karin E. Jamison, 113, 228, 229, 230, 236
Stephen Jay
Harold Jeghers, 8, 56, 57
Frederick R. Jelovsek, 271, 272
Thomas M. Jenkins
M. Harry Jennison
Shen Jiaqi, 31, 32
Carol Johnson Johns, 96
Allen H. Johnson
J. W. Johnson
Marvin E. Johnson, 255
Harry S. Jonas
Lawrence W. Jones
Albert R. Jonsen, 194
P. B. Jorgensen, 114
Desmond G. Julian, 85, 94, 107, 108, 109, 118
Ralph C. Jung, 73
Charles L. Junkerman
Maurice J. Jurkiewicz
Mehwet Kam
Rokay Kamyar, 114
Thomas Edward Kane
W. Kane
Stanley Kaplan
Jerome P. Kassier
D. Kassum
Robert Kerlan
Louis J. Kettel, 206
M. Kenton King, 221
Richard Kingston
David M. Kipnis
Joseph B. Kirsner
Rodanthi Kitridou, 234
Margaret S. Klapper
Gerald Klatskin
Suzanne B. Knoebel, 38
Malcolm Knowles, 8

Interviewees and Correspondents

Chris Kraft, 214
Richard O. Kraft, 41
Gabriel A. Kune
Gustavo G. R. Kuster, 91, 93, 168
Robin B. Lake
Frank L. Lambert, 215
Richard H. Lampert
F. Wilfrid Lancaster, 251
Donald G. Landale
Tom Landry, 166
Jeffrey Latts, 159
Peter Lawin
G. Hugh Lawrence, 117, 118
Aubrey Leatham
Joshua Lederberg, 68–71
Peter V. Lee, 207, 208
Philip R. Lee, 193, 194, 195
John Leedom
Wenzel A. Leff, 113, 115
Thomas J. Lehar
John N. Lein, 113
Michael A. Lemp
Patrick D. Lester
C. Robin LeSueur
Leo L. Leveridge, 130, 131, 257
Ceylon S. Lewis, Jr., 134, 136
Jerry P. Lewis
Walter M. Lewis
Fred V. Light, 254
Sir William Liley
Donald A. B. Lindberg, 76, 252, 266
A. J. Lindgren
G. Littenberg
Nancy M. Lorenzi, 79, 250
Leah M. Lowenstein
Robert J. Luchi
Frederick Ludwig, 38, 87, 93, 116
Joseph Lydon, 93
Andrew McCanse
Margaret McCarron, 58, 64
Robert N. McClelland
Ruth McCormick, 74
Clement J. McDonald, 269, 270
C. E. McDonnell
Walter R. McFarland

Page McGirr, 219, 222
Charles H. McKinna
Sir John McMichael, 92
I. R. McWhinney, 203
George Macer
Donald N. Mackay
Ian R. Mackay, 40, 91, 92, 108, 118, 172–177
Willis C. Maddrey, 150
Robert Mager
W. E. Malle
Susan B. Mallory
Robert T. Manning, 6, 141
Charles M. March
N. M. March
Eugenia Marcus
Alexander R. Margulis
Helen E. Martin, 209
Maurice J. Martin
Ralph B. Martin
Byron J. Masterson
Nina W. Matheson, 74, 250, 251
James L. Mathis
Manuel Martinez-Maldonado, 86
Gastone Matioli, 39
Betty H. Mawardi
Sherman M. Mellinkoff, 9, 52, 96–99, 108, 179
Robert C. Mendenhall, 157
Pat Mensah
Henry S. Metz
Thomas C. Meyer, 126
David Micaelvitch
William Millard, 129, 130, 131
George E. Miller, 143, 213
Jacqueline D. Miller, 227, 231, 234, 237
Perry L. Miller, 268
William Richey Miller
Don Harper Mills, 188
Malcolm S. Mitchell
R. W. Montgomery
Pat Mooney
Francis D. Moore, 82, 87, 89, 118, 200, 220
Dean H. Morrow

Robert H. Moser, 31, 36
James M. Moss, 42, 82, 118
Edward Movius
Richard H. Moy
Donald R. Moyes
John F. Mueller
John H. Mulholland
W. V. Murowsky
Alvin I. Mushlin, 168
Jack D. Myers, 265, 266, 267
Richard Nabours
Frederick Naftolin
Richard H. Nalick
William D. Nelligan
Eugene C. Nelson
Victor Neufeld
Charles H. Nicholson
John T. Nicoloff
Lilia F. Nikolaeva, 122
Robert A. Nordyke
Jackson Norwood
Sir Gustav Nossal, 173
Celia M. Oakley, 163
Claron L. Oakley, 125, 126
Byron Oberst, 254
Richard L. O'Brien, 37
Alton Ochsner, 37
Frederick C. O'Dell, Jr., 93
Kunio Okuda, 92, 201, 202
Wesley M. Oler
D. E. Olson
Claude H. Organ, Jr., 111, 119, 121
Edwin L. Overholt, 134
Irvine H. Page, 3, 39, 65, 81, 196
R. H. Palmer
Robert L. Palmer, 116
P. J. H. Pansegrouw
James L. Parkin
Richard P. Parkinson, 144
William Parmley, 105
Joseph Paterno, 166
E. Mansell Pattison, 8
Stephen G. Pauker
Beverly C. Payne, 153, 185
Meredith J. Payne
Gee Pei, 240

Robert G. Petersdorf, 42, 43
Hans E. Peterson
Jon T. Peterson
Roger Peterson
Donald Petit, 114
Thomas A. Petro
Ronald J. Pion, 129
Nicholas Pisacano, 186, 187
Lynn Pittier, 244
Gerald I. Plitman, 32, 38
Hiram C. Polk, Jr.
Bernard Portnoy
Barbara Quint, 249
George J. Race, 113
Robert C. Rainie
Robert E. Rakel, 197
Eli A. Ramirez-Rodriguez, 66
Elizabeth Ramirez-Rodriguez, 240
K. J. Rao
Samuel I. Rapaport, 117, 140
C. Thorpe Ray, 137
Joe Redding
Frank Reed, 253
Peter L. Reichertz
J. S. Reinschmidt
Richard J. Reitemeier, 200, 223, 224
Ralph D. Reynolds
Telfer Reynolds, 59, 160, 162, 217
William A. Reynolds
Richard D. Richards, 105
Robert Richards
Benjamin M. Rigor
Jesse D. Rising, 111
Brooke Roberts
James M. Robertson
Carroll H. Robie
L. Rodney Rodgers, 141
Jonathan E. Rodnick, 203, 204
John Romano, 162
Robert Rosati
Donald H. Rose
Margaret Rose
Noel R. Rose
Robert M. Rose
Edward C. Rosenow, Jr., 58
Joseph F. Ross

Interviewees and Correspondents

Herbert J. Rothenberg
Edward Rubenstein, 114
Ian E. Rusted
Robb H. Rutledge
David C. Sabiston, Jr., 15, 42, 93, 266
David L. Sackett, 33, 34
Alfredo A. Sadun, 4
Murray Salkin, 218
Paul J. Sanazaro, 2, 185
Marilyn Sanders
Jay P. Sanford
Ragheb Sawires, 113
John L. Sawyers
Irwin J. Schatz, 210
Robert Scheig
DuWayne Schmidt
Harold M. Schoolman
Alvin Schultz, 82
M. Roy Schwarz, 128
Milton H. Seifert, Jr.
Donald Wayne Seldin, 39, 42, 44
Hugh Shade
Edward Shapiro, 93, 105
Om Sharma
Dame Sheila Sherlock, 140, 232, 243
Edward Shortliffe, 45, 262, 264
Linda D. Shortliffe, 229, 233, 234, 237
Jerry M. Shuck
A. A. Siddiqui
Mark E. Silverman
George M. Simpson
Maureen Sims, 232
Marjorie S. Sirridge, 235
S. E. Sivertson, 157
Harold Skalka
J. Orson Smith
Lloyd H. Smith, Jr., 58, 63, 138, 140
Robert B. Smith, III, 65, 164
Ronald E. Smith
William A. Sodeman, Sr.
Eric W. Sohr, 248, 249
Jane Somerville, 164

Walter Somerville, 106, 163
Eli Sorkow
Robert D. Sparks, ix–xi
Robert L. Spears
Harold M. Spinka
John A. Spittell, Jr.
Eugene A. Stead, Jr., 3, 10, 15, 146–149
William Stead
Knight Steel
David Steinman
G. Gayle Stephens, 203
W. Eugene Stern
Roger Stickney, 219, 222
Margaret T. Stockstill
Gene H. Stollerman
Daniel C. Stone, 37, 107
Patrick B. Storey, 112
C. F. Stout
John S. Strauss
Jeffrey K. Stross
Patricia J. Stuff
James M. Swain
Donald M. Switz, 38, 248
Lee R. Talbert
Dorothy Tatter
Annabel J. Teberg
Jack E. Tetirick, 82
John Thayer
Joe Theil
Leigh Thompson, 133, 134
George W. Thorn, 102, 103
David Torin
Gary Toule
Richard Treiman, 85, 167
Donald Trunkey
Suzanne Trupin
Susan B. Tully, 231
Philip A. Tumulty, 52–55
Marvin Turck, 141
Fred Turrill, 41, 94, 220
Edmund E. Van Brunt, 272
Stanley van den Noort
Joseph P. Van der Meulen, 31, 57, 134
J. Van Dyke

John F. Viljoen
Richard W. Vilter
Jean-Louis Vincent
Robert Volpe, 85
Kenneth Walker, 24
Gary L. Walkup
Marsha Wallace, 122
Betty Wallerstein, 241
Ralph Wallerstein, 138
Lila Wallis
Alexander J. Walt
Richard F. Walters
Waltman Walters
Paul H. Ward
William C. Waters, III, 9, 40, 134, 140
David E. Waugh
Lawrence L. Weed, 10, 28, 165, 247, 256
Paul F. Wehrle, 40, 101, 118
Laurel Weibel, 228, 234
Max H. Weil
Horst D. Weinborg
John M. Weiner
James M. A. Weiss
Claude E. Welch, 5
Murray Wexler
G. M. Whitacre
G. E. Wiebe, 114

George D. Wilbanks
Hibbard E. Williams
Martha E. Williams, 250
Warren Williams, 105, 154, 155, 191, 216
John Williamson, 33
Robert J. Williamson, 87
Marjorie P. Wilson, 90, 227, 234, 235
George Winokur
Francis C. Wood
Thomas C. Wood, 82
Sherwyn M. Woods
Frank Woolsey
Harold Wooster
Eton W. Wright
Kerry E. Wylke
Milford G. Wyman
James B. Wyngaarden, 141, 142, 144
Rosalyn S. Yalow
Sadahiro Yamamoto, 85
Myron Yanoff
J. Young, 116
Lawrence E. Young
Martin Zane
Bruce E. Zawacki, 164, 168, 194
Samir M. Zeind
Israel Zwerling

Name Index

Abrahamson, Stephen, 120
Adler, Mortimer, 7
Alford, Bobby, 137
Arnon, Amos, 158
Askey, John Martin, 138

Bain, Ruth M., 83, 232, 235
Baker, Duke H., 60–62, 65
Bakhtiar, Lailee, 228, 229, 234
Balchum, Oscar, 92–93
Balint, Michael, 201, 203
Bardsley, William, 221
Bargen, J. Arnold, 200
Barnett, George DeForest, 97
Barondes, Jeremiah, 157–158
Barr, David, 204
Bauer, Julius, 140
Beeson, Paul, 88, 117
Behnke, Roy, 11–12, 86
Bellows, John, 258–259
Bennett, Bill, 204, 206
Berge, Kenneth, 87, 116
Berne, Clarence J., 161
Bernstein, Lionel, 255
Bessman, Alice, 232, 237
Best, Peter, 113
Bethune, John E., 75
Billings, John Shaw, vii, 32–33
Bird, Daniel, 117
Bird, Majorie, 244
Blackburn, John, xxvi
Blankenhorn, David, 62, 65, 78
Blois, Marsden S., 265
Bloomfield, Arthur, 97

Blumberg, Baruch S., 3, 104
Bogdonoff, Morton, 146
Bohannan, Paul, 220
Bowey, Walter, 223
Bowler, Francis L., 182–183
Brashear, Richard H., 60–62
Braude, Robert, 74
Braunstein, Mark, 253
Braunwald, Eugene, 45, 48–51
Brayton, Donald, 128
Brem, Thomas H., 84
Brook, Robert H., 214
Brooks, Dorothy, 240
Brown, Bernice Z., 232, 236
Brown, Janis, 128
Buchanan, Barbara, 231
Buck, Francis S., 221
Budd, William, 153
Burk, Genevieve, 232
Burns, Joan, 240
Burns, Thomas, 134–135
Byyny, Richard, 40, 86

Caldwell, Kathryn S., 128
Callister, Thomas, 37, 41
Caplan, Richard, 112, 114
Castle, C. Hilmon, 125
Castle, William, 138
Caton, Cathleen, 218
Chambers, Kit, 231, 235, 236, 240, 242
Chambers, Wallace, 85
Cherny, Walter, 201
Cheshier, Robert, 66, 251
Christakos, Arthur C., 201

Churchill, Winston, 91–92
Clark, Gail, 232
Cleaveland, Clifton, 134
Clever, Linda, 137
Codman, E. A., 166–167
Cogan, David Glendenning, 4
Confucius, 32
Cooper, William, 155
Covell, David, 38, 91, 92
Cox, Alfred, 239
Craddick, Joyce, 187
Creek, Jean, 85–86
Cross, Harold D., 11, 165
Cury, Hiram, 158

Da Costa, Jacob M., 31
Dale, Andrew, 88
Davis, William, 121
DeBakey, Lois, v, ix–x, xviii, 1, 33, 193
  acknowledgments by, xix–xx
  afterword by, 275–277
  preface by, xiii–xv
DeBakey, Michael E., xix, 3, 6, 14–23, 137, 167, 193
DeBakey, Selma, xix–xx, 33
de Dombal, F. T., 261
Diddie, Kenneth, 58
Donaldson, Rose, 213–214
Dooley, James, 102
Douglas, J., 244–245
Doyle, Arthur Conan, 57
Duggan, Eileen, 228
Durant, Will, 138

Ebbin, Allan, 37
Eichna, Ludwig, 51
Eimerl, T. S., 158
Elgart, Marvyn L., 204
Elgee, Neil, 65, 85
Ernst, Richard E., 62
Essin, Daniel and Cecelia, 241, 244

Farber, Saul J., 5, 138, 139, 140, 141, 198
Farinola, Gerard, 113
Feder, Aaron, 106

Feinstein, Donald, 116
Felch, William, 181–182, 183–184
Feray, Cotton, 221–222
Field, Richard, 37, 141, 144
Fifer, William, 186–187
Fox, Arthur, 140
Frame, Boy, 5
Franklin, Benjamin, 91
Friedman, William F., 49
Fries, James F., 263
Fry, John, 154–155, 164

Gage, Mims, 137
Geyman, John P., 203, 204, 205
Given, Charles W., 253
Glaser, Robert, 195
Gonnella, Joseph, 94–95, 215
Goodell, Brian, 94, 144
Gordon, Alan, 42, 141, 239
Gordon, Babs, 239
Gotto, Antonio, 135, 137
Green, Lawrence, 37, 253, 270
Greenberger, Norton J., 5, 9, 38, 150–151, 159, 162
Gregorius, Beverly June, 229, 236
Grignon, Janet, 244
Grossman, Mort, 98

Halle, John, 101
Hamburg, David A., 68–69
Hamburger, Jean, 3–4
Hamman, Steven, 220
Hammond, Louis, 148
Harper, Harry, 28
Hart, Louise, 244
Hart, William, 219
Harvey, A. McGehee, 97, 98, 178–180
Harvey, Paul, 106–107
Harvey, Proctor, 206
Haymond, H. Ralph, 91, 141
Herrick, W. W., 81–82
Highman, Lawrence, 114
Hippocrates, x, 81, 108, 276
Hoffman, Daniel, 113
Holmes, Oliver Wendell, 7, 112
Houle, Cyril O., 8, 125
Houy, James D., 129
Howard, Sidney, 141

Name Index

Howell, Ted, 58–59
Hubbard, Bill, 50–51
Hunter, Thomas, 194
Hurst, J. Willis, 6, 9, 11, 24–30, 146

Ignatius, Joseph, 41
Inui, Tom, 158

Jacobs, Donald, 114
James, D. Geraint, 243
Jamison, Karin E., 113, 228–231, 236
Jeghers, Harold, 8, 56, 57
Jelovsek, Frederick, 271, 272
Johns, Carol Johnson, 96
Johnson, Marvin, 255
Johnson, Samuel, 3
Jonsen, Albert, 194
Jorgensen, P. B., 114
Julian, Desmond, 85, 94, 107, 108, 109, 118

Kamyar, Rokay, 114
Kettel, Louis J., 206–207
King, M. Kenton, 221
Kipling, Rudyard, 27
Kitridou, Rodanthi, 234
Knoebel, Suzanne, 38
Knowles, John, 5
Knowles, Malcolm, 8
Kornberg, Hans, 135
Kraft, Chris, 214–215
Kraft, Richard, 41
Krebs, Hans, 135
Kuster, Gustavo, 91, 93, 168

Lambert, Frank L., 215
Lancaster, Wilfrid, 251
Landry, Tom, 166
Lantz, K. Holley, 157
Latham, Peter Mere, 111, 153, 181, 225
Latts, Jeffrey, 159
Lawrence, Hugh, 117–118
Lederberg, Joshua, 68–71
Lee, Peter V., 207, 208
Lee, Philip, 193–194, 195
Leff, Wenzel A., 113, 115

Lein, Jack, 113
Leonard, George B., 247
Leveridge, Leo L., 130–131, 257
Levine, Maury, 8
Levine, Sam, 147
Lewis, C. S., 134, 136
Lewis, Dean, 98
Lewis, Howard P., 204, 206
Lewis, Thomas, 33
Light, Fred V., 254
Lindberg, Donald A. B., 76, 252, 266, 268
Locke, John, 2–3
Longcope, Warfield T., 199
Lorenzi, Nancy M., 79, 250
Ludwig, Frederick, 38, 87, 93, 116
Lusted, Lee B., 261–262
Lydon, Joseph, 93

Mackay, Ian R., 40, 91, 92, 108, 118, 172–177
Mackenzie, James, 153–154
Maddrey, Willis C., 150
Manning, Phil R., v, ix–x, xix–xx, 81, 261
  acknowledgments by, xvii–xviii
  afterword by, 275–277
  introduction by, xxv–xxviii
  preface by, xiii–xv
Manning, Robert, 6–7, 141
Martin, Helen E., 209
Martinez-Maldonado, Manuel, 86
Matheson, Nina, 74, 77, 250–251
Matioli, Gastone, 39
Maugham, W. Somerset, 7
Mayo, Charles, 93, 133
Mayo, Will, 93
McCarron, Margaret M., 58, 64
McClelland, Robert, 40
McCormack, J. N., xxvi
McCormick, Ruth, 74
McDonald, Clement, 225, 269–270
McGirr, Page, 219–222
McMichael, John, 92
McWhinney, I. R., 203–204
Mellinkoff, Sherman M., 9, 52, 96–99, 108, 179
Mendenhall, Robert C., 157
Meyer, Thomas, 127, 157

Millard, William, 129–130, 131
Miller, George E., xxvii, 8, 143, 213
Miller, Jacqueline D., 227, 231–232, 234, 237
Miller, Perry L, 268–269
Mills, Don Harper, 186
Moore, Carl, 221
Moore, Francis D., 82, 87, 89, 118, 200–201, 220
Moorhead, Robert, 158
Morehead, Mildred A., 213–214
Moser, Robert H., 31, 36
Moss, James, 42, 82, 118
Moynihan, Berkeley, 6
Mushlin, Alvin, 168–169
Myers, Jack D., 265–266, 267

Nikolaeva, Lilia F., 122
Nossal, Gustav, 172–173

Oakley, Celia, 163–164
Oakley, Claron L., 125–126
Oberst, Byron, 254
O'Brien, Richard, 37
Ochsner, Alton, 17, 37–38
O'Dell, Frederick, 93
Okuda, Kunio, 92, 201, 202
Organ, Claude H., Jr., 111, 119, 121
Osler, William, vii, 2–3, 6–7, 32, 35, 37, 39, 73, 164, 222–223, 239
Overholt, Edwin, 134

Page, Irvine H., 3, 39, 65, 81–82, 196
Paget, James, 241
Palmer, Robert, 116
Paracelsus, vii
Parkinson, Richard, 144
Parmley, William, 105
Pasteur, Louis, 4
Paterno, Joseph, 166
Pattison, E. Mansell, 8
Paullin, James Edgar, 147
Payne, Beverly, 153, 183
Paz, Octavio, 11
Pei, Gee, 240–241
Pepper, O. H. Perry, 138
Petersdorf, Robert G., 42, 43

Petit, Donald, 114–115
Pickles, William N., 153
Pion, Ronald J., 129
Pisacano, Nicholas, 184–185
Pittier, Lynn, 244
Plitman, Gerald, 32, 38
Pollack, Seymour, 207

Quint, Barbara, 249–250

Race, George, 113
Rakel, Robert E., 197
Ramirez, Eli A., 66
Ramirez-Rodriguez, Elizabeth, 240
Rankin, W. S., xxvi
Rapaport, Samuel, 117, 140
Ravitch, Mark, 98
Ray, Thorpe, 137
Reed, Frank, 253–254
Reid, Robert A., 157
Reitemeier, Richard J., 200, 223–225
Reynolds, Telfer B., 59, 160, 162, 217
Richards, R. D., 105
Rising, Jesse, 111
Rodgers, Rodney, 141
Rodnick, Jonathan, 203, 204
Romano, John, 162
Rosenow, Edward, 58–59
Rubenstein, Arthur, 40
Rubenstein, Edward, 114
Ryan, Francis, 71

Sabiston, David C., Jr., 15, 42, 93–94, 266
Sackett, David, 33–35
Sadun, Alfredo, 4
Salkin, Murray, 218
Sanazaro, Paul, 2, 183–184
Sarton, George, 45–46
Sawires, Ragheb, 113
Schatz, Irwin, 210
Scheff, David, 213
Schultz, Alvin, 82
Schwarz, M. Roy, 128
Seldin, Donald W., 39, 42, 44, 45
Seneca, 133
Shapiro, Edward, 93, 105–106

Name Index

Shaw, George Bernard, 2
Shen Jiaqi, 31–32
Sherlock, Sheila, 140, 232, 243
Shortliffe, Edward H., 45, 262–263, 264
Shortliffe, Linda D., 229, 233, 234–235, 237
Sims, Maureen, 232, 234
Sirridge, Marjorie S., 235
Sivertson, S. E., 157
Slocum, Harold, 62
Smith, Lloyd H., Jr., 58, 63, 138, 140
Smith, Robert, 65, 164
Sohr, Eric, 248–249
Somerville, Jane, 164
Somerville, Walter, 106, 163
Sparks, Robert D., ix–xi
Starfield, Barbara, 213
Stead, Eugene A., Jr., 3, 9, 10, 15, 146–149
Stephens, G. Gayle, 203
Stephens, Lorin, 85
Stevenson, Robert L., Jr., 214
Stevenson, Robert Louis, 236
Stickney, Roger, 219, 222
Stollerman, Gene, 199
Stone, Daniel, 37, 107
Stone, Jerry, xx
Storey, Patrick, 112
Switz, Donald M., 38–39, 248

Tetirick, Jack, 82, 85
Thayer, William, 98
Thompson, Leigh, 133, 134
Thorn, George W., 102, 103
Treiman, Richard, 85, 167
Tully, Susan, 231
Tumulty, Philip A., 52–55, 98
Turck, Marvin, 141
Turrill, Fred, 41, 94, 220

Van Brunt, E. E., 272
Van Der Meulen, Joseph, 31, 57, 134
Vilter, Richard, 7
Volpe, Robert, 85

Walker, Kenneth, 24
Wallace, Marsha, 122
Wallerstein, Betty, 241, 244
Wallerstein, Ralph, 138, 241, 244
Waters, William, 9, 40, 134, 140–141
Weed, Lawrence L., 10, 28, 165, 173–174, 175, 247, 256
Wehrle, Paul, 40, 101, 118, 121
Weibel, Laurel, 228, 234
Weiss, Soma, 147
Welch, Claude, 5
White, Paul Dudley, 28–29, 148, 159
Whitehead, Alfred North, xxv, 7, 10
Wiebe, G. E., 114
Wilbush, Joel, 174
Williams, Martha, 250
Williams, Warren L., 105, 154, 155–157, 191, 216
Williamson, John, 33, 213
Williamson, R. J., 87–88
Wilson, Marjorie Price, 90, 227–228, 234, 235
Wood, Thomas, 82
Woolsey, Frank, 127
Wyngaarden, James B., 141, 142, 144

Yamamoto, Sadahiro, 85
Youmans, John B., xxvi–xxvii
Young, J., 116

Zawacki, Bruce E., 164, 168, 194–195

Subject Index

Abstract services, 40–41
AMA (American Medical Association), 130, 195
AMA-GTE network, 255, 258
American Medical Association (AMA), 130, 195, 259
Analysis of practice, 8, 20–21, 153–180, 181–191, 203–204, 253–254
Appointments, overbooking, 216
Attributes, ideal, 3–6, 15–23, 25–26, 70, 97, 134–144, 276
Audiotapes, 125–126, 203–204
Audit of patient records, 164–165
  analytical, 8, 165

Bibliographies, 78–79, 249–250
Biographies, clinical, 203
Boolean search, 249
Bulletin boards, electronic, 259

Card files, topic word, 61–62
Central index, 61–62
Chart audit, 165
Clinical
  biographies, 203
  computer programs, 262–271
  experience, 20–21
  problems, 157–159, 162–164
  skills, 199–207
Clinicopathologic conferences, 118
Colleagues, learning with, 82–95
Collegial
  conversations, sites of, 88, 91–94

Collegial (*continued*)
  network, 9, 71, 81–95, 234–235, 251–252
  problems, 82, 85–88, 188
  relationships, women, 234–235
Communication, interactive, 127–128
Community discussion groups, 128–129
Companionship in medicine, 9
Compassion, 6, 19, 22, 25–26
Computer
  aids to learning, 247–260
  assisted instruction (CAI), 129–130
  clinical programs, 262–271
  collegial network and, 251–252
  diagnostic guidance, 261–274
  future practice and, 247
  indexing articles, 248–249
  messaging, 252
  practice analysis, 253–254
  reprint files and, 65, 248–249
  therapeutic guidance, 261–274
Conferences, 22, 111–123
  clinicopathologic, 118
  curbstone, 87
  death, 118
  formal, 111–123
  hospital, 117–118, 121
  teleconferences, 127
Consultations, 101–109, 176, 252
Continuing education, every page
Correspondents and interviewees, 279–286
Cost-containment, 107
Courses, 111–123
Cumulative data, 159

293

Curbstone conferences, 87
Curiosity, 3–5, 15–16, 70, 97
Currency, maintaining, 21–22, 31–47, 69–71, 111–123, 203, 207, 210

Data bases, bibliographic, 73, 77–78, 249–250
Death conferences, 118
Decision-analysis, medical, 176
Decision-support system, data in, 261–274
Diagnosis, computer guidance in, 261–274
Discipline, 5, 17–18, 275
Discussion groups, 91–92
  community, 128–129
Doctor-patient relationship, 199–211

Economic problems in medicine, 193–198
Education, continuing, every page
Electronic
  data bases, 73
  journals, 250–251
  mail, 252, 259
Errors, 164, 180, 188, 217–218, 223–225
Ethical problems in medicine, 193–198
Examinations, physical, 204, 206–207, 215–216
Experience, 2–3, 6–9
  clinical, analysis of, 20–21
  notes on, 163–164
  profiting from, 153–154
  reading and, 32

Family relationships, 15–16, 25, 239–245
Files
  alphabetical, 60
  card, 61, 62
  indexing, 59–60
  numerical, 60
  reprint, 56–60, 65–66
  subject, 61–62
Films, 128
Flow sheets, 217

Follow-up of patients, 218
Fulfillment, 1–12, 22–23, 235–237

Group practice, 85–86

Health professionals, learning from, 94–95
History, patient, 215–216
Hospital
  conferences, 117–118, 121
  physician-practice in, 186–187

Ideal traits, 3–6, 15–23, 25–26, 70, 97, 134–144, 276
Incompetence, 188
Index
  central, 61–62
  computer, 248–249
  diagnosis, 156
  files, 59–60
  patient charts, 154–157
  patients, 28–29
  reprints, 60–66
Index Medicus, 77, 79
Individual involvement, 194–195
Information
  center, personal, 57–67, 248–250
  computers and, 254–259
  libraries and, 57–67, 73–80, 247–250
  network, 82
  retrieval, 73–74, 77–80, 254, 258
  sources, 10
  telephone, 126
Institutional medical libraries, 73–80, 250–251
Instruction
  computer-assisted (CAI), 129–130
  physician, misunderstanding of, 219
Insurance companies, data collected by, 186
Interviewees and correspondents, 279–286
Interviews of physicians, xiii–xiv, xix

Subject Index

Journals
  electronic, 250–251
  reading of, 31–47

Knowledge, medical, unrelated problems, 213–226

Laboratory data, 216–217
Language in medicine, 19
Learning
  colleagues and, 82–95
  computers as aids to, 247–260
  consultants and, 106–107
  delight of, 15–16
  from experience, 2–3, 6–9, 153–154
  from formal consultations, 101–109
  from health professionals, 94–95
  from mistakes, 164
  from puzzling cases, 180
  from teaching, 26, 133–145, 149
  lifelong, 2, 49–51, 97–99, 147–149, 179–180
  personal responsibility for, 179–180
  programs, independent, 128–129
  self-directed, 8, 53–54, 120, 179–180
  teaching and, 26, 133–151
Librarians, 251
  medical, 74, 77
Libraries, medical, 57–67, 73–80, 249–251

Mail, electronic, 252, 259
Malpractice suits, 186
Medical
  consultations, 101–109, 176, 252
  data banks, computerized, 176
  decision-analysis, 176
  knowledge, problems unrelated to, 213–226
  librarians, 73–77, 251
  libraries
    institutional, 73–80, 250–251
    personal, 57–67
  problem-solving, 176
  records, 102, 173–176, 217–218
    audit of, 164–165
    education and, 174–176

Medicine, every page
Mistakes, 164, 180, 188, 217–218, 223, 225
Morbidity and mortality rounds, 117–118
Motivation, 70
Murphy's Law, 213

National Library of Medicine, xviii, 73, 77–78
Network
  collegial, 9, 71, 81–95, 251–252
  information, 82
  "old girl," 234, 235
  telephone, 87–88
Noncompliance, patient, 218–220
Note cards, 159, 162–164
Note-taking
  journal, 248–249
  reading and, 35, 37

Office record review, 164–165, 184–185

Patient
  audit, 165
  cards, 159, 162
  charts, indexing, 154–157, 173–177
  data, 158–159, 186, 216–217, 222
  denial by, 219–220
  follow-up of, 20–21, 218
  history and physical examination of, 204–207, 215–216
  inattention of, 219
  instructions, misunderstanding of, 219
  interesting, indexing of, 28–29
  learning from, 173–177
  management programs, 130
  noncompliance, 218–220
  overbooking appointments with, 216
  records, auditing, 164–165, 184–185
  relationship with physicians, 199–211
  teaching and, 204
  transposition technique, 106
Photographs, list of, xxiii

Physical examination, 204, 206–207, 215–216
Physician profiles, individual, 182
Physicians, *see also* Practice
  academic, 86, 134–144
  as managers, 215
  attributes, 3–6, 15–23, 25–26, 70, 97, 276
  clinical skills, 199–207
  colleagues, 9, 81–95, 222–225, 234–235
  compassionate, 6, 19
  continuing education, every page
  courses and conferences, 111–123
  denial of significant data by, 222
  discipline, 5–6, 17–18
  education and, 182–185
  effectiveness, limiting factors, 220–222
  errors, 164, 180, 188, 217–218, 223, 225
  experience, 2–3, 6–9, 153–154
  factors limiting effectiveness of, 220–222
  family relationships of, 15–16, 25, 239–245
  fulfillment, 1–12, 22–23, 235–237
  ideal attributes, 3–6, 15–23, 25–26, 70, 97, 134–144, 276
  inattention of, 220–221
  interviews of, xiii-xiv, xix
  lifelong learning, 2, 49–51, 97–99, 147–149, 179–180
  network, 9, 71, 81–95, 251–252, 259
  nonmedical problems, 213–226
  patients and, 199–211
  practice analysis, 8, 20–21, 153–180, 181–191, 203–204, 253–354
  priorities, 11
  problem, 188–189
  reading, 18, 31–47, 69–71
  referral, 101–109
  satisfaction, 1–12, 22–23, 235–237
  self-education, 8, 22, 49–51, 179–180, 204
  teaching and, 21–22, 134–144
  women, 227–237
  writing and, 19–20, 29–30
Practice, *see also* Physicians
  analyzing products of, 20–21, 189, 253–254

Practice (*continued*)
  audit, 213–218
  clinical skills, 199–207
  group, 85–86
  information needed, 254–259
  priorities, setting of, 11
  problems unrelated to medical knowledge in, 213–226
  profile, 181–182, 253–254
  questions arising in, 254–258
  satisfaction from, 1–12, 22–23, 235–237
  solo, 86
Practitioners, full-time, 141, 144
Priorities, setting, 11
Problem orientation, 175
Problem-solving, medical, 176
Problems, nonmedical, 213–226
Procedural audit, 165, 213–218
Procedures, new, 207, 210
Publications
  proliferation of, 33
  reading of, 18, 31–47
  scientific, 21
Puzzling-case books, 180

Questions, framing of, 10–11, 26–27, 105

Radio program
  one-way, 127
  two-way, 127–128
Reading, 18, 31–47, 69–71, 151, 240–241
  general, 31–32, 39–42
  library and, 41, 57–67, 73–80, 250–251
  media and, 41–42
  on individual patients, 45
  note-taking and, 35, 37
  practice-related, 42, 45
  principles, 32–39
  relating, to experience, 32
  retreat, 38–39
  scheduled time for, 37–39, 240–241
  scientific publications, 21
  screening for, 32–35
  solving specific problems by, 42, 45
  specific, 39, 42–45

Subject Index

Reasoning by physicians, 18
Recording data, 158–159
Records, 173–176, 217–218
Referring physicians, 101–109
Reporting of errors and omissions, 223, 225
Reprint files
  alternatives to, 66
  computers and, 65, 248–249
  decimal system, 60
  indexing of, 60–66
  personal, 58–60, 65, 69–70, 99, 248–249

Sabbatical leaves, 122
Satellites, television, 128–129
Satisfaction, 1–12, 22–23, 235–237
Scientific publications, 21 (*See also* Reading; Libraries)
Screening for reading, 32–35
Self-assessment, 41, 112
Self-directed learning, 8, 53–54, 120, 179–180
Self-discipline, 5, 17–18, 275
Self-education, 8, 53–54, 120, 179–180
Seminars, 201, 203
Social problems in medicine, 193–198
Solo practice, 86
Study groups, 91–92

Teachers, effective, attributes of, 134–138
Teaching
  benefits of, 133–145, 204
  learning and, 26
  learning from, 133–151
  patients and, 204
  writing and, 29–30
Technology in continuing education, 125–132, 252, 259
Teleconferences, 127
Telephone
  information, 126
  network, 87–88
Television satellites, 128–129
Textbooks, medical, 57–58
Therapy, computer guidance in, 261–274
Tracing outcomes, 166–169

Videodiscs, 130–131
Videotapes, 128, 203–204

Women–physicians
  collegial relationships and, 234–235
  continuing education and, 227–237
  single, 235
  time pressures on, 227–231
Writing, 19–20, 29–30